MASTERING
LEPTIN

MASTERING LEPTIN

THE KEY TO ENERGETIC VITALITY, YOUTHFUL HORMONAL BALANCE, OPTIMUM BODY WEIGHT, AND DISEASE PREVENTION!

BYRON J. RICHARDS, CCN
with MARY GUIGNON RICHARDS

Wellness
Resources
books

NOTE TO READERS

The information presented in this book is for educational and informational purposes. It is not intended as a diagnoses or treatment of any medical condition. The information given is not medical advice nor is it presented as a course of personalized treatment. Before changing any medical treatment or before discontinuing any course of medical treatment you may now be undergoing, you should consult your physician. The reader should not stop prescription medications without the advice and guidance of his or her personal physician. Any application of the material set forth in the following pages is at the reader's discretion and sole responsibility.

MASTERING LEPTIN

Published by Wellness Resources Books
A division of Wellness Resources, Inc.
www.wellnessresources.com, www.masteringleptin.com
6200 Excelsior Boulevard, Suite 103, Minneapolis, Minnesota 55416 U.S.A.

Cover Photograhy and Copyediting by Kathy Hetherington
Cover design and Interior design by Tiffany M. Richards

Printed in the United States of America

International Standard Book Number: 0-9727121-0-0

Library of Congress Control Number: 2002117389

*This book is dedicated to
those who wish to take charge
of their health and help their friends
and family to do the same.*

For the latest updates on leptin, visit:
www.masteringleptin.com

CONTENTS

PART 3 - SOLVING THE HORMONE PUZZLE

INTRODUCTION

The information in this book represents one of the most significant advancements in our understanding of health to come along.

As a clinician and health educator on the leading edge of applied clinical nutrition, we have had the opportunity to help many thousands of people achieve a better level of health. We have been a place of last resort for many individuals over the years, those unable to receive help for their problems from the traditional Western medicine approach.

We solve tough problems. This also makes it much easier to help people who are not having difficult issues. Certainly, the consumer demand to understand natural options for health has never been higher.

The information in this book is truly groundbreaking. We can say this because we work day in and day out on the front lines. We know what is going on in our field. We know what is being told to the public and what is being taught to our peers.

The significant undertaking of reading, understanding, compiling, and coordinating thousands of current studies, including the most recent and up-to-date ones, makes this work truly unique. Its usefulness will be broadly realized; the number of individuals in search of the answers to help them with their health and finding solutions here, will be countless. This has been our mission, our purpose for tackling this tremendous undertaking, to help as many people as possible to live healthier, thus happier lives.

The general public lacks a workable way to figure out what to eat, not to mention how to lose weight and keep it off. America is getting fatter and sliding down a path of poor health. There exists an ever growing epidemic of increased obesity and diabetes that our society has never before seen. Overall health problems are getting worse; disease is more rampant than ever. Real solutions are lacking.

This problem is about to change with the release of this book. The discovery of leptin in 1994 marked a major change in traditional theories of health. Leptin is a powerful hormone; it controls and permits other hormones to function – or not function.

The discovery of leptin and what it means, now backed by undeniable science, puts to rest some of the oldest arguments about the nature of disease itself. It is now found that malfunctioning genes and leptin, overburdened by a variety of stressors, are the actual cause of disease.

Restoring these genes and related hormonal rhythms back to a condition of healthy function will dramatically improve the quality of health of any person who chooses to follow this path. If enough individuals in society follow this path, then health care costs will plummet and the "diseases of aging" will greatly decrease.

There is no longer a need to look for the cause of these diseases. There is only a need to work out the best approach to solving them.

Mary and I have been working with people to help them solve health issues for over 20 years. We have wanted to write a book for many years, but have not had the time. Between developing and running a busy practice, raising children, as well as everything else that goes on in life, it just was not practical. Several years ago, we finally decided we would make the time to write our book; we knew it was the right time.

I am very proud of how Mary has taken care of herself over the years. It is not that she has had a stress-free life, far from it. She runs our busy business, has raised four children ages 16-26, and has helped me more than anyone could ever imagine.

Our cover picture was taken four months after Mary's fiftieth birthday, yet she looks much younger. She is full of energetic vitality, has no hormonal issues at transition, is at her optimum body weight and maintaining it, and has never had a disease or significant illness.

This is a true testament to the workability of what we are teaching. The principles in this book work in the real world; they help solve real problems. Even healthy people will benefit by applying the information in this book, by slowing down the rate of aging and preventing disease.

Our initial idea for a book was to write on the subject of aging without wear and tear. A big part of this was going to be about getting to a proper body weight and staying there. We have a tremendous amount of knowledge and experience in these areas.

As we began to put this book together and document how our program works in terms of the scientific rationale, it became clear we would need to tackle the monumental task of explaining leptin to the general public, a task that has not been done before.

There are over 5,000 published scientific articles on the subject of leptin. Many of these studies seem conflicting and are rather confusing. One minute leptin was good, the next minute it was bad.

Leptin was a big problem for a fat mouse, yet it was not really a problem for overweight people, or was it? Was it causing diabetes or preventing diabetes? Was it causing cancer or preventing cancer? Was it causing heart disease or preventing heart disease? Was it causing hormonal problems or was it the problem itself? Was it helping pregnancy or causing infertility? Or did it not matter one way or the other?

The complexity of the contradictions was overwhelmingly interesting and intriguing. Thus began a journey that will forever change the way we view health.

In a sense, it felt as if we had struck gold. Everything began to come together, like a complex puzzle falling into place. As we figured out the complexity of leptin, we could apply it to everything we had learned in the past 20 years. We now understood even more clearly the specific nature of weight problems, hormonal problems, fibromyalgia, thyroid problems, metabolic syndrome X, heart disease, and cancer. We saw the true significance of this information we had uncovered.

Mary and I have been an inseparable team for over 20 years. We are an example of the whole being greater than the sum of its parts. In this book, I have done the highly technical research, study, and compilations. Mary has helped to turn it into plain English, ensuring its clarity, applicability, and usefulness. Her unique skills and experience have enabled her to develop an uncanny knack for combining compassion and intelligence in an appropriate way of teaching people to become more empowered with information that can improve their lives.

Writing this book was a difficult and sometimes grueling task, as the information regarding leptin is highly technical and complex and does not follow simplistic cause and effect thinking. While we may wish our bodies worked in simplistic ways, they do not.

Health is a reflection of an elegant and harmonic symphony of well-coordinated rhythm and timing. A healthy body is reflected in the efficiency and quality of millions of simultaneous and synchronized events. Leptin is the guiding energetic regulator that permits this to happen properly.

We have gone to great lengths to provide the appropriate scientific references to document this information and these discoveries, with over 700 scientific studies referenced in our book. Enjoy and learn from an amazing array of up-to-date scientific findings at the cutting edge of modern science, including studies from as recent as a week prior to this printing.

With the evaluation and interpretation of this breakthrough science and placing it in its applicable context, this book will become a useful tool for every reader.

Our main goal for undertaking this project is to help the general public make constructive changes to a wide variety of issues that directly affect health, to become more educated about their health, and to be better able to take charge of it.

With the introduction of the term Health Asset Manager™ as an essential concept in health self-care, we teach the importance of taking charge of one's health, thus making it possible for an improved quality of life.

This information directly relates to overcoming our societal issue of obesity. However, it is a great deal more than that. It is the essence of the quality of all areas of health.

Our extensive documentation makes this book an excellent reference tool for any student or health professional who wants to get up to speed on the subject of leptin, its importance and role in overall health, and how to master it.

It is our hope that our readers will pass a copy of this book along to their physicians. This information is not known – not known by the general public and not known by doctors and other health-care practitioners. With the knowledge we now have, it seems inconceivable that a doctor can do an ongoing good job without understanding the many ramifications of leptin to health and disease and the numerous medications they prescribe on a daily basis. The information on leptin is of primary importance to every aspect of medicine and quality of medical care.

The time we have put into this book causes us to remember why we never had time to write a book in the first place. Nevertheless, we managed to finish our project.

We are very proud to be the first to explain the diverse nature of leptin and how important *Mastering Leptin* is to the health and well being of every man, woman, and child.

As a gift to you, it is both Mary's and my wish that this book brings you more knowledge and useable health information, so that you and your loved ones may live a healthier and happier life, now, and into the future.

Byron Richards
December 2002

PART 1

The Scope of Leptin

The Most Powerful Hormone in the Human Body

The twentieth century saw Americans transform from fit to fat. Scientific advancements enable many Americans to live longer but not necessarily healthier. Heart disease, cancer, obesity, diabetes, osteoporosis, and serious age-related mental decline, including Alzheimer's, are problems that plague our society and show no signs of improvement.

The cost to treat these problems is staggering in terms of the money spent on care, the burden placed on caretakers, rising health-care costs, the lost productivity of the ill individual, and the personal loss of quality of life.[1]

Surgeon General David Satcher calls obesity in America an epidemic. Two out of three American adults are classified as overweight or obese, compared with one in four in the early 1960s. A person is obese when they weigh over 20 percent more than maximum healthy body weight.

Our nation's health-care costs jumped to $1.424 trillion in 2001, up from $1.310 trillion in 2000. Health-care spending averages about $5,000 per person. Prescription drug spending comprises $140 billion of total health spending, obesity accounts for $117 billion per year. The prescription drug and obesity costs are directly related to individuals not keeping themselves in a healthy condition of natural balance. There are major diseases associated with these costs. This is preventable disease!

When individuals fail to make good personal health choices during the course of their life, it affects more than just themselves and their families. There is a consequence to society that is reflected by the significant economic burden of preventable health costs.

A recent study published in the *Journal of the American Medical Association* shows that the consequence of an individual overweight is worse than previously known, causing significantly reduced life-span. If a person is overweight at age 40, it shortens life by three years. If a person is obese at age 40, it shortens life 6-7 years. If an overweight person also smokes, it shortens life by 13 years. If obesity starts at a younger age, the problem is even worse. The life of a 20-year-old obese male is shortened by 13 years.

Health officials plead with the public to eat better and exercise more, a plea falling on deaf ears. The need for a real solution to these problems has never been more important.

THE SCIENTIFIC BREAKTHROUGH SOLUTION

Somewhat quietly, at the end of the twentieth century, a hormone called leptin was discovered. The immense importance of this hormone was not immediately recognized. In fact, all that it does is not yet fully understood.

One thing is very clear, mastering leptin transforms the subjects of weight management and disease prevention to an astounding new level, opening the door for solving many major health issues that have not yet been successfully improved for the majority of Americans.

THE POWER OF LEPTIN

Leptin is the hormone secreted by fat cells contained in white adipose tissue. It is the most significant hormone there is in understanding the function of the human body.

Leptin is essential for survival. It has a regulating effect on other hormones, not in a passive way but as a prime controlling signal. Leptin tells thyroid hormones, adrenal hormones, pancreatic hormones, and sex hormones how to perform. Leptin can function without any help from these other hormones, but the other hormones cannot function properly without leptin.

The significance of this new information reveals that leptin is the single most important hormone known to man. Interestingly, it was not discovered until 1994, and it has not been written about in its comprehensive role for broad public knowledge.

Leptin is secreted by white adipose tissue, the undesirable fat that accumulates on the abdomen, buttocks, and thighs. What was once considered something to liposuction out of the body is now seen as a most important endocrine organ. This is a rather amazing turn of events.

LEPTIN PROBLEMS

Leptin is responsible for bizarre and erratic behavior and cravings related to food, including the inability to attain and maintain a healthy body weight. Leptin is essential for survival; without it, the human race would have perished from starvation long ago. However, in the land of food on every corner, it is also the hormone that fuels addictive and compulsive behavior. It is the reason why individuals will "start their diet tomorrow."

The food pyramid, as well intentioned as its creators may have been, will be seen as an eating method that induces serious health issues. There is one healthy way to eat. It is a way that maximizes the efficient function of leptin. All this information is new. Low-fat diets are incredibly destructive as are high-fat diets. Understanding leptin finally puts to rest the conflicting diet information that is currently running rampant in society.

Problems with leptin set the stage for serious health issues. In addition to obesity, this includes anorexia, immune problems, bone loss, gastrointestinal problems, liver problems, cognitive problems, nerve problems, heart disease, and cancer.

Leptin is a hormone, it carries on communication in the body. Leptin-related problems occur as a result of a breakdown in communication. In some cases, this means not enough leptin; in other cases, this means too much leptin.

When leptin problems are magnified, there is a serious risk for disease. Leptin problems cause excess internal friction, meaning that cells in general begin to "overheat" or become overly stressed. This sets the stage for serious disease.

SUMMARY

If one desires to be healthy while growing older, it would be wise learn what leptin is all about. We are entering into a new era of health and wellness, wherein the understanding of genes and molecules can be translated into tangible and realistic ways to improve health.

There is no need to wait for some startling drug discovery to improve life. The information is already available, and the tools for improvement already exist.

2

Be a Health Asset Manager ™

Q uality of health is an individual's most important asset. Everyone should know enough about health to stay on a good track and have appropriate solutions in the event that health problems arise. Individuals need to be able to think for themselves, make correct decisions, and take effective action.

In terms of health, this requires an ability to understand one's own body and to have enough knowledge to implement solutions to keep on a healthy track. This is the bare minimum of expertise required to stay in charge of one's own health.

Understanding leptin will help improve health IQ. There is no simplistic and false premise such as "good" and "bad" cholesterol. Too many Americans are illiterate on the subject of health, a sad state of affairs directly contributing to out-of-control health care costs and burdens. Many Americans have a poor ability to implement even rudimentary health data and to translate it into correct action.

There is only one solution to these problems, on both an individual and a society-wide basis, and that is for individuals to learn to become much more responsible for their own health. This means having the knowledge and skills to manage the most important personal asset, health. We call this becoming a Health Asset Manager.™

DO NOT BECOME PART OF THE PROBLEM
People are continuing to get fatter and unhealthier. Three hundred thousand Americans a year die from obesity-related issues.[2,3] It does not matter how much public-health officials warn us about the need to exercise and eat better; the majority of people in America cannot seem to get on track and stay there.

In order to improve personal health, one must be able to think with health data. This requires a whole set of self-assured ideas relating to health and the ability to implement those ideas. Without intelligent decision making relating to health, our country's health care woes and costs will continue to spiral out of control.

Empowering oneself with useful knowledge is the first step to becoming a competent Health Asset Manager.™

ON THE CUTTING EDGE OF SCIENCE

Much of the information in this book is new even to health professionals. There is a new health paradigm that will evolve from this information, one focusing on solutions that are in the best health interests of the individual.

There must also be a framework in one's mind for evaluating this health information. If every time there is a health problem, all one does is "follow the advice of my doctor," then that is the individual's personal health paradigm. Such advice may be good or bad, but that is the extent of the person's thinking.

In the new health paradigm, individuals will need to take charge of their own health. This is a much greater level of personal responsibility, especially in non-emergency situations. This means understanding options, doing personal research on the pros and cons of any important decision, fitting the information discovered into a workable way of thinking about optimum health, and initiating life skills adequate to implement knowledge so as to get healthy results.

Scientific health discoveries are happening at a breakneck pace. It is sometimes years before essential discoveries are implemented in day-to-day health care. Many traditional ways of looking at health information are quickly becoming obsolete.

For example, there is a tremendous amount of new and astounding scientific information about what is happening at the cellular level in terms of molecules, genes, and disease processes. Virtually all drugs on the market today have been approved for safe use without ample or any consideration to this important science. It already costs drug companies millions of dollars to bring a drug to the market. Now that there is new science that places new meaning to "safe," what should be done to verify safe use of current drugs?

These are political and financial questions wherein the forces in place will not wish to revisit the safety of already approved medications. In many cases, it is not difficult to figure out which medications should be on the dangerous list. At the conclusion of this book, it will be clear why any medication that causes weight gain as a side effect or makes insulin resistance worse, and there are many, is a contributing causative factor to major diseases as a person uses them over time. As a consumer, it places new emphasis on actually needing a medication before simply taking it on an ongoing basis.

THE FUNDAMENTALS OF BEING A COMPETENT *HEALTH ASSET MANAGER*™

Here are the key points about thinking with health data and making good personal health decisions. These are a common set of useful ideas to guide decisions and integrate information in a productive way. These tools for thinking with health data will enable processing health information more effectively, meaning that there is a better likelihood of taking care of an individual's most important personal asset, their own health.

Individual responsibility for health decisions.
Gone are the days of relying on anyone else but oneself, at least in the final analysis. Information and education are the keys to personal empowerment. Asking intelligent questions and not robotically following instructions will be a hallmark of this approach.

There usually is one individual in the family, frequently the mother, who will learn this way of thinking and act as a valuable resource for other family members as part of their health team. The advantage is that this individual has only the best health interest of the other family members in mind.

The quick-fix mentality is replaced with proactive health behavior.
Society is currently conditioned to believe that there is a drug for everything. For example, there will never be a single drug that stops bone loss. An individual is not going to arrive at age 55, discover there is a bone-loss issue, take a drug, and solve the problem.

The handwriting has been on the wall for over 20 years. Stress, lack of fitness, not enough sleep, overeating, under eating, and lifestyle abuse are among the many factors that contribute to the problem. Problems with leptin are a major cause of bone loss.

The solution involves learning to master leptin. Following a healthy lifestyle is the underlying foundation in this new way of looking at health. This is a life-long commitment to a healthy lifestyle.

Relational thinking will dominate over cause and effect thinking.
Virtually all of Western medicine is based on cause and effect thinking. Name the illness or disease, and name the drug. Medicate the problem, or operate on the problem. Apply as many such treatments as possible to increase the statistical chance of improvement. This has caused a long list of specialists to evolve that scrutinize cause and effect in narrow areas of health, frequently ignoring consequences or relevant information in other aspects of health.

This way of thinking is important for specific problems that have defined causes, a small percentage of actual health issues. Due to our lawsuit-happy culture, it leads to progressively invasive methods, trying to find a cause that frequently does not exist. It also leads to excessive and harsh treatments for problems just to be on the "safe side."

It is evident that the human body functions in a complex and interrelated way, wherein multiple issues happen at the same time, and, in many situations, the "cause" is an inability of the body to tolerate the effects of multiple stressors. This results in symptoms that defy cause and effect thinking.

The ability to figure out what these interrelationships mean is an important factor in having "health intelligence." Leptin is the key hormonal signal that crosses virtually all areas of body function. It is the key that unravels the great mysteries of health.

Healthy function and efficiency are far more important than number management.
A great deal of emphasis is currently placed on using drugs to force certain numbers on lab tests into range. This includes blood pressure,

cholesterol, and clotting times, to name a few. In the new way of looking at health, numbers that are out of range are a symptom of an imbalance in the body, not the cause of a problem. Improving numbers by improving healthy function will be a sign of a skilled health practitioner.

Drugs will be used primarily as temporary solutions, as needed, until healthy function can be restored. By asking the doctor how long to take a medication, or what else can be done so the medication is not needed, or how willing the doctor is to work on employing other solutions to either not go on the medication or to eventually get off the medication, one can quickly tell if this is the type of doctor wanted on their health team.

When a doctor can helpfully and intelligently answer such questions, there is the confidence that their training and areas of expertise include a more synergistic and functional understanding of health. This gives individuals more options for integrating a variety of strategies to improve issues and get on a healthy course of action.

It will be decades before the general medical profession has this level of knowledge and expertise, even though it is fundamental for them to do a good job. In the meantime, this places an even higher priority on Point No. 1, individual responsibility for health decisions.

Function will also have greater meaning than lab test numbers in general. For example, the clear symptoms of a poor metabolism will take on more importance than "normal-range thyroid scores." The solution will not be giving out thyroid hormone; the solution will be resolving the stressors on metabolism that cause the hypothyroid symptoms. Leptin issues will be recognized as the prime cause of the great majority of slow metabolic conditions.

It will also be imperative to determine how efficiently the body is working. For example, it is not as important how many immune cells there are, compared to how well the immune cells work. The properly trained and well-armed immune cell will take considerable priority over an immune cell that cannot get the job done. Understanding leptin provides key working knowledge as to the cause of immune deficiency, cancer, and autoimmune problems.

There is no reason for any doctor in the United States not to become an expert in this subject. Leptin affects all aspects of medicine and every medical specialty as a primary causative issue.

There are many shades of gray.
The difference between optimum health and a disease are many levels of progressively less efficient function. Traditional medicine is based on the belief that a person is either healthy or diseased. This form of logic has little to do with current scientific discoveries relating to disease. It is an old way of thinking about health, whose time has passed.

For example, on one end of calorie burning is optimum function. On the other end is the diabetic. In between are a thousand shades of gray that represent various levels of less efficient calorie metabolism. Leptin is the key to understanding how a person becomes diabetic. This is true for both type I diabetes and especially type II diabetes.

Individuals need to learn what symptoms go with what problems. Part of health intelligence is the ability to see a small problem developing and take effective action to return it to a more optimal function. This is a life skill, not a paper and pencil test. Only when a large number of individuals personally have this skill will current disease trends improve. It is important to catch problems at an early stage rather than letting them evolve into more complex issues.

A greater importance on saving for older age.
The quick-fix mentality and excessive stress lifestyles will be replaced by a more prudent understanding of the long-term consequences of current actions on future health. Everyone knows they need to save money for retirement; this is called financial reserves. Some people do it better than others. It takes some restraint not to spend everything on a current "want" so as to have stability in the future.

The same concept applies to being a competent Health Asset Manager.™ An important aspect of health is that every part of the body has reserves of different types that provide stability to health. When reserves run low, then health problems are prevalent and risk factors skyrocket. There are many types of reserves that relate to health: antioxidant reserves, mineral reserves, alkaline reserves, and energy reserves, to name a few. Stress demands tend to drain health reserves just as financial problems drain savings.

Any person who needs caffeine or antidepressants to function has a clear warning that energetic reserves are lacking. Building up reserves that have been drained takes time, minimally 3-6 months. It is also a lifelong commitment to doing things correctly, similar to managing a regular savings plan.

The skill with which a person builds and maintains important health reserves determines the quality of health that is established for a lifetime.

Even decisions made early in life affect one's overall reserves in the long run. It is never too late and seldom too early to begin being a good Health Asset Manager.™

Timing is everything.
Timing is the most powerful principle that will align health-related decisions. Timing influences optimum health as a dominant principle. When one eats is often more important than what one eats.

Getting the body into rhythm is far more important than any single symptom that may be viewed as a problem in terms of permanently resolving that symptom. Leptin responds to specific rhythmic patterns and is a fundamental hormone in regulating body rhythms.

These principles also apply to forward-thinking physicians. The emerging field of chronotherapy shows that the timing of medication administration is of profound importance to cardiovascular health,[4,5] cancer treatment,[6] mental health,[7,8] sleep disorders,[9] asthma,[10,11] and will eventually relate to many aspects of medicine.[12,13]

When the body is working in harmony, it has much less internal friction and much less wear and tear. Leptin is doing what it is supposed to be doing instead of being a primary underlying issue at the root of diseases that plague our society. There is little or no reason that most Americans could not maintain vibrant health until age 100.

SUMMARY

Every individual faces numerous health decisions on a day-to-day basis: the food that is eaten or not eaten, the exercise completed or not, the procrastination on starting a healthy lifestyle pattern, and the list continues. At the end of the day and the end of the week, look back and see what was actually done. Only in this way can there be an objective view of what the entire mind, subconscious plus conscious, has set as priorities.

True health intelligence is based on the ability to translate useful information into constructive behavior. This means having a clear understanding of health information. It also means having the skills to take charge of life and the subconscious mind. This means learning to master leptin.

3

What is Natural Balance

*H*omeostasis is a key principle of health. It is defined as an ability of the body to establish stability, regardless of the stress it is under, by regulating internal physiologic responses. Homeostasis is the key to being able to bounce back, to recover, and to tolerate stress of any type. It is the essence of natural balance.

Problems with leptin involve the loss of natural balance regulating food intake, fat storage, and metabolic rate throughout the body. In essence, leptin either allows or restricts energy production, making it of prime importance.

If individuals fail to understand what this means personally, proper health-related decisions will be difficult to make. When individuals or health practitioners do not understand natural balance, they focus on symptom suppression and number management. Such approaches are not necessarily in one's best interest.

THE WESTERN MEDICAL VIEW

During the evolution of Western medicine, homeostasis was considered to be a divine principle, something that is always there. This was an essential belief underpinning the entire paradigm of Western medicine. A great majority of the protocols used today in Western medicine are still based on this assumption.

These beliefs support the idea that almost anything can be done to the body to eradicate a disease or germ and it will automatically bounce back to normal. Unfortunately, modern molecular science proves that this is not the case.

During the evolution of Western-medicine thinking, the "cause" of disease was considered to come from outside the individual. The classic example is germs. This led to treatments involving antibiotics to eradicate the cause, immunizations to bolster defense against the cause, and surgery to remove the cause.

The thought is, diseased cells, like cancer cells, must be eradicated at all costs. A "successful" treatment is the complete removal of the offending, diseased cells. It is then considered that once these cells are removed, natural balance will simply reappear in a healthy state.

Cancer treatment involves drugs, surgery, radiation, chemotherapy, and anything else that aids the goal of complete eradication of the cancer. Since modern medicine is unable to determine the 100 percent eradication of all cancer cells, the guiding approach is to do as many therapies as possible, for as long as possible, to increase the statistical chance that all cancer cells are killed. Drugs are frequently used as a follow-up to treatment in an effort to regulate metabolism in such a way as to hopefully prevent a recurrence of the problem.

Little or no attention is given to why cancer occurred in the first place, what is fueling it in the present, or how to restore natural balance in such a way as to prevent it from coming back. It is much easier to do the treatments and drugs, hoping that the physical body can tolerate the treatment long enough to kill the cancer. It is common knowledge that many forms of cancer are resistant to current medical therapies.

This type of medical thinking evolved with the creation of immunizations and was reinforced with the discovery of antibiotics. A whole medical economy and vested interests have grown around this thinking, facilitating the use of drugs and/or surgeries. It has a degree of workability and has enough of a track record to pass as standard medical care. This does not mean it is the best care or best option; it is simply an agreed upon level of care.

KEEP ALL BODY PARTS IF POSSIBLE!

In 2001, over 600,000 gall bladders were removed. Many times these surgeries were performed even though a person did not experience a significant problem. The rationale is that because the gall bladder has stones in it, it is diseased. The gall bladder is seen as the cause of a problem or a potential cause of a problem.

Insurance pays for this operation, and it is considered safe because an individual can live without a gall bladder. Little attention is given to why a person forms stones, how to clean up a gall bladder that makes stones, what happens to the overall natural balance of a person with a poorly functioning gall bladder, or what happens to natural balance in a person without a gall bladder.

It is easier and more cost effective to take out the gall bladder and send the person on his way with little advice about what to do now. While it is true the person may need such an operation, it is also common that there are other options.

Surgery should only be performed when truly needed. Unless the person takes charge, they are caught up in the automatic gall bladder removal production line. The female reproductive system is another favorite surgical target. A basic rule of natural health is to try as much as possible to keep all body parts.

MALFUNCTIONING NATURAL BALANCE

It is currently inconvenient for Western medicine to think of homeostasis in any other terms than as an always operational and healthy system. However, what if a malfunction of the homeostatic system is the cause of a health problem? What if the inability to bounce back or self-regulate causes problems?

In reality, new discoveries show that this is the prime cause of virtually all serious diseases. What we formerly considered to be "causes" are stressful irritants that strain homeostasis until the body breaks down. Science now shows that various stressful irritants change the natural defense systems so they begin to work against the body and cause disease.

Leptin is the essential hormone that controls energy balance and metabolism in the human body. Problems with leptin are issues that disrupt the natural balance of homeostasis and are, therefore, the cause of a great majority of health problems.

The homeostatic system cannot be surgically removed. Leptin cannot be removed from the human body. A malfunction in the homeostatic system cannot be killed with a drug. When an imbalance causes anxiety, the nervous system can be drugged to a point where it cannot generate anxiety; however, drugs only suppress symptoms while the underlying problems worsen.

Blood pressure can be forced down with medication, but then what has been done to general circulation? Cholesterol can be lowered with drugs, but what has been done to the liver and overall steroid synthesis in the human body? Hot flashes can be stopped with estrogen but will excess estrogen cause cancer?

Current Western medical dogma, the day-to-day in the trenches drug-dispensing paradigm, does not want to have to evaluate these complexities. They want to employ a system of standard medical protocols focusing on the use of drugs and surgeries, relying on test scores to indicate the need for or correct response to the therapy that is used. They want to believe that homeostatic systems in the human body will be unharmed no matter what they do to them. The new science shows this method of practicing medicine has significant shortcomings.

HOW THE WESTERN MEDICAL VIEW TOOK POWER

The debate over the cause of disease is not new. In the nineteenth century, it played out in the French Academy of Science with the classic battle between Antone Bechamp and Louis Pastuer. Bechamp believed that the cause of disease was deterioration in the internal health of the person, a breakdown of homeostasis or natural balance. Pastuer believed the sole cause of disease was germs from the outside.

Pastuer's research led to the first marketable drugs for immunizations and the birth of the pharmaceutical industry. His ideas were backed by considerable money, that is why today his name is known and Bechamp is not recognized.

The discovery of penicillin in the 1930s ushered in the antibiotic era. Penicillin is a poison derived from fungus, a poison that kills bacteria. The seemingly instantaneous results of this antibiotic sealed the fate of the eclectic and other natural medical ideas.

Western medicine ideas became the dominant theme in health care with huge money and legal forces placed behind their implementation and competitive survival. At the time of their evolution, the science supporting them seemed to provide an acceptable level of workability.

The discovery of penicillin led to massive pharmaceutical research looking for more antibiotics. Research quickly showed that most of the new antibiotics being developed kept killing the tested animals as the drugs were too toxic. Most of this research has never been made public.

Today, germs have built resistance to most antibiotics, and a major health crisis has resulted since stronger antibiotics are simply too toxic for humans to consume. Even if an individual is very healthy and never uses antibiotics, there is still a chance of being infected with one of these superbugs that has been created due to the overuse of antibiotics. These new superbugs are very hard to get rid of once they settle into a person's system. Just when the illness seems to be over, the bug flares up again and there is a reoccurrence.

One drug that evolved in the early antibiotic research was cyclosporine, allowed for use as an anti-rejection drug for transplant surgery. The drug was originally intended as an antibiotic but was too toxic to give to the general public. It found a market niche because it poisons the immune system to a point where the immune system will not reject a donor organ. This drug currently has a needed role in transplant surgery; if not for that role, it would not be on the market at all.

Unfortunately, long-term use of this drug invariably results in a significantly increased risk for heart disease[14] and cancer[15] due to the effects of this poison in the body. When doctors employ their common practice of using drugs for unapproved use, major problems can occur. When cyclosporine is used in this manner to treat autoimmune skin problems, the result can be a fatal cancerous fungal infection.[16,17]

This book makes it clear that when mastering leptin, many autoimmune problems will simply go away. Older therapies that rely on toxic immunosuppressive drugs will no longer be a mainstay approach. There is a huge difference between poisoning the immune system and returning the immune system to natural function.

THE MEDICATION TRADE-OFF

There is a price to pay for almost any medication. That price is based on the toxicity of the drug as well as how that drug may deregulate natural function in the process of trying to produce a "desirable" result. Some undesirable side effects may be noticed in a matter of days or weeks; others are more insidious and may slowly emerge over a period of years.

What constitutes a desirable result depends on the situation. Medical emergencies require drugs to facilitate care. A heart recovering from a heart attack requires medications to ensure it does not have to work too hard while it regains strength. There are numerous appropriate uses of medication. Most of them involve short-term use for a definable amount of time. They are used to help get the body back on track so that it can function on its own. It is like using a cast to allow a broken bone to heal. Once the bone is healed, the cast is discarded. Few would argue the use of any medication in this context. Even antibiotics have an appropriate use combating acute infections.

In the case of drugs and ongoing use, negative effects are cumulative and progressive over time. For example, let us say a doctor wants to lower cholesterol with medication. A statin drug is given to lower the cholesterol to an acceptable number. Since this medication interrupts natural signals to synthesize steroidal hormones in the body, and since steroidal hormones help regulate homeostasis, especially the ability to adapt to stress, what will be the effect? It will vary dramatically from person to person. Some will feel miserable right away. Others will lose 5 to 15 percent efficiency in their natural-balance system. They do not feel the same, but they accept it.

After a number of years on a cholesterol-lowering medication, this lack of efficiency has a domino effect on many other systems in the body that are not directly related to steroid synthesis, only indirectly related because the body is not working as well, and so a new symptom or problem crops up somewhere else. This requires a new medication to address that symptom, and the cycle goes on and on. This type of medical symptom and number management approach is definitely in the interest of drug companies and not in the long-term health of individuals.

The human body is not composed of drugs. It is made up of proteins, carbohydrates, fats, water, vitamins, minerals, and numerous cofactor substances that facilitate healthy function and structure. These substances work together in an effort to maintain natural balance. The human body performs millions of self-regulatory steps every minute in an attempt to deal with stress and maintain natural balance.

Drugs are powerful, forcing self-regulation to take a back seat and thereby forcing natural balance to take a back seat. It is impossible to predict all consequences of any drug taken for a long period of time. Furthermore, the current guidelines for safe use of drugs need major re-evaluation in light of new scientific discoveries regarding the cause of disease so as to warn consumers of the potential life-threatening risks of long-term use of numerous medications.

SCIENCE FORGES NEW GROUND

Molecular medicine has opened a new Pandora's box. The very scientists looking for the causes of diseases and seeking to improve treatments are proving the unthinkable! They are showing that the causes of cancer, heart disease, and age-related diseases are changes in the body's own normal regulatory communication systems. The same exact gene and hormonal signals that are essential for survival are used against the person to cause cancer and heart disease. This is an amazing discovery; one that alters the way health care should be viewed on a fundamental level.

This is great news for individuals who are truly interested in their own quality of health. These discoveries translate to realistic and practical steps that can be taken by anyone to dramatically improve their quality of health and reduce their risk for serious disease, regardless of their genetic risk factors.

SUMMARY

This book is written for those who want to better understand their own health options and those who are interested in truly improving and maintaining their quality of health. It teaches the key principles of self-care, the essence of being a Health Asset Manager.™ It is about thinking with health-related information, empowering individuals to be in charge of their own health, and to be responsible for the final decisions on their personal care.

The stressors inherent in modern society are enough to throw any person's health out of balance. It is easy to get off track to the point where symptoms are bad enough that doctors recommend a drug. This is especially true in the baby-boomer generation that is growing older. Ask questions and learn to take charge; knowledge is power; there are options.

This is a book about employing health options in their proper context towards the goal of managing health in a way that keeps the quality of health in tact. The bottom line is the result of improved quality of health.

4

Fat and Leptin - The New Reality

The old view of fat was that it primarily acted as a place for the body to store extra calories. No higher level thinking or more prestigious purpose was given to fat; it simply became the undesirable extra weight that many people carried around.

That view of fat changed dramatically and forever in 1994 with the discovery of leptin,[18] and with this discovery, the basis of Western medicine theory of the last 100 years will need to change.

Leptin is a hormone that is secreted by fat cells in white adipose tissue (Figure 1). Leptin was found to be a signal to the brain, having a primary influence on body weight. However, it was soon discovered to be involved with insulin, cardiovascular health, reproductive function, sex hormones, immune function, adrenal function, stress, thyroid function, bone health, cancer, and inflammation. In fact, it has a major determining role in many aspects of healthy function.

Even more important, when the hormone falls out of natural balance and loses its ability to communicate efficiently, health problems follow. The concept of fat as a storage place has been transformed to fat as a major endocrine organ, such as the thyroid gland, adrenal glands, and sex glands.[19]

THE SUBCONSCIOUS ANTI-STARVATION PRINCIPLE

While there is an optimum body weight for health as well as our own personal opinions, the subconscious brain has its own ideas about how much the body should weigh.

The subconscious brain does not care about body weight from the point of view of how the body looks. The subconscious brain has no idea when a person thinks they are fat or at the right body weight. The subconscious brain cannot see the body in the mirror. In fact, the subconscious brain does not even know how much fat is actually stored. Yet, the subconscious brain is in primary control of eating behaviors.

The brain is concerned with surviving, especially on a subconscious basis. The brain is concerned about replenishing the body back to a proper amount of fat for survival. If the body is in a state of natural balance, it has the ability to normalize itself at a reasonable weight.

The brain senses how much fat is on hand by a system of communication with fat cells. The hormone signal secreted by fat cells is called leptin. When the brain senses that leptin levels are normal, then there is no need to store extra calories as fat. These are core survival issues programmed into the essence of the human survival genetics. These impulses are much more powerful than a person's willpower; a reason why abnormal cravings reflect leptin problems.

On the one hand, leptin is quite good. It is how the human race has survived in response to times when there was little food. In today's society, there is a new problem called "food is everywhere." From a genetic and evolutionary point of view, we do not have a lot of experience with chronic overeating. As it turns out, the subconscious brain gets very confused by this behavior. The brain no longer properly senses the leptin message; it becomes leptin resistant. Once this problem sets in, a person keeps eating and gets fatter, and the confused metabolism responds as if it is starving.

Worse yet, excess leptin reinforces the problems that set the stage for the onset of cardiovascular disease, cancer that may not respond to treatment, and the diseases of aging.

The bottom line is that a fundamental principle of survival is turned against the individual and ends up causing major health problems, one of which is being overweight. This is a breakdown of natural balance.

THE DISCOVERY OF LEPTIN

There is a type of mouse called an *ob/ob* mouse. It is always hungry and cannot stop eating. It gets to be three times the weight of a regular mouse. It also becomes type II diabetic and has great difficulty reproducing. Scientists

What is Leptin?

Figure 1

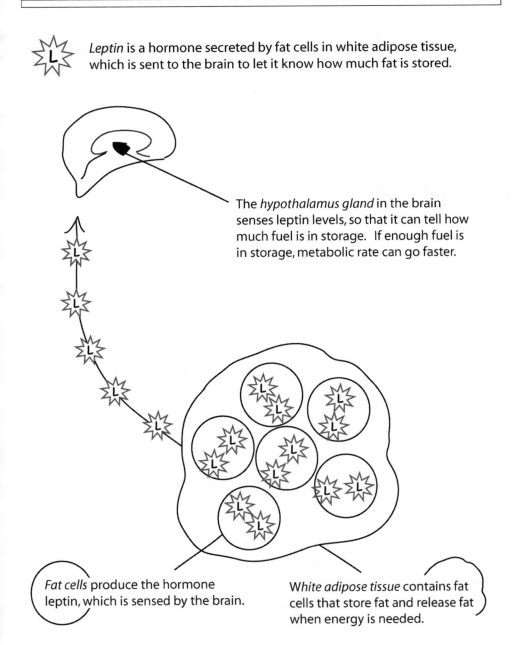

Leptin is a hormone secreted by fat cells in white adipose tissue, which is sent to the brain to let it know how much fat is stored.

The *hypothalamus gland* in the brain senses leptin levels, so that it can tell how much fuel is in storage. If enough fuel is in storage, metabolic rate can go faster.

Fat cells produce the hormone leptin, which is sensed by the brain.

W*hite adipose tissue* contains fat cells that store fat and release fat when energy is needed.

figured out that this mouse was missing a signal to stop eating, and leptin turned out to be the missing hormonal signal.

Since the discovery of leptin in 1994, intense scientific research has been going on around the world trying to figure out exactly how leptin works. As it turns out, the issue is incredibly complex. With each passing month, the jigsaw puzzle takes on new meaning. Enough is known to force a revolution of the entire scientific basis of medicine.

To understand why this is the case, let us back up and go through the story a bit slower, placing it in the context of the attainment of natural balance and proper body weight.

ENERGY BALANCE

The energy needs of the human body are critical to the function of every cell, to every body part, and to humans as a whole. Thus, establishing adequate energy and maintaining energy balance are fundamental to survival.

Generally speaking, a person is going to be in one of three situations regarding energy balance and food intake:

1) **Energy Deficit** – Not enough intake of energy in the form of food relative to the need for energy. Examples include malnutrition, starvation, anorexia, bulimia, and the low-calorie diet employed in an effort to lose weight (Figure 2).

2) **Energy Excess** – The consumption of too much food. This frequently promotes the storage of calories as fat.

3) **Energy Balance** – Body weight stays the same as the amount of calories consumed is about the same as the amount metabolized into energy. A person may be overweight or normal weight.

A primary purpose of the hormone leptin is to coordinate the metabolic, endocrine, and behavioral responses to starvation.[20] This hormone has a powerful influence on the subconscious mind that is programmed at a genetic survival level, completely taking over eating patterns if the circumstances from its point of view dictate that it should.

In our genetic evolution, there were many times when there was not enough food. This induced an energy-deficit state. In order to survive, calories stored in fat were broken down and used as fuel. When this happens, leptin levels drop and metabolism slows down to conserve stored energy. This slower metabolic rate is implemented to match the limited supply of food.

In our evolution, when food was found, eating a higher amount of food would resume. The amount of food a person eats in one meal cannot restore depleted fat reserves from a prolonged period of reduced calorie intake. However, after eating a number of meals, the fat cells begin to replenish their reserves and the hormone leptin begins to increase. Once the leptin levels rise to a certain point, the fat cells are replenished. The message goes out to stop eating so much. The hormone leptin is core to the survival of our species. It is very powerful. (Figure 3)

So far, this seems like a relatively straightforward proposition. When leptin is low, one will be hungry and want to eat. When enough food is eaten over a period of days or weeks, then leptin will be higher, signaling the brain to reduce appetite.

The *ob/ob* mouse does not make any leptin due to a mutation of the gene that synthesizes leptin; thus the mouse is always hungry and eats endlessly. When the *ob/ob* mouse is given leptin, it quits overeating and loses weight. Indeed, this is how leptin works in a person's body that is in a good and healthy state of natural balance.

This sounds like the weight-loss miracle everybody is awaiting. Why have the drug companies not made a leptin pill and given it to every overweight person? It seems like an ideal drug. It would certainly apply to the quick-fix mentality of the American public. It would appeal to the cause and effect thinking of Western medicine. A blood test could check for leptin; it could be given as a prescription until the blood level is normal and the person no longer wants to overeat. Everyone's weight-loss problem would be solved. Rest assured, the drug companies wished it were that easy.

EFFICIENCY AND RESISTANCE - DOMINANT HEALTH PRINCIPLES

Almost all overweight individuals have high leptin levels. That is right; most overweight people have too much leptin!

Leptin Function when Dieting

Figure 2

When on a low calorie diet, the body goes into a survival mode and slows the rate at which stored fat is used for energy.

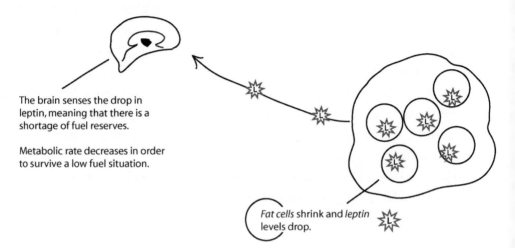

The brain senses the drop in leptin, meaning that there is a shortage of fuel reserves.

Metabolic rate decreases in order to survive a low fuel situation.

Fat cells shrink and *leptin* levels drop.

Leptin Function when Food is Available

Figure 3

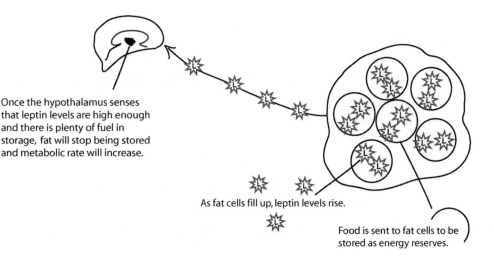

When food is available, it heads to fat cells to replenish depleted reserves.

Once the hypothalamus senses that leptin levels are high enough and there is plenty of fuel in storage, fat will stop being stored and metabolic rate will increase.

As fat cells fill up, leptin levels rise.

Food is sent to fat cells to be stored as energy reserves.

When a person gets thrown out of natural balance, the brain does not sense leptin levels correctly, literally building up resistance to the hormone (Figure 4). This problem steadily gets worse as a person gets older.[21]

The main target for the leptin message is the hypothalamus gland of the brain. In overweight people who have difficulty controlling the amount of food they eat, their body is insulin resistant and their brain is leptin resistant. There are too many of these hormones circulating, and they are not productive.

In a normal situation, the white adipose tissue is trying to make a phone call to the brain. The message traveling over the phone line is a hormone called leptin. The amount of leptin in the phone call tells the brain how much fat is in reserve, this information allows the brain to regulate energy for the rest of the body.

Virtually all overweight people do not make this phone call properly. There is plenty of leptin; it just does not get through to the brain. The fat cells make repetitive phone calls, and the brain does not answer. The net result is that the brain thinks the body is still starving and continues to order the storage of fat, even though there may be plenty of fat already in storage.

The problem is not having too much or too little of the hormone leptin; the problem is leptin not working efficiently. So how is the problem of leptin resistance corrected?

A drug company tries to follow the cause and effect sequence of leptin activity in the brain to locate a receptor or some other change in signal that leptin induces. A drug may be formulated to target something closer to the "cause" of the problem. Drug companies are currently in a mad race to the market with drugs that affect neuropeptide Y, melanocortin receptors, and leptin receptors.[22]

These drugs will seek to reduce the desire to eat. There is no doubt this will be the next class of "hot" weight-loss drugs appealing to the quick-fix mentality. There is also no doubt that such drugs will have many side effects that disrupt natural balance and will cause numerous health problems in individuals who use them.

If an individual is truly interested in managing their own health, they will ask a few basic questions. Why do I have leptin resistance? How did the problem get started in the first place? Can I eat in such a way that will improve the problem? What options do I have that will correct the problem and

Leptin in Overweight People

Figure 4

Leptin resistance occurs in overweight people. The brain thinks there is not enough fat in storage and continues to fill fat cells with fuel.

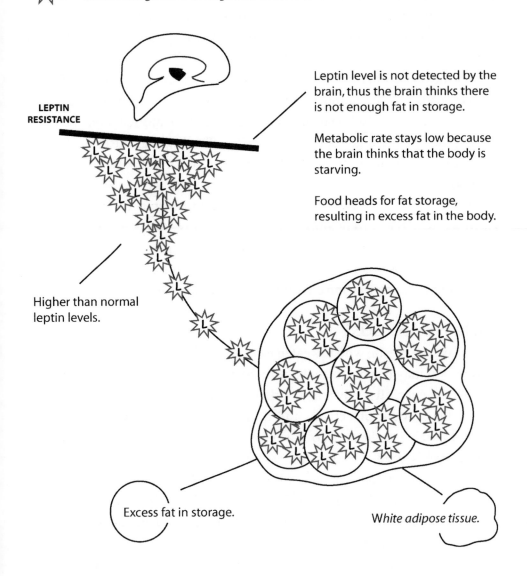

LEPTIN RESISTANCE

Leptin level is not detected by the brain, thus the brain thinks there is not enough fat in storage.

Metabolic rate stays low because the brain thinks that the body is starving.

Food heads for fat storage, resulting in excess fat in the body.

Higher than normal leptin levels.

Excess fat in storage.

White adipose tissue.

forever change my weight issues and health risks by fixing the source of the problem?

These types of questions go against the grain of traditional Western medicine thinking. For example, obesity is considered a disease. A primary cause of obesity is leptin resistance. However, leptin resistance cannot be surgically removed. It cannot be medicated out of existence. It is a functional problem of homeostasis; a problem of the natural balance system in the body gone awry.

Furthermore, obesity causes other diseases such as heart disease. Thus, a primary cause of the number-one killer in America is a problem in energy homeostasis. It is also clear that leptin resistance is a direct contributor to cancer, the second-largest killer in America. The leading causes of death in America are primarily the result of disruption of natural balance in the human body.

The answers to these questions about leptin resistance are not simple. However, with the current amount of science that is available, it is possible to have a major impact towards permanently improving these issues. There is no quick fix; leptin is not a quick-fix hormone in the first place. The time invested in learning this information may be a life saver.

BASIC WEIGHT LOSS

Let us take the person who has eaten too much and gained a few extra pounds. This person may be able to cut back on eating, increase exercise, and take off the extra weight. It really was not that difficult. As long as they keep up a reasonable amount of activity and do not go overboard with eating, they maintain their weight and do not have to think too much about it. Their energy level is good, and they feel healthy.

Such a person does not have a significant problem with leptin resistance. When they gained their extra weight, they were pushing the leptin system into a condition of imbalance, but their health was good enough that they got things under control by watching food intake and increasing exercise.

As we get older, leptin resistance becomes much more of an issue. It provokes insulin resistance, in a somewhat chicken and egg manner, and the two lock each other into place. A third problem develops – resistance of fat cells to the stimulation of the sympathetic nervous system, a problem called adrenaline resistance. The metabolism of the fat cells becomes sluggish, making it easier for them to accumulate fat and more difficult to eliminate stored fat.

Fat cells have a tendency to become larger in size and readily multiply as we age, and leptin resistance fuels this undesirable state of affairs. In this situation, we keep gaining weight. We can follow a diet for a while, but we find that it is all too easy to eat and gain the weight back, sooner or later. Such a person has a major problem with leptin resistance. This is typically reflected as being 15 or more pounds above an ideal weight. While this happens more easily as a person ages, aging is no excuse.

THE PERSON WHO EATS LITTLE AND STRUGGLES WITH WEIGHT

Another example of leptin resistance is the person who has a history of struggling with leptin-resistant weight issues and now eats very little in an effort to maintain a more optimum body weight. Such a person may be at a reasonable weight, from their point of view, but they have low energy and poor immune response. This person lives in a state of energy deficiency. They frequently sleep all day. Their entire metabolism is in slow motion. They are prone to fatigue and have abnormally low energy.

They maintain their body weight by hibernating. They may make themselves exercise, but it does not feel refreshing. They are afraid to eat because they know they will get fat. This forces leptin levels to be lower for the time being. In some cases, this can develop into full-scale anorexia. However, when food is eaten, the tendency is to gain back excessive weight unless the person learns the secrets of leptin management.

On the other hand, there are people who eat very little and cannot lose weight. Such individuals may go into rapid weight gain when they eat moderately. They can be significantly overweight and unable to lose weight even on a relatively low-calorie diet. Their body thinks it is starving even though it is not; therefore, their metabolism slows down.

In essence, they are also hibernating. If they try to reduce their calorie intake to a very low level to lose weight, they run out of energy just like the person described in the previous paragraphs. When they start eating again, they gain even more weight.

These types of individuals think they may have thyroid problems. In some cases they do. However, in the majority of cases, the thyroid problems, or low-thyroid symptoms, are caused by leptin resistance and improperly functioning leptin signals. The thyroid gland is simply experiencing the brunt of the problem with poor leptin function.

SUMMARY

It is a survival instinct to replenish the supply of fat. This will never change. The primary problem that people get into and cannot get out of is a major breakdown in communication between the white fat cells and the brain. This problem is called leptin resistance.

Leptin resistance means that the brain cannot correctly judge when stored fats are at a proper level. It can keep a person significantly overweight because the subconscious brain is not sure there is enough fat on hand. Worse yet, the brain may be enforcing orders on a subconscious basis to replenish the fat even though the stores of fat are overflowing.

Under the influence of leptin, a primary role of white adipose tissue acts as a reserve of fuel. Leptin controls how the body restores fuel after a period of food deprivation or illness. The fact that fat is much more than a storage bin is quite fascinating. Fat cells talk directly to the brain, and in response, the subconscious brain commands eating behavior. In some cases, this may completely override willpower.

Fat cells carry out many types of communication. This makes understanding them a more complex issue. In addition to leptin, scientists have identified at least 15 other major communication signals coming out of fat cells.[23] This is discussed later. At this point, we know that fat is involved with immune function, cardiovascular function, kidney function, liver function, reproductive function, thyroid function, adrenal function, and toxins. Its involvement in these issues is not a passive role.

Due to this new understanding, white adipose tissue has gone from the lowly status of being a storage bin, to being a primary player in eating behavior, metabolism, cardiovascular disease, and cancer. White adipose tissue is a major endocrine organ in human metabolism. Leptin is the most important hormone discovered to date.

5

How Fat Communicates

The brain remains commander and chief of the human body and the prime regulator of communication going on in the body. The brain relies on accurate perception of leptin to set the appropriate metabolic rate.

It has been known for many years that the sympathetic nervous system is the primary stimulant to the metabolic activity of white adipose tissue.

The sympathetic nervous system is the aggressive side of the nervous system. In a positive sense, the sympathetic nervous system enables an individual to be focused, communicative, and motivated towards a goal.

Sympathetic nervous system activity correlates to the "left brain" view of the world, more orderly, organized, and assertive. The left brain handles 5-9 pieces of data at a time; it is time and sequence oriented. The classic Type-A personality is driven by sympathetic nervous system activity.

However, many individuals who have a dominant left-brain orientation to the world are not classic Type-A personalities. Such individuals are usually direct and straightforward with communication so as to organize and implement plans.

Typical left-brain stress responses are anger, frustration, agitation, or irritation. Generally, these feelings are expressed.

By comparison, the more relaxed side of the nervous system is called the parasympathetic nervous system. It correlates to the "right brain" view of the world, more spatial and adaptive in nature.

The right brain handles millions of pieces of data at once and sees relationships between data. This side of the brain likes pleasure and sensory stimulation and tries to avoid or deny pain. The classic Type-B personality is driven by parasympathetic nervous system function.

Typical right-brain stress reactions include sadness, guilt, resentment, or denial. These feelings are frequently not expressed.

SUBCONSCIOUS ACTIVATION

Under stress, the sympathetic nervous system takes over, at least on a subconscious basis. This is called the fight or flight response. A classic Type-A personality is more likely to fight, whereas a classic Type-B personality is more likely to be afraid or flee. Regardless of personality type, the release of sympathetic nervous system adrenaline is a survival impulse.

For example, a person is driving down the street, and someone pulls out almost causing a collision; the reaction is to quickly avoid the accident. The heart races, and the body is jittery. There is no time to stop and think about what to do. A perceived threat to survival enters the conscious awareness that is monitored by the hypothalamus gland in the brain, the bridge between conscious and subconscious. In the presence of perceived danger, the hypothalamus gland takes control of the body. It causes nerves to release adrenaline, stimulating the metabolism and body into fast reaction for survival.

This is an example of how the subconscious brain takes over control of conscious thought processes to facilitate survival.

LEPTIN IS A SUBCONSCIOUS PERCEPTION

The perception of leptin occurs on a subconscious basis. It is "hard-wired" into survival calculations, especially stress-related issues. It controls metabolic rate, the use of energy, and eating behavior.

When the hypothalamus gland perceives leptin correctly, then metabolism can run at a proper pace and stress can be handled in an appropriate way.

When leptin is not perceived correctly, major problems with energy and metabolism occur.

LEPTIN AND THE STRESS RESPONSE

While some emergencies only last a split second, others last for longer periods of time. A person needs to be able to maintain energy long enough to deal with the stress. This is one reason why white adipose tissue is metabolically stimulated by the sympathetic nervous system. Under such stimulation, white fat cells begin to release their stores of energy so that an emergency demand can be met over a prolonged period of time. This mechanism of white adipose tissue stimulation has been recognized since 1929.[24]

Since this early time, scientists have shown that there are different types of receptors in fat cells for adrenaline. For example, fat around the midsection has more of one type of receptor than fat in other areas. This is why some people gain weight around the midsection and others gain it on the hips and thighs. When a certain type of receptor has trouble getting the message, fat accumulates more readily in that area of the body as the metabolic rate of those specific fat cells slows down.

We have mentioned that leptin is a long-term regulator of body fat reserves, acting to restore fat reserves in an effort to recover from starvation or calorie restriction. When leptin is low, a person wants to eat; when leptin is high, a person does not want to eat, assuming everything is working properly. This is a longer-term issue, gauging fuel supply over a period of weeks or months.

Leptin is also under short-term control of the sympathetic nervous system. This is because the 911 call that goes out for the emergency need of the body takes priority over long-term storage goals. Thus, a quick burst of sympathetic nervous system activity depresses leptin production.[25]

The main point to understand is that the sympathetic nervous system drives the metabolic rate of white adipose tissue. This is a direct line of communication from the nervous system to fat. This communication is directed by the hypothalamus gland in the brain, the subconscious control center and the overall 911 commander and chief of the human body.

FAT COMMUNICATES

The primary hormone made by white fat cells is leptin. Leptin talks directly to the hypothalamus gland of the brain. When leptin levels are high in the properly functioning person, it tells the brain to decrease food intake and increase sympathetic nerve activity, thus increasing metabolic rate and direct stimulation to metabolism of white adipose tissue.[26]

As sympathetic nerve activity increases and metabolic rate increases, leptin is lowered signaling the need to accumulate more stored energy. This completes a circle of communication between fat cells and the brain. This is how metabolism works when a person's body is in a state of natural balance and an example of a homeostatic system in the human body relating to the natural balance of energy. It has its own built-in checks and balances. The ebb and flow of these communication signals are fundamental to having an appropriate appetite.

A BREAKDOWN IN COMMUNICATION

When there are problems with leptin, there is a breakdown of proper communication. Low leptin levels cause a person to have no appetite, resulting in too much weight loss and the loss of bone density. High leptin levels cause a person to eat frequently or rapidly gain weight from whatever is eaten.

This is the opposite of how the hormone behaves when it is working properly. There is a disruption of the normal communication between the brain and fat cells. Not only does this cause confusion relating to the subject of eating, the consequences to the rest of the body are of major importance. It is not a desirable state of affairs to have a primary endocrine organ, white adipose tissue, in a state of poor communication.

In addition to the daily eating patterns, it is also appropriate to view this circle of communication in the context of how a person does on a month-to-month basis. If not enough food is consumed, then leptin tends to stay low, decreasing sympathetic nerve stimulation and metabolic rate and increasing appetite. This results in the hibernation effect that enables humans to survive prolonged periods of reduced food availability. Metabolism consequently slows down to conserve body fat to survive.

When enough food is consumed, the leptin level rises, telling the brain to quit eating and increase metabolic rate. This enables the body to have an energetic metabolic drive. There is a higher level of leptin, meaning there is adequate fuel on hand so the body can work at an optimum rate and does not need to be in starvation mode. This is how the leptin hormone behaves when it works correctly, not during times of leptin resistance.

When there is leptin resistance, the brain does not hear the phone call from fat cells telling it there is enough fuel in storage. Consequently, the fat cells keep accumulating weight because neither the brain nor the fat-cell troops have a sense of what is actually happening (Figure 4).

In an effort to stimulate metabolism, the brain releases adrenaline. This is magnified by too much stress. Such adrenaline should stimulate fat cells to release energy that should cause weight loss. However, when adrenaline is too high too often, fat cells develop adrenaline resistance. From a fat cell's point of view, it is like being yelled at too often. After a while, the fat cells go numb to the adrenaline, and adrenaline resistance develops. This causes metabolism of fat cells to stay locked in a "hibernation metabolic rate." It also causes weight gain around the middle, high blood pressure, and sleep problems (Figure 5).

TIMING AND LEPTIN

In addition to the influences and communication between the brain and fat cells, leptin levels follow a daily pattern. Leptin levels are highest during the first few hours of sleep and fall to their lowest level in the morning.[27] They peak before the adrenal steroid cortisol that is highest at 6 a.m., and they are not tied to cortisol production.[28] A person who is in a good rhythm and pattern will not be hungry before bed because the brain correctly senses the higher level of leptin, thus appetite is off in terms of cravings for food.

On the other hand, a person who craves food before bed has leptin resistance, meaning that the brain does not sense the leptin signal to not eat even though it is naturally highest at this time. A major clue that a person is heading down a pattern of leptin resistance is out-of-control eating after dinner. This is a more serious problem than previously realized.

Furthermore, a meal that has too many high-glycemic index carbohydrates can cause the normal night pattern of rising leptin to occur 7-9 hours earlier than it should, completely throwing the body out of proper rhythm.[29] Therefore, eating too many sweets will cause leptin levels to rise at the wrong time. Once a person has leptin resistance, this leads to overeating, especially at night. For example, if a person has a sweet roll, muffin, or orange juice for breakfast or too many cookies at lunch, there will commonly be a leptin-resistant urge to eat after dinner that evening.

Adrenaline Resistance

Figure 5

1. Sympathetic nerves release adrenaline based on normal behavior, exercise, and stress.
2. Under excess stress or leptin resistance, there is excess adrenaline released by the sympathetic nerves.

Normal Adrenaline Release

CAUSES

Behavior: Focused and motivated drive. Assertive.
Exercise: Anaerobic exercise, physical demands.
Stress: Anger, frustration, irritation, anxiety.

NORMAL ADRENALINE - stimulates fat cells to release fuel for energy

Energy

Fat is burned for fuel/ energy requirements. Leptin level decreases.

Energy

Excessive Adrenaline Release

ADRENALINE RESISTANCE

CAUSES

Too much assertive behavior, stress, or physical output.
Leptin Resistance - Adrenaline is released excessively in an effort to stimulate a sluggish metabolism.

EXCESS ADRENALINE

Side Effects

Due to lack of stimulation from adrenaline, fat cells are not burned for fuel. Stored fat accumulates. Leptin level increases.

1. Weight gain around the middle.
2. Cardiovascular distress, including high blood pressure.
3. General inflammation, wear and tear.
4. Difficulty sleeping.

THE BRAIN SETS LEPTIN RHYTHM

It is interesting to note that the control of the daily pattern of leptin secretion comes from the biological clock in the brain.[30] Even though the hormone itself is produced in fat cells, it responds to a rhythmic signal coming from the brain. In the previous section, it was described how the sympathetic nerves were involved in communication to fat cells and how fat cells talked back to the brain. Now there is an additional feature of this communication system, meaning that there is a daily timing pattern essential for proper leptin function. This daily timing pattern is under control of the brain, like the conductor of an orchestra.

This opens the door to understanding why leptin is the cause of so many health problems. Leptin levels are crucial to survival instinct, the fundamental core level of energy. Without fuel, nothing in the human body works. Leptin is the most important hormone signal gauging fuel supply. Just as driving patterns are altered to go to a gas station when the car's fuel gauge says it is on empty, so it is that leptin levels command powerful urges relating to food consumption.

When the rhythmic pattern of leptin secretion is disrupted, the brain has trouble with energy regulation in general, and other timing patterns in the body are thrown out of natural rhythm. There are numerous examples in this book that show that major health problems involve the loss of proper leptin timing, not necessarily related to the amount of leptin. Leptin levels in the blood could be at a "normal" amount; they are simply not doing what they are supposed to be doing at the right time. This is a very important point. A lab test for leptin in the blood does not reflect these problems.

LEPTIN TONE AND ACTIVE METABOLISM

In addition to the normal nighttime rise in leptin, it is also under a shorter duration pulsing regulation. In a 24-hour period, there are as many as 32 pulses of leptin activity. These relate to circulating adrenaline levels.[31] This is believed to act as a sort of tension in the regulatory system, providing the ability of the hormone to fluctuate on a gradual basis rather than have a blatant on and off switch. This leptin and adrenaline tension is essential for fast-action response to stress as more fuel is needed to produce energy in the case of an emergency demand.

In essence, this leptin and adrenaline tension provides an "energy tone" much the same as the muscle tone we feel when in good physical shape. The opposite of this "energy tone" is a fatigued or washed-out feeling.

The dominant factor that influences leptin production is the sympathetic nervous system. There is a cycle of communication between fat cells and the brain. They talk to each other in an effort to figure out the fat storage needs on a long-term basis. This long-term plan can also be put on hold for short-term energy needs to deal with stress.

REVIEWING PRIMARY LEPTIN REGULATION

The brain determines other hormone activity in the body based on the perception of leptin. The brain controls the leptin rhythm. Leptin is the most important hormone in helping the brain determine energy use in the body.

Leptin is under short-term regulation, daily regulation, and long-term regulation. It is central to body rhythms as proper timing is fundamental to the energy supply that the brain uses to calculate how much energy it can spend for any particular situation. There is a tremendous amount of complexity in this system, a phenomenal system of evolution that enables the body to elegantly distribute energy so it can survive.

These points alone explain why drug therapy will not work to solve leptin resistance. Drugs will simply block transmission and cause a blatant off or on function. They will interfere with the natural trend of the 24-hour pattern and interfere with the proper leptin tone in circulation. Drugs will also handicap the stress response and depress immune function.

Only in the case of a true genetic inability to make leptin will leptin drugs have any value, which is likely around 1 percent of obese individuals. The great majority of overweight and fatigued Americans do not suffer from such a genetic problem; they suffer from serious leptin mismanagement.

LEPTIN AND INSULIN

Leptin from fat cells and insulin from the pancreas also communicate with each other. This is similar to two department heads in a company talking to each other. Insulin production stimulates leptin production.[32] Leptin receptors are present on the insulin-producing B-cells of the pancreas, demonstrating the ability to turn off insulin production.[33]

In normal physical function, leptin and insulin have a balancing effect on food intake, energy storage, and a stable energy level. Once leptin resistance sets in and leptin levels are high, then the pancreatic B-cells do not respond to the signal from leptin to stop making insulin.[34]

However, insulin keeps stimulating leptin production at the same time insulin promotes calories to store as fat. Furthermore, the high circulating insulin causes cells throughout the body to be resistant to insulin. Thus, we see that leptin resistance sets the stage for insulin resistance, and the two problems continue to play off each other and make each other worse (Figure 6).

THE KEY TRIAD OF PROBLEMS

Hence, we see the triad of leptin resistance, insulin resistance, and adrenaline resistance as the main cause of any overweight problem (Figure 7). For example, when the fat cells in the abdominal area become resistant to adrenaline, then the individual begins to gain weight around the middle. This is a common area for weight gain in men; it also happens to women who struggle with menstrual irregularities and women at menopause. This type of weight gain around the middle is the worst kind of weight gain, the type most associated with cardiovascular disease.

More is explained about insulin resistance in Chapter 12. It is mentioned here to emphasize the issue of efficiency and metabolism. Individuals struggling with body weight have a key triad of efficiency problems. The common denominator is that the hormonal signals cannot get through to their targets; there is resistance. It is like trying to call someone on the phone, and they do not answer. The messages in the phone calls contain adrenaline, leptin, and insulin. There are various reasons why the phone calls are not answered, all of which fall under the general category of the body being out of natural balance.

Expensive lab tests are not needed to prove there is a problem. A person just has to look in the mirror and then take note of their level of energy. The problem slowly and progressively gets worse as a person gets older.

Leptin Resistance Causes Insulin Resistance

Figure 6

Leptin resistance not only occurs in the brain, but occurs in the pancreas as well.

Normal Leptin Function in the Pancreas:
Self-regulatory loop between leptin and insulin.

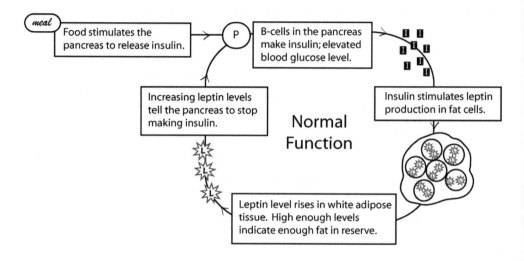

Leptin Resistance in the Pancreas, Causing Insulin Resistance
Impaired regulatory loop due to communication breakdown. Causes excess fat accumulation.

The Key Triad of Problems
at the Root of Weight Gain

Figure 7

There is always abnormal fatigue or lack of energy with this triad of problems.

Leptin Resistance:
The brain can not sense leptin, so it keeps metabolism slow and calories heading for storage. The pancreas can not sense leptin, so it keeps making excess insulin, setting the stage for insulin resistance.

Insulin Resistance:
Excess insulin production leads to insulin resistance throughout the body, as well as erratic or no energy from food.

Adrenaline Resistance:
The normal nervous system signal to stimulate fat cell metabolism is no longer received by fat cells. This causes weight gain especially in the abdominal area, the type of weight gain most associated with cardiovascular disease and reproductive organ cancer.

THE ONSET OF DIABETES

If the problem is not solved, the body may just give up trying to solve the problem. Now a person has type II diabetes. Leptin levels may or may not be elevated in type II diabetes, and they do not follow the same pattern of being elevated correlating with insulin and the amount of body fat. This may sound better than leptin resistance, but it is not. When a person has leptin resistance, at least the body is trying to return to normal balance.

Once diabetes sets in, the body is no longer able to bounce back in terms of regulating blood sugar; homeostatic energy balance is broken. The leptin levels are no longer able to correctly regulate the body. This is a poor state of affairs that is worse than leptin resistance.[35]   Solving leptin issues and restoring natural balance is possible for many individuals with diabetes; however, it is a more difficult problem to fix. Diabetes is a situation of failing to solve many warning signs of poor metabolic function on the way to developing a major problem with natural balance.

SUMMARY

Leptin is the main communication signal coming from white adipose tissue. One of its primary functions is to regulate the longer-term fuel supply of the body, ensuring that reserves are adequate for survival. The brain does not "see" body weight as one does when looking in the mirror; it knows by sensing the leptin levels. This is fine until leptin resistance sets in and fat cells continue accumulating fat, and the subconscious brain does not know the body is overweight or is storing too much fat.

As health deteriorates, especially as one is prone to gain weight and not able to get back to an ideal weight, there is a triad of problems. These involve leptin resistance, insulin resistance, and the resistance of fat cells to stimulation from the sympathetic nervous system – adrenaline resistance.

Unlocking this triad of problems, especially leptin resistance, will solve the actual cause of the problems and return the body to normal metabolic function. Taking effective action is essential before the problem spirals into a more serious issue such as diabetes and increased risk for cancer and heart disease. The cause of the problem is in the natural energy balance systems or homeostatic systems of the human body, not a disease or germ.

6

Why Dieting Does Not Work

*L*et us assume that an individual is simply overweight, not gaining or losing any weight, just too heavy. Such an individual at their heavier weight will have a faster metabolism than they would at a lighter weight. They can eat 2000-3000 calories a day at their heavier weight. They are able to metabolize that amount of calories, possibly not gaining any more weight, but they also cannot lose any weight because they are eating too much.

As they begin to cut back on calories, two things happen:

1) Initially they begin to burn stored fat for fuel as their metabolism is still set to burn the higher calorie amount.

2) As the diet continues, leptin levels begin to drop, initiating the genetic response to starvation. This in turn slows down the sympathetic nervous system stimulation of fat cells so that the body can conserve fuel. Metabolism slows down and weight loss stops.

As less food is eaten and weight is being lost, the tendency of metabolism is to slow down under the influence of less leptin and thus less sympathetic nervous system stimulation. There will be a point where no more weight loss is possible with the current diet plan because metabolism has slowed down to the new lower level of calories being consumed. A person may hit a plateau that is 15-25 pounds from their goal even though they are almost starving on a very low-calorie diet.

PREVIOUS DIETING EXPERIENCE

Such dieting problems become more severe the more often a person has attempted calorie-restriction diets in the past. This is especially true for the person who has gained and lost weight a number of times.

Their bodies can detect a diet a million miles away; even the thought of going on a diet may slow down their metabolism. Their bodies do not trust them anymore. The feast and famine principles of their genetics are in full force. As soon as there is a reduction in calories, the body slows down and starts to conserve.

A person with more serious leptin resistance has an even more difficult time. They may be quite overweight, but they may already be eating a low-calorie diet, usually 1200-1500 calories. Their weight will not budge. If they cut calories, they may lose a few pounds, but they run out of energy right away. If they increase their calories, they can start a weight gain process that they may not be able to stop. In this more serious case of leptin resistance, the body thinks it is starving even though it may be significantly overweight.

There is only so much that can be done with diet and weight loss in the conventional sense. Once metabolism slows down to coincide with the reduced number of calories in the diet, weight loss stops. Some individuals do not lose any weight, others lose a few pounds, and others may lose quite a few pounds before this happens. However, it is quite common that this happens before the weight goal has been achieved. Furthermore, as soon as a person starts to eat more food, leptin commands that calories go in the direction of fat storage.

It is a current fad in weight-loss clinics to increase drug stimulation when this plateau is hit. This is not only incredibly dangerous; it addicts the person to medication. As soon as the medication is stopped, leptin rises and weight comes back.

Keep in mind that leptin is in this for the long haul. It is the survival trait that enabled our species to go months at a time with very little food. Leptin will not be beat with a diet plan that is designed to last for only a few months. Unless strategies are learned for mastering leptin and applied as a life-long skill, failure to reach and/or maintain the goal weight is inevitable.

GAINING IT ALL BACK, AND THEN SOME

Eating little and not getting anywhere becomes frustrating. Now the individual starts to think they will just go back to eating as they did before. So, they eat more. This increase in food intake signals the end of the starvation mode, in turn causing the release of leptin. A primary survival goal of leptin is to replenish the fat stores.

The direct channel of food heading for fat storage is now opened nice and wide. The fat cells that had shrunk down in size under the influence of starvation are more than willing to fill back up and even stretch to new levels of expansiveness. In fact, they readily multiply so that additional food can be stored as fat. The older a person becomes, the more difficult the issue. Fat cells keep expanding and multiplying. If only our brain cells and muscles could perform this feat!

Leptin seems to possess some sort of "sixth sense" or "trust factor" about the individual. This is especially true the more times the dieting approach is tried and the yo-yo factor has occurred. Therefore, it is quite common that the individual gains back more weight than their original diet starting point, just to be sure that if another "diet" occurs there will be adequate stores of fat to deal with the apparent threat to survival.

Leptin has not had enough evolutionary time to figure out what to do with individuals who tend to overeat on a regular basis and then try to restrict themselves on a reduced-calorie diet. So far, its initial evolutionary response seems to be to store more fat just in case another diet is attempted.

Once the leptin management system of the individual has decided enough fat is in storage, the body starts to metabolize faster. However, for a period of time, the body is dead set on putting extra calories back into fat storage. All the weight that was lost is back, frequently along with another 10-20 pounds. This is weight-loss misery; something very real to millions of people.

THE EMOTIONAL UPS AND DOWNS OF LEPTIN RESISTANCE

The previous section defines what happens to a person who is able to start a diet in the first place. When a person has a severe case of leptin resistance, they cannot stay on a diet at all. Frequently, they make it through part of the day eating fairly well, but nighttime is usually their downfall.

During leptin resistance, there are high levels of leptin that do not communicate, thus, the brain does not receive the signal that there is plenty of stored fat even though the fat cells are trying to tell the brain that they are all filled. The brain still thinks it is in some form of starvation mode; therefore, metabolism is running quite slow.

At the same time, the brain commands the individual to eat in order to recover from the inaccurately perceived starvation. It is a vicious circle, and it leads to bizarre and erratic behavior around the subject of food.

One symptom of leptin resistance is that a person may not have a real interest in starting a diet in the first place. They know from experience they cannot beat the leptin problem. Frequently they are just happy not to be gaining more weight. Then they get a poor report, such as blood pressure, cholesterol, or triglycerides are too high or a knee replacement or back surgery will be needed if some weight is not lost. This is a motivational jolt to reality that seems to be more painful than the idea of dieting. They are stuck between the anxiety of dieting and the painful consequence of what will happen if some weight is not lost.

THE LEPTIN-RESISTANT PERSONALITY TYPE

Leptin-resistant individuals who try to lose weight can become true diet schizophrenics. They have the personality associated with being on the diet and doing fine, usually apparent for at least several hours a day and quite commonly all day until about 4-6 p.m. Then the other personality starts to come alive. The first signs of this are a grumpy and irritable personality, accompanied by a distinct feeling of a lack of energy in the head.

This internal uncomfortable feeling then becomes the excuse for going off the diet and getting some kind of quick fix to make the head or energy level feel better. These issues have little to do with willpower; the urge to eat is driven by a misguided sense of survival. This survival instinct is under the influence of leptin that is in a confused state of affairs.

This results in abnormal behavior and cravings for food. The individual will sneak food. They attempt to hide what they are eating from anyone who tries to help them. They may concoct elaborate plans to get to the food they think they need as a priority. The need to get this food fix is as bad as the craving for drugs.

There is no stopping the "bent out of shape" leptin impulse. It is a powerful survival urge that is extremely confused. There is no reasoning with someone who experiences this problem; all they want is food. Once they have eaten, they go back to their rational personality type; they even agree to try much harder on their diet, starting tomorrow.

In this upside-down situation, leptin throws the entire body out of natural rhythm. Not only does this make weight loss a difficult issue, it increases risk factors for numerous other health problems. Leptin that is not communicating properly is a prime cause of disruption of natural balance for the rest of the body.

THERE IS MORE TO FAT THAN MEETS THE EYE

White adipose tissue is composed of 30 percent immune cells. White adipose tissue is not just stored fat, that is, stored triglycerides. The more white adipose tissue there is, the greater the number of fat-related immune cells. Having extra immune cells sounds like a good idea, but with the point about how uncomfortable too much leptin can make a person feel, it is plain to see that these extra immune cells may not be on the same page with the rest of the body.

In fact, these extra immune cells inside of white adipose tissue frequently secrete extra amounts of TNFa (tumor necrosis factor alpha). TNFa in the right amount at the right time is a powerful cancer-destroying compound. However, when the body is out of balance, TNFa is another example of homeostasis gone awry. Excess TNFa contributes to cancer, heart disease, arthritis, and numerous other problems by provoking a highly inflammatory state of affairs.

It is quite common that individuals have 10-15 extra pounds of fat, and frequently much more. Thirty percent of the cells in this fat have the potential to send out highly inflammatory communication signals. These inflammatory signals set the stage for internal wear and tear and the onset of the diseases of aging. This is a serious issue.

Individuals with leptin resistance are in dire need of fixing themselves, not only to reach a healthier body weight but also to prevent life-threatening issues from taking place. Even individuals with a lesser degree of the problem need to take steps to regain natural balance to their body.

SUMMARY

The ability to go on a diet and successfully achieve an optimum weight and maintain it implies that the individual was able to overcome issues with leptin.

Most people under the age of 30 can just cut back on what they eat and exercise more and their body returns to natural balance. Leptin did not kick in as a major factor. After the age of 30, leptin becomes a significant issue for anyone trying to lose weight.

Minimally, leptin causes metabolism to slow down as one tries to lose weight, and it is the main factor that causes weight to be gained back once the diet is over. This is basic leptin survival genetics dealing with starvation issues.

More serious problems with leptin wreak havoc with weight and eating issues. On a subconscious basis, the body thinks it is starving even though it may be quite overweight. When these individuals attempt to diet, their addictions and compulsions relating to food become obvious, as they are often unable to follow a diet for any length of time.

Progressively worsening problems with leptin cause a significant increase in other health issues, many of which are serious and life threatening.

Leptin problems are the cause of dieting failure. They are at the roots of yo-yo dieting, eating little and not losing weight, and gaining weight back once a diet is over. The only solution is to learn to master leptin.

7

Addiction, Alcohol, and Leptin

*A*ddictive behavior is another major problem in our society. The *Journal of the American Medical Association* had a New Year's message for the public. One study stated that alcohol consumption and binge drinking were going up at an alarming rate.[36] Another study announced that the obesity epidemic is continuing to worsen and is a major problem for our society.[37] Their message is clear; America is getting fatter and drinking more.

It has been our observation over the years that many individuals who struggle with significant leptin resistance have a history with excessive alcohol and/or drug use. Thus, it is not at all surprising that the two trends are happening at the same time.

Individuals recovering from alcohol abuse do not like to be hungry as it triggers the cravings for alcohol. Certainly, a great deal of addictive behavior is shared by individuals who have significant food-related leptin resistance or some type of substance abuse. Since food is not illegal, we tend not to think of it in these terms, but similarities are obvious.

Our observations lead to these interesting questions:

- Does leptin resistance put a person at higher risk for alcohol or drug use?
- Does alcohol or drug use put a person at higher risk for leptin resistance?
- Exactly what is the relationship between food cravings and other drug/alcohol cravings?

LEPTIN AND ALCOHOL CRAVINGS

Researchers are discovering that there are clear correlations between leptin levels and alcohol cravings. In mice experiments, leptin administration enhanced the motivation to consume alcohol following a period of depriva-tion.[38]   The same researchers found in humans going through alcohol detoxification that those who craved alcohol the most had the highest levels of leptin.[39]

Other researchers demonstrated leptin levels were higher in chronic alco-holism, independent of nutritional status, the amount of fat the person has, or the state of liver disease. The data simply shows that the longer the person has consumed alcohol, the higher the circulating levels of leptin.[40] This indi-cates that leptin precedes other health issues caused by alcohol and may very well be the subconscious driving factor that reinforces alcohol cravings.

This also means that excess food consumption is fueled by alcohol con-sumption and vice-versa, with the cravings for each sharing a common signal of excess leptin due to leptin resistance. This leads to misguided behavior wherein the brain thinks, on a subconscious basis, that alcohol is essential for survival. Literally, this means that the need for alcohol is being confused with the need for food.

In healthy individuals who do not have leptin resistance, alcohol con-sumption lowers leptin, thus stimulating appetite.[41] Therefore, alcohol consumption, especially at night, can fuel overeating even in healthy indi-viduals, sending them into leptin resistance. The person now gains weight as well as gaining an addiction to alcohol. Many young people heading off to college in good health find that too much alcohol quickly adds pounds they did not have before and gets them stuck in a rut of addictive patterns.

This also means that a person with a history of leptin resistance may be prone to overeating at night even with mild alcohol consumption, like having a glass of wine with dinner. Many times such individuals have weak will-power on eating a proper size meal. Add a little alcohol and it is easy for them to overeat.

STRESS, LEPTIN, AND CRAVINGS

Remember, the hypothalamus gland of the brain is where this leptin signal is being processed. The hypothalamus gland is the "old brain." It seeks to regulate the chemistry reactions in the human body from the neck down. In computer terms, its circuitry is more like "hardware" than "software." Its computer program is based on survival.

Any perceived threat to survival causes a sense of instability and a stress-alarm reaction. During our genetic evolution, the scarcity of food was one of the most significant stressors on a day-in and day-out basis, thus the body's genetics are "hardwired" to deal with these issues.

In a twisted leptin-resistant way, the consumption of food and alcohol seem to have a direct effect on satisfying a subconscious threat to survival. Any time a person starts feeling stressed or threatened in some way, there is a risk for excess food or alcohol consumption resulting in "emotional" eating or drinking. Such cravings are directly wired into the subconscious hardware but unfortunately are incorrect and distorted perceptions due to preexisting leptin resistance.

A person who has never had a problem with overeating or excess alcohol consumption is much less likely to experience these craving issues. Conversely, any person who has struggled with food and alcohol cravings knows that these issues intensify dramatically under stress.

A true road to recovery from alcohol abuse would consist of a person solving leptin problems. That is to say, the individual will reach and maintain a healthy body weight and have leptin issues relating to food fully under control. This is an important key to a permanent road to addiction recovery.

LIVER DAMAGE

Alcohol-related liver damage is a huge problem in our society. Excessive amounts of alcohol cause liver inflammation resulting in the "cooking of the liver structure." The liver eventually can look like a piece of fried bacon. By the time a person has alcohol-induced cirrhosis of the liver, they have markedly elevated leptin as well as other inflammatory markers, such as C reactive protein, that induce the liver damage.[42]

Leptin is involved in a major part of the causative mechanism of inducing liver damage. This is why women, who have three times the amount of leptin as men, are more sensitive to liver damage from alcohol. As we have pointed out, leptin is elevated in alcoholics regardless of the state of liver damage; this means they are not elevated due to liver damage. Rather, excess leptin helps to cause liver damage.

In the previous chapter, we pointed out that elevated leptin causes an increase in immune-cell activity relating to the immune cells that are part of white adipose tissue. One of these primary immune signals is called TNFa, a highly inflammatory signal. It has long been known that TNFa is elevated in liver disease and is a major part of the progression of the disease.

Researchers have proven in mice that regular alcohol consumption turns up the general production of TNFa and tilts the stress response to excessively make TNFa, not only in the liver but also in white adipose tissue.[43]

This data means that regular excess consumption of alcohol turns up extra production of TNFa. We already know that TNFa is generated by excess leptin. Therefore, the current data on excess leptin and TNFa indicate that they work together to generate inflammation that causes the liver damage. Conversely, this means that if leptin and TNFa can be lowered and brought into a state of natural balance, then liver damage can be prevented and possibly even reversed.

In addition to the liver damage, the most recent study on this subject confirms the link between excess TNFa, leptin, and consequent ongoing cravings for alcohol resulting in continued consumption and further liver damage.[44]

INTRODUCING NF KAPPAB

NF kappaB is the 911 switchboard for each cell in the body. By comparison, the hypothalamus gland in the brain is the 911 switchboard for the body as a whole. NF kappaB is typically dormant inside of cells, especially when everything goes along in a routine and generally non-stressed manner.

Under the influence of cellular stress, NF kappaB is activated. It goes to the DNA of cells and tells the cell what proteins to make to meet the emergency needs of the stressful situation so that the cell can survive. Without NF kappaB, cells would not be able to tolerate any type of stress, and we all would have perished long ago.

In some cases, this essential component of survival gets hijacked and starts working against the body. As we have explained, TNFa fortifies chronic inflammation that is a primary cause of cancer, heart disease, and many other "diseases of aging."

Excess NF kappaB and TNFa coexist in the majority of serious health problems. In cases of alcohol-liver inflammation, the problem is fueled by excess production of NF kappa B and TNFa.[45] Furthermore, in order to induce liver damage from alcohol, the NF kappaB level must rise prior to the initiation of liver damage, meaning that it is a prime causative factor.[46] This damage to the liver occurs faster in women than in men because women generally have a higher percent of body fat, meaning they tend to have more leptin and can set off excess TNFa and NF kappaB overproduction easier than men.[47]

There is clear-cut science showing why the herb silymarin is so protective to the liver. Silymarin directly lowers the production of NF kappaB, specifically addressing the cause of the liver problem. Silymarin is gaining worldwide recognition as a powerful remedy for liver disease.[48]

SUMMARY

Addictive patterns, whether alcohol or food related, involve the excess leptin signal as a driving subconscious force that makes these issues difficult to manage. It is quite likely that excess alcohol and food cravings share common pathways in the brain to the point that the "need for alcohol" is confused with the survival instinct of eating.

Alcohol consumption and excess fat work together to generate too much inflammatory activity, especially in the liver. This sets the stage for liver damage. The liver is the metabolic factory of the human body. Disrupting the function of the liver cripples healthy metabolism.

Too much inflammation leads to the "overheating" of cells, promoting the excess production of NF kappaB. Chronic, inappropriate overproduction of NF kappaB is a turning point in cellular health, tilting the tables in favor of disease.

As the problems of excess fat and alcohol consumption magnify each other, they are a fast track to a poor state of health.

8

Drugs and Leptin

_E_ levated NF kappaB is a prime factor involved in the withdrawal from morphine addiction.[49] Inducing starvation as a form of stress caused animals to once again crave heroin after they had been through a prolonged drug-free period. The cravings were directly related to leptin fluctuation.[50] The mechanism of neurotoxicity from methamphetamine (METH) involves the excess production of NF kappaB causing inflammatory nerve damage.[51]

This information sheds light on the true nature of drug addiction, as well as how it accelerates the onset and increases the risk for any disease of aging, especially brain damage resulting in cognitive decline.

Amphetamine-based diet pills, known to suppress appetite, have been around for a long time. The stimulative effects of cocaine are also well known. The brain actually makes small amounts of these substances, and they have a natural stimulant effect.

The cells in the brain responding to this stimulation are called CART (cocaine and amphetamine regulating transcript). Not surprisingly, CART is a favorite target of pharmaceutical company research. CART activation suppresses appetite by interacting with the hypothalamus gland.[52] In normal and healthy metabolism, as leptin goes down, so does CART. This is because lower leptin in the brain always slows down metabolism, including CART.[53]

Diet pills and cocaine work by stimulating metabolism and depressing leptin, interfering with the leptin signal to regulate body fuel needs.[54] They are a dangerous way of bypassing normal brain regulation of energy systems, forcing stimulation on the core subconscious brain.

It has been found that leptin controls CART, and that problems with leptin resistance, a condition of leptin not being in the brain, can lead to excess CART stimulation.[55]

Addictive craving patterns are likely to exist between leptin problems and cocaine/amphetamine addiction since the hormone leptin and cocaine/amphetamine communicate with one another in the hypothalamus gland of the brain.

Excess CART activation causes too much stimulation, leading to production of anxiety that is part of the paranoia of drug addiction.[56] If such an addict has an appetite, eating food will turn off the anxiety by increasing leptin. This creates a reciprocal and cross-related addictive pattern between drug ingestion, anxiety, and food consumption, one massive confused state of addictive patterns in the subconscious mind.

This issue is further complicated by the fact that CART-related drugs, including stimulant diet pills, have no restraint keeping them out of the brain. In leptin resistance, leptin cannot enter the brain in proper amounts, even though the levels are high in the blood. Cocaine and amphetamine readily enter the brain where they can directly wreak havoc with leptin.[57] No matter how much of the drug is consumed, it will always enter the brain.

CART is a normal neuropeptide. In normal circumstances in non-drugged individuals, it is under leptin control. When cocaine or amphetamines are consumed, they bypass genetic control and have direct regulation on core issues of survival. While this may induce a temporary high, the consequence to the nervous system and overall body fuel regulation, as well as numerous other health issues, is profound. This is in part because of the neurotoxicity of the drugs via the stimulation of NF kappaB and partly because the drugs cause leptin problems.

The data on methamphetamine toxicity is quite alarming. The addictive nature of cocaine and amphetamine is becoming clear, especially the nature of addiction and the damage caused to regulatory centers in the brain and nerves in general.

A BREAKTHROUGH FOR PARKINSON'S

The correct amount of leptin entering the brain turns out to be incredibly important in protecting the brain. One of the many roles of leptin is that it seems to help body tissue grow. This applies to bones,[58] cartilage,[59] the GI tract,[60] skin,[61] and the fetus during pregnancy,[62] to name a few.

It was recently discovered that adequate leptin protects the dopamine system in the brain and is an essential component responsible for brain plasticity.[63] In fact, leptin appears to be essential for protecting the brain from excess excitation that induces toxicity, especially protecting against damage to the NMDA receptor, the receptor that is damaged in Parkinson's.[64]

An experiment wherein the neurotoxin methamphetamine was given to *ob/ob* mice and to normal lean mice showed that the methamphetamine killed the *ob/ob* mice but not the lean mice.[65] Remember, the *ob/ob* mouse has no leptin in the brain, thus no dopamine brain protection from chemical toxins.

This information shows that strategies that normalize leptin levels in the brain become a primary treatment for Parkinson's patients. Throughout this book we discuss numerous ways to normalize leptin. One key factor we will explain is calcium. High quality calcium, in the dose of 2,000 mg - 3,000 mg per day, is likely to become an integral part of the nutritional program for helping individuals with Parkinson's.

This information raises another question about the safety of Ritalin given to an overweight child. Since an overweight child has leptin resistance, and thus less leptin in the brain, their brains are more susceptible to damage not only from environmental toxins but also from any ingested amphetamine. While Ritalin is not as strong an amphetamine as methamphetamine, this is an area of concern that should be explored by health authorities.

We see that leptin is not only involved in regulation of food intake and craving issues; a proper amount of it is essential for the protection of the brain against damage.

SUMMARY

Food addiction, alcohol abuse, and drug addiction share a common communication signal gone awry – high leptin levels or leptin signals that have been destroyed by drugs. These leptin problems fuel addictive behavior by confusing the subconscious brain into believing that these substances are essential for survival.

Stress that makes a person feel unstable in some way is likely to trigger addictive behavior patterns. In part, this is because normal CART function is related to the anxiety stress response. Anxiety problems can easily be manifested in food, alcohol, or drug abuse, either leading to addictive patterns or occurring as a result of substance abuse.

In order to return health to a state of natural balance, it is essential to have leptin levels under control and in working order. Having the right amount of leptin working properly is the key to a healthy metabolism.

9

The Importance of Mastering Leptin

*M*any researchers, scientists, health professionals, and individuals have sought to uncover the keys to a healthy life. A great deal has been written about the lifestyles of healthy people. Despite all of the research and personal explorations, no clear defining principle has emerged that explains the fundamental science behind optimum health.

Our new understanding of leptin marks the defining principle of optimum health. This is because leptin controls energy regulation in the human body. Without a proper energy supply, nothing can work correctly.

Understanding leptin and learning how to manage it will make a healthy life possible for many individuals who would otherwise suffer with poor energy and poor physical health. A failure to master leptin is a fast track to increased disease risk and accelerated aging.

Mastering leptin is the only chance our society has, on an individual basis, of solving the obesity epidemic and the overwhelming health costs that are associated. It is a shortsighted individual who believes that others only harm themselves when they eat poorly. The eventual costs, in terms of health care, lost productivity, and quality of life for those related to the individual, are a staggering burden.

While the government could do a great deal more than they are to improve the quality of our general food supply, this is not an issue of needing laws to regulate junk food. That is because the cravings associated with leptin mismanagement are an individual issue. When enough individuals learn to master leptin, there will be little consumer demand for junk food, and the corporate contributors to the issue will either dry up and go away or start producing quality food that people want to eat.

We live in a world of temptation on every corner. Learning to master leptin is a true life skill. It is not easy. The reward is quality of health. It is a personal choice. It is the most important life skill of a Health Asset Manager.™

In the first part of this book, we introduced the scope of leptin. Leptin is the hormone secreted by fat cells in white adipose tissue. It communicates to the brain to let the brain know how much fuel is "in the gas tank." If there is adequate fuel, then metabolism runs along at a nice pace, and everything works normally. If fuel is running low, then metabolism slows down to conserve so as not to run out of fuel and thus die of starvation. Leptin is truly the survival principle of the subconscious mind.

Overeating leads to excess leptin production and the eventual development of the problem called leptin resistance. Once this happens, the brain no longer perceives the true amount of leptin. The brain cannot judge how much fat is in storage. Typically, this causes a person to have an extra 5-20 pounds that will not go away.

In more serious situations, the brain thinks the body is starving even though there is plenty of leptin and 25-150 or more extra pounds of fuel in storage. The individual is stuck in a pattern of leptin resistance, insulin resistance, and adrenaline resistance.

Many individuals experience problems with leptin at very young ages. Type II diabetes, formerly called adult-onset diabetes, is now common in adolescents. This is an alarming trend of society-wide leptin mismanagement.

It would be bad enough if the problems with leptin simply caused individuals to be overweight. That is only the tip of the iceberg. White adipose tissue also contains immune cells that, under the influence of leptin problems, generate massive amounts of inflammation.

This sets the stage for all types of ill health, including the early onset of virtually all diseases of aging.

The fact that these risk factors and trends can be completely stopped, simply by learning to master leptin, is a major breakthrough in our understanding of optimum health.

In Part 2 of this book, we explain key lifestyle essentials that form the foundation of leptin management. These are the important basics of how to eat so as not to upset the leptin apple cart. It is essential that individuals learn enough diet and lifestyle skills to maintain an excellent state of natural balance.

In Part 3, we explore numerous leptin issues in more depth. We explain how thyroid problems are almost always leptin problems, and by solving the leptin problem, the thyroid problems tend to go away. We explain why leptin is essential for a variety of factors in healthy function, including healing, immunity, and strong bones.

We explain how nutritional supplementation can help individuals overcome issues with leptin resistance, insulin resistance, and adrenaline resistance. These are true solutions that open the doors of good health to many individuals who would otherwise struggle needlessly.

We discuss how leptin relates to cardiovascular function and how leptin problems are a prime cause of cardiovascular disease. This opens the door to a new understanding of heart health, and it explains practical steps to take to change the actual source of the problem that makes cardiovascular disease the number-one killer in America.

We explain how the new understanding of genetic science demonstrates that disease is caused when the body's own natural defense systems are hijacked and turned against itself.

Not surprisingly, leptin mismanagement is key to fanning the flames of these gene-related problems. A lifetime of leptin mismanagement significantly increases cancer risk.

The factors behind how leptin relates to male and female hormonal function, growth hormone, stress hormones, and fibromyalgia are explained. This leads to an understanding of how leptin problems set the stage for male and female cancers.

The human body is complex. It takes some time to learn principles of leptin management and successfully apply them. The time spent is worthwhile, it more than pays for itself in terms of extended life-span and higher quality of health.

PART 2

The Five Key Dietary Rules for
Mastering Leptin

10

The Five Rules

*T*here are five key dietary rules to mastering leptin. We call these the *Five Rules*. These rules apply to almost everyone. They are essential to mastering leptin. Individuals need to learn to implement the *Five Rules* on a consistent basis in their life. Doing so establishes a solid foundation for mastering leptin.

Rule 1: Never eat after dinner. Allow 11-12 hours between dinner and breakfast. Never go to bed on a full stomach. Generally finish eating dinner three hours before bed. This rule is explained in Chapter 11.

Rule 2: Eat three meals a day. Allow 5-6 hours between meals. Do not snack. This rule is explained in Chapter 13.

Rule 3: Do not eat large meals. Always try to finish a meal when slightly less than full. Eating slowly is important. This rule is explained in Chapter 15.

Rule 4: Eat a breakfast containing protein. This rule is explained in Chapter 16.

Rule 5: Reduce the amount of carbohydrates eaten. This rule is explained in Chapter 17.

WHY THESE RULES?

Traditional dietary advice focuses on the number of calories in food. Calories come in the form of fats, carbohydrates, and proteins. These substances can potentially become energy, or if the body cannot metabolize them for one reason or another, they may become stored fat.

No progress will be made on weight loss or maintaining a high quality of health if the body is abused with too many calories or improperly timed consumption of calories. Any type of calorie can become toxic to the body if it is consumed inappropriately.

Defining "inappropriate" is no small task. One glance through the dieting section of any bookstore quickly reveals there are as many diets as there are possible food combinations. However, understanding leptin places a whole new perspective on appropriate eating. The *Five Rules* are fundamental to eating so as not to upset leptin balance.

It is certainly wise to eat fresh, organically produced, high-quality foods whenever possible. This includes foods free of chemicals, preservatives, food coloring, partially hydrogenated oils, hormones, antibiotics, and mold toxins from being stored too long.

THE IMPORTANCE OF THE *FIVE RULES*

The *Five Rules* are not a special diet. They are a lifestyle that promotes health. They are designed to be used as an effortless dietary lifestyle pattern throughout life.

Some individuals can violate the *Five Rules* and seem to get away with it. This will catch up with them sooner or later. Minimally, this is like rowing a boat against the current. It is a harder way to go. The *Five Rules* are a safe and effective way to maintain a healthy eating pattern over the course of a lifetime.

Some individuals do not have the physical ability to follow the *Five Rules*. This does not mean the rules are wrong, it simply means the individual needs to get in better shape. Individuals know they should exercise; some are physically not able to or do not find the time, both leading to poor fitness. It is the same with the *Five Rules*. Working on a path to better "eating fitness" is essential for any person so they can implement the *Five Rules* into their life.

There are ways to vary the *Five Rules* and still maintain healthy metabolism. Elite athletes may need to eat more often simply to get the number of calories they need. Diabetics have malfunctioning "hormone switches" and end up using food to compensate for a "broken metabolism." There are a variety of special circumstances that require tailoring the *Five Rules*. However, the principles underlying the *Five Rules* are workable concepts to help keep one's body in natural balance and enhance the proper communication of leptin.

This is why an individual needs to learn to be a competent Health Asset Manager.™ Individuals need to understand why a rule is a rule so they can think intelligently with the information and apply it to their life.

Oddly enough, the *Five Rules* are so helpful that 80 percent of the population could robotically follow them without knowing why they work, and they would be healthier. This includes resolving long-standing issues with body weight.

As our goal is to teach individuals to become a Health Asset Manager™, this part of the book explains the *Five Rules* in great detail, including the science behind them.

WHAT DO CRAVINGS MEAN?

Once on the path to implementing the *Five Rules,* the next important issue is to stay on that path regardless of what happens in one's life. There are a variety of factors that induce food cravings, and they need to be managed effectively in order to stay on track.

There is tremendous knowledge and scientific research regarding food cravings and addictive eating patterns and compulsions. Understanding how these factors relate to each individual and how to manage them effectively is a key skill of the Health Asset Manager.™

In Part 2 of the book, we explain the fundamentals involved and solution strategies for stress eating and other craving issues. Part 3 of the book offers additional information regarding disease and more advanced strategies for stubborn patterns. These issues can and must be solved.

SUMMARY

Understanding and implementing the five key dietary rules for mastering leptin is the foundation of health and getting one's body into natural rhythm. It forms a stable frame of reference for other hormonal and energy patterns in the human body. The *Five Rules* are the fundamentals for efficiently extracting energy from food; being able to transform the calorie potential in food to real energy – energy that can be felt!

Master these rules and build the foundation of optimum health from the view of dietary stability for health. This is not simplistic dietary information. These dietary principles are essential for healthy, disease-free living.

11

Maximum Primary Fat-Burning Time

When leptin is out of balance, it interferes with the ability of the body to burn fat for fuel. The number-one sign there is a problem with leptin resistance is overeating at night. This is the single most important symptom that leptin is really out of control.

It is common that an individual can do a fairly good job of eating correctly until about 6 p.m. After that, the "other eating personality" takes over, the one driven by leptin resistance. This alter personality is reinforced by alcohol consumption and/or stress. The failure to obey the erratic impulses of this other personality makes the individual feel tired, grumpy, and irritable. Only when they eat will they feel better, or so they think.

THE 24-HOUR LEPTIN PATTERN

In order to unravel this issue, it is important to understand what is taking place. Leptin levels rise at night. They follow a 24-hour pattern of natural rhythm or natural balance. They peak in the evening hours and are the highest the first two hours of sleep. They gradually fall during the evening and reach their lowest level around noon, then begin to rise again.

When leptin works properly, a high leptin level tells a person they are full and not to eat. Therefore, it is completely natural not to be hungry after dinner or before bed. There are a variety of reasons for this, one of which is that the body has other functions to do other than digest food during sleep.

A person with leptin resistance also has higher levels of leptin at night, but the brain is not able to perceive the message. The result is that the brain thinks the body needs to store more fat as a priority in order to survive; a conclusion that is terribly incorrect. This aberrant conclusion is reinforced by core survival instincts stronger than conscious thought.

This is why a person with leptin resistance has trouble looking in a refrigerator after dinner and not eating. It is why their conscious self may try to ensure there is no food around the house to eat. There is no way a person can win a direct confrontation with leptin-resistance urges. The only way to win this battle is to prevent leptin resistance from happening in the first place (Figure 8).

The first step is to understand what is supposed to be done and why. The next step is to implement various strategies to keep leptin under control and working correctly for optimum balance and health.

THE *FIVE RULES* - Rule 1

Never eat after dinner. Allow 11-12 hours between dinner and breakfast. Never go to bed on a full stomach. Generally finish eating dinner three hours before bed.

Any person with active leptin resistance finds this rule somewhat inconceivable to follow. Even people who do not have active leptin resistance may have a variety of reasons why they cannot follow this rule. Some examples include:

1) If I do not eat before bed, I cannot get to sleep.
2) If I do not have a nighttime snack, I wake up hungry in the middle of the night.
3) If I do not eat before bed, I wake up with a headache or I feel queasy.

Just because someone cannot follow this rule does not mean the rule is wrong. Anyone who cannot follow this rule has a significant problem with blood glucose metabolism, liver function, and/or leptin resistance.

Most people agree that it is good to go for a long walk or a 3-5 mile jog. Many people do not have the ability to do this. Reasons vary and may include lack of energy, lack of desire or drive, or physical problems such as a knee problem, just to name a few. Regardless, if the person is fit enough to do the exercise and get a good response, they will be healthier. The same

Normal Leptin Function after Dinner

Figure 8A

Leptin Resistance

Figure 8B

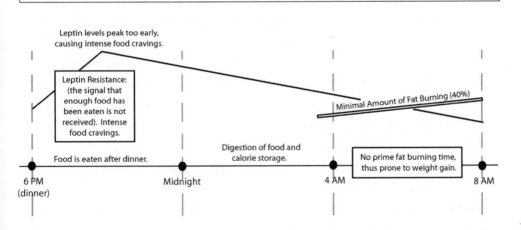

principle applies to not eating after dinner and going 11-12 hours between dinner and breakfast.

There are many reasons why this is a key rule of weight loss and overcoming leptin resistance. It is fundamental for establishing healthy patterns of hormones in the human body. Improperly timed eating can disrupt thyroid hormone, growth hormone, adrenal hormones, sex hormones, and melatonin, and it throws the body out of rhythm to set the stage for serious diseases.

If physicians or public-health officials informed people of the extreme importance of not eating after dinner, the health-care costs of our country would decline. It may be the most important and under-appreciated principle relating to any type of health problem.

PRIME FAT-BURNING TIME

Sleep is the only time a person loses any significant and consistent weight from their white adipose tissue stores. This only works well when no food has been eaten for 11-12 hours.

In general, the body burns a certain amount of sugar and fat at the same time. When a meal is eaten, the sugar and fat are readily available from the ingested food. After three or so hours, the sugar entering the blood is produced by the liver. A certain amount of sugar is released into the blood, otherwise the brain will not function well and blood sugars will be low. This principle applies whether awake or asleep.

Most of the fat burned during the day either comes directly from the food eaten or is already in the blood. The majority of calorie metabolism during the day is mostly from readily available energy supplies. Intense exercise may dip into actual fat stores, but for the most part, the goal of daytime fat metabolism is to keep the system running smoothly so stored fat can be burned at night.

During the night, the body gradually begins to burn a higher portion of fat for fuel. Nine hours after finishing dinner, it is quite likely that the readily available fats have been used, and the body will dip into the fat savings account. Therefore, 9-12 hours after dinner are the prime fat-burning hours in terms of accessing the fat stores in the buttocks, thighs, and stomach.

If anything is eaten before bed, this prime fat-burning time is shut off! This principle is not going to change; it is a fact of biochemistry.

SUMMARY

In order to lose weight properly and healthfully, natural balance must be restored to the leptin communication system. Since leptin is highest at night, this points to nighttime eating patterns as a key indicator of health.

Individuals with significant leptin resistance are not able to control their eating at night and so have a deviation in their behavior in the evening hours on the subject of food. The first step is to simply recognize that this is an important part of the problem.

Ideally, a person should not eat after dinner and should go 11-12 hours before eating breakfast. A person in good health feels satisfied eating this way and is in an improved state of natural balance.

12

Leptin and Insulin, Birds of a Feather

*I*ndividuals with leptin resistance also have problems with insulin resistance. This fact has been well established in scientific literature, and it has been proposed that excess amounts of insulin are a prime contributing factor of leptin resistance that leads to obesity.[66] It is also clear that the triad of insulin resistance, leptin resistance, and adrenaline resistance lead to high blood pressure.[67]

It is essential for adrenaline resistance to exist, that is, fueled by leptin resistance and insulin resistance, before a person has a breakdown of their blood glucose regulation ability and becomes type II diabetic or what is known as adult-onset diabetes.[68]

In order to reduce adrenaline resistance and leptin resistance, one approach is to reduce insulin resistance. This is because whatever a person does to improve any one of these three problems has a synergistic positive impact on the other two.

There is so much confusion on the subject of insulin and eating that it is truly mind-boggling. The fact that so many health professionals and "dieting experts" recommend snacking and eating frequent small meals is a real disservice. Besides overeating at night, this is the primary reason why so many Americans are overweight. Even if the snack is low in calories or a "healthy snack" such as an apple, it becomes a problem.

Eating between meals changes powerful hormonal signals that prevent the breakdown of fat, gum up liver metabolism, and induce calories to head for fat storage. This fact is a primary feature governing how food can induce stressful problems with hormone balance. Taking the time to understand why this is the case is important to learning the skill of mastering leptin and being an effective Health Asset Manager.™

HOW INSULIN WORKS

The pancreas secretes two hormones that regulate blood sugar: insulin and glucagon. These two hormones play crucial roles in how the body regulates fuel utilization. Imbalances in these two hormones cause vicious circles of hyperglycemia followed by hypoglycemia, resulting in the inability to lose weight.

Insulin is released in response to a rise in blood glucose from food that has been eaten. Insulin signals the body to refuel and possibly to store extra fuel in the form of fat. The primary function of insulin is to promote the storage of calories. The big question is – where will the insulin store the calories?

Normally, insulin is secreted in two phases. The first phase occurs when food is eaten; it is an initial burst of insulin for the first ten minutes from readily available insulin in the pancreas. This is followed by the second phase where the pancreas synthesizes more insulin.[69] Insulin normally peaks about 30 minutes after a meal and then gradually returns to baseline over the next three hours. This is an important rhythm; it has a normal pattern, and this pattern is very important.

Beyond immediate energy needs, ideally the liver takes about 60 percent of the blood glucose from a meal and stores it in the liver as glycogen, fuel to be used later.[70] Insulin also promotes the storage of amino acids in the liver that are used to help sustain energy 5-6 hours after the meal.[71]

Muscles throughout the body, depending on how much they have been used, are also stimulated to take up blood sugar and store it as glycogen for future use. If muscle tissue breakdown has occurred, as from exercise, then insulin is also a key signal that enables muscles to take up protein to rebuild themselves. The use of muscle is essential for conditioning the body to use insulin and glucose correctly.[72] Thus, in an ideal situation the other 40% of calories are taken up directly by muscles and other body tissue.

In the ideal situation insulin is promoting storage of calories into the liver and body tissues, especially muscle. It is not promoting excess calorie storage into fat cells.

When muscles are not used enough, meaning that a person is too seden-tary or a meal is too large, then insulin facilitates the storage of extra calories as fat. Insulin helps carry glucose into fat cells where it is converted into glycerol to help form triglycerides, the type of fat in storage. [73]

Insulin turns on the enzyme lipoprotein lipase that tells fat cells to grab circulating triglycerides in the blood and store them in fat cells. [74] Insulin also inhibits enzymes that cause fat to break down. [75] Thus, insulin levels that are too high are a primary reason why calories are stored as fat, and why fat is not broken down to be used as fuel.

If there is excess fuel from an oversized meal or a lack of physical activity, that extra fuel is likely to be stored as fat.

HOW GLUCAGON WORKS

The counter balance to insulin is another pancreatic hormone called gluca-gon. It is stimulated by the fall in blood glucose and is a natural defense against blood sugar dropping too much. It is the main fuel regulator that helps a person to go 5-6 hours or longer without needing to eat.

Glucagon orders the liver to quit storing fuel and to begin making fuel. The liver does this in two ways:

1) It converts the stored fuel called glycogen back to glucose, a process called glycogenolysis.
2) It makes sugar from other compounds, including protein, and glyc-erol from stored fat and lactic acid, a process called gluconeogenisis.

In the process of breaking down stored fat, fatty acids are liberated. The liver does not generally take these up; primarily the muscles take them up directly to be burned as fuel.[76] It should be rather obvious that if muscles are not used then there is no demand for these fatty acids. The next time the person eats, insulin rises and the fatty acids now circulating in the blood are turned back into triglycerides and put back in storage. To lose weight, one needs to exercise.

In a healthy person, insulin and glucagon take turns. It is all about tim-ing. Insulin is used to refuel the body; glucagon helps sustain energy between meals. It is a survival system that ensures a steady supply of glucose to the brain and nervous system, essential to maintain energy and health (Figure 9).

Our survival genetics enable us to go long periods of time with little food. There are enough carbohydrates stored in the liver and muscles to last only 24 hours. After that, the body breaks down muscle protein as the primary fuel for up to a week.[77] Once skeletal muscle is significantly lost, then fatty acids become the primary fuel. This is why fasting for weight loss is not advised; too much protein is lost from the physical structure before the body ever gets to the stores of fat, a dangerous and unhealthy thing to do.

Factors that disrupt the balance of insulin and glucagon create major havoc in the body, setting the stage for weight-gain issues. An obvious example is that of insulin-dependent diabetes mellitus (IDDM) or type I diabetes. In this case, the pancreatic B-cells that make insulin are destroyed for one reason or another. Since the rising level of insulin is the key signal that turns off glucagon, the liver is under constant orders to synthesize more sugar in the absence of insulin. This causes blood sugar levels to raise dangerously high, the condition known as diabetes.

It is much more common that individuals encounter a problem called type II or non-insulin dependent diabetes mellitus (NIDDM). This is often referred to as adult-onset diabetes. This is a situation of excessive insulin production due to insulin resistance. This type of diabetes now includes teenagers due to their excessive dietary abuse and inactivity.

Any person who progressively gains weight and has trouble losing weight is at serious risk for developing type II diabetes. Before the actual diabetes occurs, it is preceded by a condition known as insulin resistance.

Insulin Pattern After Meals

Figure 9

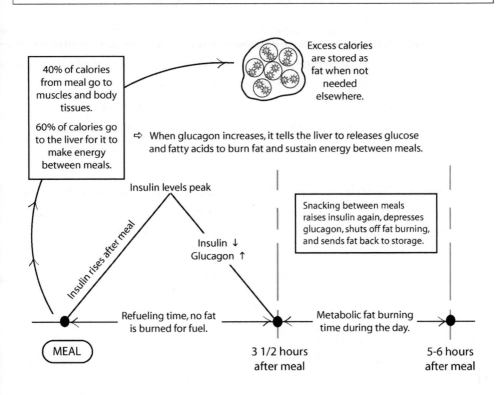

40% of calories from meal go to muscles and body tissues.

60% of calories go to the liver for it to make energy between meals.

Excess calories are stored as fat when not needed elsewhere.

⇨ When glucagon increases, it tells the liver to releases glucose and fatty acids to burn fat and sustain energy between meals.

Insulin levels peak

Insulin rises after meal

Insulin ↓
Glucagon ↑

Snacking between meals raises insulin again, depresses glucagon, shuts off fat burning, and sends fat back to storage.

Refueling time, no fat is burned for fuel.

Metabolic fat burning time during the day.

MEAL

3 1/2 hours after meal

5-6 hours after meal

INSULIN RESISTANCE

Insulin acts like a taxicab carrying passengers (glucose) to various destinations. Generally, the body synthesizes insulin whenever food is eaten and for as long as food is eaten.

Let us say that we overeat or eat between meals. Insulin, acting in its taxicab role, takes its passengers to the liver, muscles, and other places to be dropped off. However, the cells have no need for the fuel. At first they politely tell the taxicab to go someplace else. As time goes by, they see the taxicab coming and lock the doors, literally turning off and, in some cases, eliminating the receptors for insulin on the membranes of cells. This is called insulin resistance.

Insulin resistance is a self-preservation issue for cells. If the cells did not reject the calories, they would enter the cell and cause the cell to become cemented. If sugar cannot be used, it caramelizes or hardens structures, similar to leaving spilled honey on the counter for a few days.

Over the years, insulin resistance causes major problems in the balance between insulin, glucagon, and fuel utilization.

LIVER INSULIN RESISTANCE

In addition to every cell of the body, the liver also develops insulin resistance. This causes the liver to not store the 60 percent of fuel it typically stores from a meal, meaning that calories that are eaten head in the direction of fat storage.

This problem is magnified when a person eats too often. Not only does the liver fail to store calories properly, eating too often causes the liver to retain the calories it has in storage. The bottom line is that frequent eating clogs the liver's fuel system. Fatigue is a common symptom of a person with a clogged liver.

When a person eats too often, especially meals high in sugar, the liver goes into a chronic stimulation of VLDL synthesis (very low density lipoproteins), the form of cholesterol most associated with cardiovascular disease. This delivers an excess of fatty substances to muscle wherein they clog muscle tissue and make it resistant to glucose. This is a typical way that many individuals start on the path to insulin resistance and elevated cholesterol,[78] and consequently leptin resistance. This means the foremost reason for elevated cholesterol, from a dietary point of view, is snacking between meals, not the cholesterol content of food.

Liver fuel is the first fuel released under stress; it is essential to meet a current energy demand. If there is reduced storage of fuel in the liver, an individual is easily tired by stress and susceptible to irritability and moodiness. Individuals with insulin resistance have some level of fatigue and irritability.

Liver insulin resistance also makes it difficult for the person to go 5-6 hours without eating or to sleep properly through the night, as it is the liver's consistent release of stored sugar, under the direction of glucagon, that stabilizes blood sugar between meals and prevents hypoglycemia.

When there is insulin resistance in the liver, the liver decides to turn calories into fat at an increased rate, thus causing the person to become overweight.[79]

During leptin resistance and insulin resistance, the liver gets confused and misunderstands the messages. Excess leptin becomes involved with the normal pathway of insulin in the liver, confuses the liver as to the state of fuel on hand, and has the net effect of turning down glucagon, the hormone needed to activate the liver's metabolic drive.[80] This helps a person continue to gain weight even though they have plenty of fat in storage.

When a person has insulin resistance, the calories from a meal have a difficult time getting into muscles.[81] Such muscles are weaker, contributing to fatigue issues. Therefore, insulin resistance is a combination of a lack of physical fitness and a lack of liver fitness. Just as we know how it feels when our muscles get out of shape, fatigue and getting hungry too often are key signs of an out-of-shape liver.

HIGH BLOOD SUGAR

The extra calories that are not used need to go somewhere. In part, they are stored as fat, leading to progressive weight gain. Since blood-sugar levels tend to stay higher than normal during insulin resistance (hyperglycemia), the flexible structures of the body are exposed to the caramelizing effects of sugar. This makes the body age faster. It causes the circulatory system to stiffen leading to conditions such as high blood pressure. It causes capillaries in the eye to stiffen leading to circulation problems in and out of the eye resulting in all manners of eye problems. It causes nerves to harden, leading to a variety of neurological issues including mental decline and memory loss.

Properly functioning leptin is essential for normal glucose uptake and utilization in the liver, both in the fed and fasted state.[82,83] Leptin resistance causes high blood sugar following a meal, leading to hypoglycemia 3-5 hours after the meal.

SYNDROME X

It is quite common that insulin resistance results in the combination of weight gain, high cholesterol with low HDL, high triglycerides, and high blood pressure – a combination called Syndrome X. Syndrome X, also called metabolic syndrome, is recognized as a precursor to serious disease.[84] Leptin resistance is a prime cause of Syndrome X, a major factor in the onset of cardiovascular disease.[85]

Syndrome X is a serious problem because fat infiltrates structures that should not have excess fat; this includes the liver and heart. This sets the stage for lipotropic disease, meaning diseases of excess fat accumulation in all the wrong places.[86] Insulin resistance causes the liver to accumulate excess fat. The first sign of this problem is weight gain around the midsection.

IS INSULIN BAD?

On the surface, it may appear that insulin is a bad guy. After all, it is the main hormone that helps the body store fat. When levels are elevated, a person is prone to increased risk of heart disease, hypoglycemia, hyperglycemia, and developing non-insulin-dependent diabetes. On the other hand, when there is no insulin, a person becomes diabetic in a hurry.

This apparent conflict provides an important point about how the body works. Timing is everything. When insulin is secreted at the right time and in the right amount, the body runs like a fine-tuned engine.

As mentioned earlier, insulin is secreted in two phases. The initial phase comes from stored granules in the pancreas, followed by a second phase of insulin production by pancreatic B-cells. When a person does not eat between meals the pancreas has time to prepare for a meal by getting some insulin ready. When the meal is eaten, this already prepared insulin is released and, in turn, tells the pancreas that more insulin is needed. This causes the B-cells to go into a high level of insulin production that peaks about one-half hour after the meal is complete.

As a person develops insulin resistance, the first phase of insulin secretion does not occur. Part of the reason for this is eating too often; therefore, the pancreas does not have enough time to prepare insulin for the next meal.

This sluggish initial insulin response to a meal is followed by a prolonged release of insulin in the second phase, leaving higher insulin in the blood for longer periods of time thereby increasing the storage of fat and preventing the breakdown of stored fat.[87] This inability to release insulin in the first phase response is considered to be the first sign that a person is on the path to becoming type II diabetic.[88]

The prolonged and inefficient insulin release suppresses glucagon from being released 3-4 hours after the meal, thereby blunting the healthy function of the liver and setting the stage for hypoglycemia. As blood sugar drops, the ability of the body to sustain blood sugar is suppressed, as the liver cannot synthesize blood sugar well enough to maintain normal energetic function. The individual then becomes hypoglycemic, or has low blood sugar symptoms, 3-4 hours after the meal. This sets up the vicious circle of hyperglycemia followed by hypoglycemia, leading to excess eating in an attempt to prop up the blood sugar.

In this common situation, a person uses food to maintain energy. This is not a normal reason to eat. Eating is done as a quick fix to solve the symptoms of out-of-balance insulin and glucagon. Even if a person feels better for a while, the body does not use the calories efficiently, and weight gain and a poor energy level are common results.

It is not that insulin is bad; it is an issue of the right amount of insulin at the right time. The problem of insulin resistance is an example of how poor timing throws one's energy level out of sync.

To make matters worse, it is not just insulin and glucagon that are in a state of imbalance. This out-of-sync fuel utilization has a negative domino effect on hormones throughout the body. There are problems dealing with stress; thyroid hormone is deregulated; growth hormone is depressed; and estrogen imbalance locks in the problem. All of these problems occur in a generally simultaneous way; in a more or less chicken and egg proposition, each problem makes another problem worse and vice versa.

There may be no disease, such as thyroid disease, that can be defined in traditional medical terms. Yet, a person may have the symptoms of hypothyroid function. The entire functional system of the human body becomes less responsive and less functional.

SUMMARY

Insulin and glucagon must function in natural rhythm in order to have an efficient metabolism. Developing and maintaining muscle and liver fitness is essential for preventing problems with leptin.

Individuals with insulin resistance are generally tired and hungry, many times shortly after eating. Such individuals do not extract proper energy from the food they eat; instead food acts as a block on metabolism because it forces hormonal signals into a state of imbalance. Even worse, more food is eaten at the wrong times in an effort to solve unpleasant hypoglycemic symptoms that are a result of the out-of-balance situation.

These issues pose a huge metabolic Catch-22. No drug can fix the problem. Only a return of true health can set the body's systems back on track. It can be done. The *Five Rules* are essential ways to eat to avoid stressing the balance between insulin and glucagon. Rule 2, explained in the next chapter, is the functional test of insulin and glucagon efficiency.

13

Space Meals for Maximum Benefit

*E*ven though leptin is primarily involved with long-term fuel issues, it still has a secondary communication system to support short-term energy needs. We know that leptin and insulin are in a process of communication, similar to cross communication between two department heads as opposed to a direct order from the boss/ brain. Insulin production stimulates leptin production.[89] It has also been proven that leptin receptors are present on the insulin producing B-cells of the pancreas, demonstrating the ability to turn off insulin production.[90]

This forms a circle of self-regulatory checks and balances that is another example of natural energy balance in the human body. In normal physical function, leptin and insulin have a balancing effect on food intake, food storage, and a stable energy level.

Once leptin resistance sets in and leptin levels are high, the pancreatic B-cells do not respond to the signal from leptin to stop making insulin.[91] Not only is the brain developing leptin resistance, so is the pancreas. However, insulin keeps stimulating leptin production while at the same time insulin is encouraging calories to be stored as fat.

This is why leptin and insulin are frequently in a high state together with neither hormone working efficiently. A key step in avoiding this difficult problem is following Rule 2 of our *Five Rules*. This rule is constantly violated by many who provide weight-loss advice, contributing to the societal obesity problem.

THE *FIVE RULES* - Rule 2
Allow 5-6 hours between meals. Eat three meals a day. Do not snack.

The first three hours after eating, the body refuels under the influence of insulin, like filling up at a gas station. Insulin is the carrier of calories to other locations throughout the body. During this storage time, weight loss is not possible.

Three hours after eating, insulin levels should be lower. As it falls, glucagon rises. This is a true fat-burning time. It is when the liver, the metabolic factory of the body, kicks into high gear. During this time, the liver maintains blood sugar through a combination of using its own stored sugar called glycogen and converting protein and fat to fuel as needed. Fats in the blood begin to burn, thereby clearing out stagnant calories.

Not eating between meals is exercise for the liver; it is just as essential as exercising the muscles. Anyone knows how it feels to be physically out of shape. The same thing happens to the liver when there is snacking between meals. The liver needs to have time to generate energy. It needs to deplete its stores of glycogen. If a person eats sporadically throughout the day or has a series of consistent small meals, that process is blocked. This is a fast track to insulin resistance. It synthesizes excess amounts of cholesterol, even if the food eaten contains no cholesterol.

The majority of fat that is broken down between meals is taken up directly by the muscles, thus the importance of exercise. If a person does not exercise, the demand for fatty acid use in the muscles is negligible. Even if fatty acids are freed from triglycerides to be potentially burned for fuel, they are not used anywhere near the rate they could be if muscles were more active. The next time a person eats and insulin goes up, these free fatty acids turn back into triglycerides and head back to fat storage.

The "need" to snack, reflected by dropping energy levels between meals, is a sign of how out of shape the pancreas/liver/muscle system is. When a snack is eaten, insulin levels rise, fat burning is shut off, and calories go back to storage. True enough, some of that fuel will prop up the dropping blood-sugar levels, but if the system were in proper condition, blood-sugar levels would not have dropped in the first place.

Snacking causes the pancreas to become fatigued. Remember that insulin is released in two phases; the first phase is from stored granules of insulin in the pancreas. Snacking between meals is like a repetitive strain injury to the pancreas. The pancreas does not have time to get itself ready for the next meal, meaning time to prepare stored insulin granules for the first part of the insulin response to a meal. This causes an exaggerated second response, meaning that insulin stays elevated past the three-hour point, in turn depressing glucagon and causing hypoglycemia. These two issues, no first-phase insulin response and a prolonged second-phase insulin response, are the hallmarks of insulin resistance. Eating too often causes them. Another cause is eating too much.

The prolonged insulin response shuts off fat burning so no weight loss is possible. Because the prolonged insulin response is inappropriate, it also interferes with the release of glucagon that is essential to get the liver into motion. As blood sugar drops, glucagon is not released because insulin is still too high. This causes the low blood-sugar situation that makes a person want to snack. This is the vicious Catch-22. There will be no weight loss if energy crashes between meals or the person eats between meals.

Some individuals may need to gradually work their eating in the right direction. They may need to have four meals a day, four hours apart. As they increase their exercise and improve the condition of the pancreas, adrenals, muscles, and liver, they will gradually be able to move to the three-meal a day plan without having energy drops between meals.

If 5-6 small meals a day are needed to maintain energy, the metabolic situation is not in good shape. Eating very small meals may cause some weight loss, but metabolism will likely slow down before the weight goal is achieved. Even a low calorie snack increases insulin release, thus fat-burning mode ceases or never begins. Only by increasing the amount of time between meals will proper weight loss take place.

Many children, teenagers, young adults, intense bodybuilders, and athletes can seemingly violate this rule without any apparent consequence. This is because their demand for calories to aid body growth and repair is quite high. This genetic gift tends to disappear after age 30. However, it is alarming the number of children who are overweight and too inactive, thus having hormonal balance problems that used to only be present in the over-30 age group.

After age 30, if this rule is violated, there will be a tendency to slowly and progressively gain weight. If it is truly impossible to make it five hours without eating, the following may apply:

1) There was not enough eaten at the previous meal.
2) There were too many carbohydrates eaten at the previous meal.
3) There needs to be a gradual improvement in physical fitness.
4) There was poor digestion of the food eaten so there was little or no energy from it.
5) There are sluggish and congested liver problems with weak adrenals. The gall bladder has commonly been removed by this time as well.
6) Metabolism is exhausted; the individual has fibromyalgia.
7) Normal blood-sugar regulation is broken, meaning the individual is likely diabetic.

SUMMARY

The fundamental problems of day-to-day fuel regulation lead to a combination of insulin resistance, leptin resistance, and adrenaline resistance. This combination precedes the onset of high blood pressure and type II diabetes. There is a high risk for serious heart disease, cancer, and other disease as well.

The timing of the release of insulin determines if insulin is "good" or "bad." When meals are properly spaced, the pancreas has time to recharge and get prepared for an efficient insulin release following a meal. This initial insulin surge, followed by pancreatic synthesis of more insulin, enables a proper peak of insulin about half an hour after a meal is complete. It then gradually declines over the next few hours.

Insulin acts as a taxicab for calories, taking them to places they need to go to refuel, in the case of glucose, or assist in repair, in the case of protein.

Once insulin returns to its baseline level, 3-3½ hours after the meal, the liver maintains blood glucose. The liver secretes glucose from sugars it stored from the previous meal or it synthesizes sugar from protein, fat, and/or lactic acid. This provides the base of blood glucose needed to fuel the brain as well as provide the essential base for burning fatty acids. Proper function enables a person to not become hypoglycemic between meals.

When a person eats the next meal, rising insulin tells the liver to quit making sugar and start storing sugar. This is a natural rhythm taking place. Major body organs work in a particular way for a period of time and then get a break. The entire system has natural checks and balances, some that enable a person to get extra bursts of energy as needed to meet the demands of any type of situation.

This system slides out of balance by eating between meals; even a "healthy" snack is a problem. It does not matter how many calories are eaten; the snack causes insulin to rise. This interrupts the liver's synthesis of sugar, causes the liver to become clogged with fat and develop insulin resistance, and causes fats that were breaking down to go back into storage.

Eating between meals also causes the liver to excessively secrete cholesterol and initiates insulin resistance for the whole body. When this takes place, usually by the mid-thirties for almost anyone who keeps stressing their metabolism by snacking, problems with leptin resistance take hold. If nothing is changed after that, health rapidly declines.

Individuals who think they must eat between meals for their head to be able to function have significant liver, adrenal, and blood glucose metabolism problems. The actual problems need to be fixed so that eating patterns become healthy ones.

An apple a day may keep the doctor away, but not if it is eaten between meals. Snacking between meals or eating small, frequent meals are counterproductive ways to eat. Those who master leptin will learn to space meals 5-6 hours apart and eat nothing between meals.

14

Inheriting Leptin Problems - Are Your Parents Overweight?

*T*here are several factors that set up a person for problems with leptin resistance. These problems are programmed into the developing brain, sometimes while in the womb and sometimes as an infant. Such individuals may or may not develop leptin issues, but the likelihood is high. This is especially true if the individual violates any of the *Five Rules* on a regular basis.

Only a very small percent of obese individuals have an inability to make leptin, similar to the problem of the *ob/ob* mouse. The overweight issue is a problem of leptin resistance, 99-percent of the time.

There is environmental programming that influences how leptin is set up in an individual's metabolism. These factors come courtesy of one's parents. If parents are overweight, their children are at a higher risk for developing leptin resistance due to programming that took place while they were in the womb.[92] Children born to such parents may develop problems early or they may not manifest until middle age.

Additionally, it is being reported that overeating as an infant sets the stage for later-life obesity, high blood pressure, and heart disease.[93] This is especially true of bottle-fed infants who are prone to getting too many calories.

This factor is alarming because pediatric advice for many years has been to fatten up an underweight baby. In the past, low-birth weight babies have been forced to eat more than normal as standard medical advice. This advice turns out to be wrong as it programs the leptin resistance issue into the developing brain at a very young age, setting the stage for later-life problems.

A combination of overeating and early brain programming sets the stage for leptin-resistance problems.[94] If one's parents were prone to being overweight or if one gained a lot of weight early from bottle-feeding, then the risk for this problem is much higher. It is essentially easier for this individual to fall into leptin resistance than someone else. However, any person who overeats can induce leptin resistance regardless of family history. Once there is a personal history of leptin resistance, there is a higher risk for slipping back into the problem.

Being aware of family genetics and predisposition to the problem is important for individuals so they can take more care not to head down a path of leptin resistance.

15

Preventing the Super-Sized Waistline

*T*he fastest way known to cause leptin resistance is to overeat.[95] Once there is a pattern of excess food consumption, leptin resistance and insulin resistance will be in hot pursuit. When they get locked into metabolism, it is difficult to get on top of them with willpower. This is because their signals are core subconscious signals, programmed into the instincts of survival.

The first two rules of our *Five Rules* place emphasis on the timing of eating and how improper timing fuels an out-of-balance situation that leads to overeating. That is why the first two rules are of extreme importance.

A key time for leptin-resistance overeating is at night for most people. However, since leptin-resistant people arrange their eating to fit their life, they may become excessive during the day if their schedule allows it or if they are under some type of stress.

This brings us to the third of our *Five Rules*; another one to learn on the path to becoming an effective Health Asset Manager.™

THE *FIVE RULES* - Rule 3

Do not eat large meals. Always try to finish a meal slightly less than full. Eating slowly is important.

The amount of food that should be eaten at any one meal depends on how active a person is that day. If one is physically active, more food may be eaten. If one strenuously exercises, more may be eaten. However, most people eat meals that are much too large.

Unfortunately, when food is eaten by a person who is leptin and insulin resistant, the efficiency that allows the body to easily convert food to energy is woefully lacking. Calories can easily head for fat storage, and the person complains of fatigue as a routine fact of life.

There is no such thing as a leptin-resistant person with a great energy level, that is, energy naturally present all day without artificial stimulation such as caffeine or nicotine. In such individuals, excess food acts as a roadblock that obstructs the metabolic pathways in the human body. Since food is essential for survival, this is a perplexing state of affairs.

SHRINK AND TONE YOUR STOMACH

One reason individuals eat too much is because the size of their stomach becomes stretched from eating large meals. Thereafter, they have to keep eating large meals to feel full.

In order to get on a healthy eating track, the physical size of the stomach needs to become smaller. This cannot be accomplished if a bag of popcorn is eaten as a snack or a lot of bread is eaten with meals. These foods simply enlarge the size of the stomach. Even if thinking the popcorn is not such a bad "little meal" at night to satisfy food cravings, it makes one want to eat more at following meals because it stretches the stomach.

Start cutting down on portion sizes, especially carbohydrates. Skip extra bread with meals. Begin to train the stomach to shrink in size. Do some stomach crunches to obtain better abdominal tone.

Stop eating before feeling full. If having a larger meal, have it at lunch when there is more time to metabolize it during the day. Also, try to keep the eating time to 30-45 minutes when possible as this causes insulin to rise for a definable amount of time. Individuals who eat a meal and then go back in an hour for dessert are more likely to get an excess insulin surge, resulting in calories heading in the direction of fat cells for storage.

BIG MEALS CAUSE HYPERGLYCEMIA

It does not matter what the ratio of fats, carbohydrates, and protein is if the meal is too large. A big meal causes excess secretion of insulin to deal with the excess calories resulting in hyperglycemia; that is, high blood sugar.

Hyperglycemia from a meal that contains too many calories causes a person to feel fatigued within 45 minutes of eating; sometimes it even causes cravings for more food. If the meal was really overdone, this fatigue may be extreme and a nap is required or the head feels heavy. This is a common feeling after the classic Thanksgiving dinner. This issue is prevalent with many individuals all year long.

Hyperglycemia from a large meal is a major stress to the body. It usually results in a rebound hypoglycemia 3-4 hours after eating. The potential energy from food is derailed because the hormones regulating the ability to use that fuel are thrown into a state of disarray by the large meal. The calories are headed for fat storage.

Individuals are frequently surprised to find that they notice increased energy from eating less food. This is because the smaller meal helps insulin and glucagon act on calories in the proper way, leading to energy production. This is a clear example where smaller is better.

American restaurants typically serve excessive portions, even offering super-size options. These large portions are not necessary and are detrimental to health.

SLOW DOWN

When out to dinner with a group of friends, look around the table and see who finishes their meal first and then look at their waistline. Nothing more needs to be said.

It takes ten minutes for the brain to receive the signal of being full. A lot of food that is not needed can be eaten in those ten minutes.

Take the time to chew food well. This not only helps the digestive system immensely, it enables the brain to turn off hunger signals without eating as much food.

Have conversation, relax, slow down, and enjoy the meal. If food is chewed for a longer time, there will be the same amount of pleasure in terms of taste while eating much less food.

If prone to being a fast eater, learn to take a five-minute break in the middle of the meal. The satisfaction of feeling full will be felt sooner. There is no need to eat as much.

Many leptin-resistant individuals cannot seem to inhale food fast enough. While some younger people can eat fast and get away with it, this will not last long. Leptin resistance is knocking at the door. After age 30, eating too fast invariably involves eating too much, and metabolism cannot keep up.

SUMMARY

This point is simple but important in the road to mastering leptin. Eat too much as a lifestyle pattern and be on the fast road to leptin resistance and increased risk for any disease. Meal size, including portion control, is essential for a balanced body free of leptin and insulin problems.

Eating slowly, relaxing during the meal, and having enjoyable conversation are all great ways to learn to eat less food.

16

Getting off to a Good Start -
The Importance of Protein

*E*ach calorie is potential energy that can be extracted from food. Theoretically, protein and carbohydrates contain the same number of calories. They contain four calories per gram whereas fat contains nine calories per gram.

If fuel regulation is inefficient, then the potential energy of a calorie does not become actual energy that is used, it gets stored as fat. While it is fine that a person is aware of the number of calories they eat, it is equally important to eat in such a way that improves energy and enhances any type of calorie to be used more efficiently.

The type of food eaten has a different effect on the liver regardless of the amount of calories in that food. The liver is the metabolic factory of the body, the most important organ in regulating the use of calories. When the "liver factory" sees fats or carbohydrates coming, it does not need to change these substances much before they are useful to the body. Fats and carbohydrates increase the liver's metabolic rate by only 4 percent.

On the other hand, protein is a very complex calorie. Proteins form the backbone of the genetic signaling system. Everything in the body is made of protein. The liver must take proteins from the food and assemble them into the various needs for the body. Sometimes the liver will attach fats or carbohydrates to proteins, but it is the complexity of protein that drives the liver factory into action.

Dietary protein is the raw material that tells the liver to get in gear. Without adequate protein, the work cannot get started, and metabolism will sit still. It is like a carpenter waiting for the nails and plywood to show up at the job site.

THE *FIVE RULES* - Rule 4
Eat a breakfast containing protein.

Metabolism can increase by 30 percent for as long as 12 hours from a high-protein meal, the calorie-burning equivalent of a three or four mile jog.[96]

A high-carbohydrate breakfast such as juice, cereal, waffles, pancakes, or bagels does not enhance metabolic rate. It may trigger a problem with insulin resistance as a lot of insulin is released in response to the carbohydrates, causing energy fluctuations and sugar cravings during the day. High glycemic carbohydrates can shift normal leptin release earlier in the day. If there is leptin resistance, this fuels overeating throughout the day and especially at night.

The two signs of a poor breakfast are:

1) Being unable to make it five hours to lunch without food cravings or energy crashing.
2) Being much more prone to leptin resistance later that afternoon or evening. This sets in motion strong food cravings resulting in poor eating habits.

A high-protein breakfast helps metabolism turn on, and it stabilizes hypoglycemia or low blood sugar reactions later in the day. A high-protein meal helps prevent leptin fluctuations later in the day. Protein enhances the release of glucagon, helping to blunt the excess insulin response that causes insulin resistance. Eggs are a good breakfast, just not smothered in butter and cheese.

We use high-efficiency whey protein for quick and easy breakfasts. Any lean protein can be eaten at breakfast along with a moderate amount of carbohydrates. Avoid fruit juice at breakfast; this is too much sugar for anyone who has a problem with insulin or leptin resistance.

This rule becomes even more important the older a person becomes. This is because there is less ability to tolerate stress. A poor breakfast adds to the wear and tear of the body and induces an unstable energy level before the day is over. Fatigue later in the day, from a poor breakfast, is noticeable once a person begins to pay attention to how they feel later in the day based on what they ate for breakfast.

As far as children are concerned, there is some variance in this rule. Some children can do just fine on a high-carbohydrate breakfast. However, those with learning difficulties, ADD, ADHD, depression, mood fluctuations, and/ or are overweight, do best eating a high-protein breakfast. This is especially true if a child has parents who struggle with leptin resistance.

Eating no breakfast is an extreme version of a poor breakfast. This forces the body to run on energy reserves and tends to leave the liver struggling with a shortage of proper raw materials. Even if a person can get through some of the day eating this way, it will not be long before this pattern of eating catches up with them in terms of energy issues, mood swings, poor eating patterns, and overall increased wear and tear on the body.

Some individuals simply do not feel like eating breakfast. Their digestive system is too full of toxic waste from the inadequate job of house cleaning that was done the night before. It may be two or three hours before they can even think about eating a normal-size breakfast. A bowl of oatmeal may work well for them as it is a higher-protein grain. They may just have to have a little something to not feel queasy, and then eventually have the high-protein meal. This problem improves as their overall level of toxicity decreases.

PROTEIN AND FLUID RETENTION

Protein has a significant effect on fluid-retention issues. Adequate protein helps make a primary blood transport protein called albumin. Many nutrients are carried on albumin. Albumin circulates in the blood. The heart forces nutrients and water out of capillaries and into the tissue delivering oxygen and nutrition.

However, water must be drawn back into circulation, otherwise the body becomes dehydrated. This is accomplished by the osmotic force of albumin, which attracts water from tissues back into capillaries. If there is not enough protein, albumin levels drop, and the body loses its ability to maintain water in circulation. Instead, water accumulates in the tissues causing edema. Adequate protein intake helps solve fluid-retention problems by ensuring there is a proper amount of albumin.

GRADUALLY INCREASE PROTEIN INTAKE

In cases where individuals have not been eating enough protein, it is best to gradually increase the amount of protein, especially if a person is in poor health or significantly overweight. It is also important to improve physical fitness at the same time protein in the diet is increased. This is because muscles use protein to repair themselves. Additionally, the increased energy to exercise stimulates many enzymes to be used that are protein dependent.

If a person is in poor fitness and eats too much protein too fast, they will feel irritable and fatigued because the liver cannot process the protein due to a poor state of liver fitness. There is an important relationship between liver function, physical activity that results in improved fitness, and protein intake. This is especially important for individuals recovering from a prolonged period of poor health.

By gradually increasing protein and exercise, the liver is able to channel the consumed protein into a health-promoting direction. Muscle strength, muscle fitness, and the ability to exercise longer improve, and the liver is in better working order. Protein is the calorie that can wake up a sleeping metabolism, as long as increased protein intake is done in a way that benefits health.

SUMMARY

It is not just the amount of calories that are eaten that influences the ability to lose weight. The type of calorie and the timing of eating are just as important. One essential principle is to eat enough protein to help the liver stay metabolically active.

Eating a solid protein breakfast provides a stable base for energy, mood, and blood sugar throughout the day and evening. It helps keep the body in a calorie-burning mode, a mode that can burn fat for fuel. When energy crashes during the day, frequently due to a lacking breakfast, then metabolism and weight loss come to a grinding halt.

A great number of metabolic problems can be solved or avoided by eating a breakfast that consists of ample protein.

17

Eat Like a Pyramid, Look Like a Pyramid

*T*he food pyramid places much too much emphasis on eating carbohydrates relative to protein. This leads to carbohydrate snacking between meals or eating meals that contain an overabundance of carbohydrates.

While the designers of this pyramid are certainly not in favor of overeating, the pyramid plan subconsciously causes individuals to overeat. This is because this style of eating causes imbalances in insulin and glucagon, in turn inducing leptin resistance and out-of-control overeating.

Therefore, the pyramid designers can preach portion control all they want; they just cannot get individuals to do it very well with this type of diet plan; people tend to overeat.

Our *Five Rules* are far more important than what the food pyramid may have to offer. There is nothing very innovative about the food pyramid. People agree with eating a variety of food. Most agree with not overindulging on fat, junk food, and sweets. These basics are already known.

The problem with the food pyramid is that the amount of carbohydrates in this diet plan causes individuals who are heading in the direction of insulin resistance and leptin resistance to worsen. This is because it promotes excess insulin release that in turn promotes fat storage and higher circulating insulin leading to insulin resistance and leptin resistance. Furthermore, there is no warning not to snack, an issue that really gets a person going in the wrong direction.

The food pyramid contributes to and, in some cases, directly causes problems with leptin resistance, especially for those age 30 and over. A person is literally pulled down the dark alley of leptin resistance by inducing insulin resistance as the amount of carbohydrates suggested in this plan is consumed.

Even though the carbohydrates eaten may have little fat, the liver becomes congested and synthesizes excess fat due to the pitfalls of the pyramid plan.

Unfortunately, because this plan makes leptin resistance worse, it increases the rate of the onset of major diseases in our society, including obesity. This is not good public-health policy.

THE *FIVE RULES* - Rule 5
Reduce the amount of carbohydrates eaten.

Carbohydrates are easy-to-use fuels. The body takes money from its purse or wallet, the food on a plate, before it dips into the savings account, the hips, thighs, buttocks, and midsection. Carbohydrates in the diet are the main signal for insulin secretion. If there is a problem with insulin resistance and leptin resistance, as is the case with most overweight individuals, then cutting back on carbohydrates helps reduce the amount of insulin produced and tends to cool off the problem as well as settle down the leptin resistance.

Some carbohydrates are needed in a healthy diet or the thyroid turns off, electrolytes become deregulated, muscles weaken, growth hormone is not released correctly, fat is not burned efficiently, there is an unsatisfied feeling after a meal, the heart becomes stressed, and the digestive system goes on the blink. We certainly do not advocate a no-carbohydrate diet.

In general, many Americans eat twice the amount of carbohydrates they are able to metabolize, a main reason why more than 50 percent are overweight.

When the amount of carbohydrates is reduced, the amount of fat or protein needs to increase in order to have enough calories to function. Finding the right balance for each individual takes time and paying attention to the body. Every meal of the day does not have to be the same. The goal is to be able to go 5-6 hours between meals with a good energy level and be able to lose weight or maintain proper body weight.

EMPLOY THE 50/50 TECHNIQUE
In most cases, just getting the protein and carbohydrates into better balance goes a long way towards assisting weight loss. This is easily done with the visual 50/50 technique. Look at meals and see a palm-size piece of protein (a

4-6 ounce portion for women; 6-8 ounce portion for men). Try to keep the total carbohydrate physical size the same physical size as the protein, a 50/50 visual. This way there is no calorie counting. Compare the protein (chicken, meat, turkey, eggs) to the carbohydrates (bread, rice, potatoes, fruit, desserts). Eat any amount of vegetables; however, eat corn, carrots, and peas in moderation.

If dessert is on the menu, plan to skip the bread, rice, and potatoes in the meal. If carbohydrates are eaten during the meal, then plan on only one bite of dessert.

The consumption of too many carbohydrates causes leptin to rise too high at the wrong time of the day. For example, a person with leptin resistance who eats a sweet roll, muffin, juice, or bagel for breakfast, with little or no protein, will have trouble with overeating later in the day. If such a person eats too many carbohydrates at lunch, they will be ravishingly hungry by dinner.

Such individuals have a lack of energy later in the day and insist on eating a larger meal so they feel good. In this situation, calories are not being used efficiently, and misguided leptin signals enforce eating behaviors. It is amazing to these individuals that when they quit eating the excess carbohydrates, they have a better sustaining energy level and mood.

SOME CARBOHYDRATES ARE IMPORTANT

Carbohydrates are a primary fuel source for the body. The other primary fuel source is saturated fat. A debate could easily be made over the preferred fuel source, but that issue is not critical to weight loss. The important point is that carbohydrates are easy to use for fuel.

Excess consumption of carbohydrates prevents the body from dipping into fat reserves for energy. Excess consumption also turns into fat quite easily even though there are no fat grams in the carbohydrates. This is because under the influence of excess insulin, the body stores excess calories as fat. At the same time, excess insulin inhibits the breakdown of stored fat. When the liver also has insulin resistance, it is prone to directing calories to fat storage as well.

On the other hand, carbohydrates are especially important for muscle function; without enough carbohydrates, muscles lose their water content and become dehydrated, weak, and/or develop cramps. As part of their role in maintaining proper hydration of the body, they have a direct influence on electrolytes. Diets too low in carbohydrates can eventually lead to kidney and cardiovascular distress. A person with leptin resistance may already have strained kidney and cardiovascular function, thus a diet too low in carbohydrates may aggravate these issues.

A physically active person who uses their muscles frequently has a higher need for carbohydrates and has an increased ability to metabolize carbohydrates. If a physically active person does not eat enough carbohydrates, they lack sustainable muscle energy. Performance suffers.

SUMMARY

The basic approach for weight loss is to visually balance the amount of protein (4-6 ounces for women, 6-8 ounces for men) with the amount of carbohydrate eaten. There is generally an amount of fat naturally occurring in the protein.

Active individuals with no weight issues can certainly eat more carbohydrates than this, as they have an ability to metabolize them. As an individual loses weight and maintains a good weight for a period of time, along with a good level of physical activity and energy, the ability to metabolize carbohydrates improves.

In order to keep weight off after losing it, it is important to exercise and maintain the goal weight while slowly increasing the carbohydrate amount. Too many carbohydrates too fast after losing weight causes rapid weight gain. Once there has been a problem with insulin resistance and leptin resistance, it is easy to get back in a poor pattern.

Being a Health Asset Manager™ means that one must pay attention to the trend one's body is in and learn to manage that trend effectively. A Health Asset Manager™ who has mastered leptin has the knowledge and life skills needed to keep weight off after losing it.

18

The Secrets to Accessing Fat-Burning Mode

The whole purpose of the *Five Rules* for mastering leptin is to create energy and metabolic efficiency in the body. An individual has the ability to correctly extract real energy from the food they eat. If an individual is overweight, then employing the *Five Rules* helps normalize body weight. These rules also keep a normal-weight individual from gaining weight, especially as they grow older.

When the *Five Rules* are employed in an effort to lose weight, they help an individual enter fat-burning mode. This is a metabolic ability to dip into the stores of fat without the body slowing down into the hibernation mode because it thinks it is starving.

HOW TO ENTER FAT-BURNING MODE

Stored fat is called a triglyceride; it contains three fatty acids and one glycerol – a carbohydrate. In order to induce the body to go into fat-burning mode, it is necessary for the body to break down stored fat, the savings account of stored energy. This requires that there be a relative deficiency in the easiest to use fuels in the diet; these are carbohydrates and saturated fats.

If there is a deficiency in all fuels, metabolism slows down and stored fat is conserved. For most people, there should be slightly higher protein relative to fat and carbohydrate in order to lose weight.

When eating in accordance with our *Five Rules* and gradually reducing easy-to-use fuels, that is, saturated fat and carbohydrates, a person enters fat-burning mode.

THE FLUID-RETENTION PROBLEM

If fluid retention is present, weight loss becomes difficult. When the body clicks into fat-burning mode, the first thing it does is dump 3-6 pounds of stuck fluid, and only then does it get down to the business of burning fat.

When a person loses weight or maintains their ideal weight, they do not have a fluid-retention problem. Individuals who struggle with weight loss may be 2-4 pounds lighter after a strenuous workout, but all they did was dump the water that was embedded in their connective tissue. After their next meal or later that night, they are right back where they were prior to the exercise as their body has regained the water it lost during the exercise.

There is a simple test to help determine if too many carbohydrates are eaten. Stand on the scale first thing in the morning and then stand on the scale at night. If an individual weighs over two pounds more at night than in the morning, one of our *Five Rules* of eating has been violated. If Rules 1-4 were followed, then too many carbohydrates were eaten that day.

Gradually decrease carbohydrates in the diet until there is less fluid retention, and a fat-burning mode will begin.

ONCE YOU ACCESS FAT-BURNING MODE, STAY THERE!

Following our *Five Rules* and accessing fat-burning mode creates a wonderful feeling of energy and well-being. However, when a person has been in fat-burning mode for a few days and feels great, it does not mean their underlying issues with leptin resistance are solved.

There may be numerous temptations that divert an individual from fat-burning mode. Such temptations cause one to violate one or more of our *Five Rules*. Beware; fat cells lurk in the wings ready to refill themselves at a moments notice. This is the opposite of fat-burning mode.

While it may not seem like that big of a deal to occasionally go out of rhythm, it unfortunately is. If a person is in a good fat-burning mode and then violates one of the *Five Rules*, fat-burning mode will stop.

However, even if the individual goes back to the *Five Rules* the next day, it may take 2-5 days for fat-burning mode to resume. During that time, the individual will have to wrestle with the additional urges of leptin resistance and previous compulsive eating patterns that did not exist when they were in fat-burning mode.

Unfortunately, when a person tries to lose weight and is in a good pattern, any violation of the *Five Rules* can cost 2-5 days of progress. Once in fat-burning mode, stay there!

SUMMARY

The whole purpose of healthy eating is not calorie restriction and deprivation. These approaches simply result in yo-yo dieting and endless problems with fluctuating leptin. The issue is one of improving the metabolic efficiency in response to food. Most Americans need to eat less, and when they do it right, they will find they have more energy on less food.

Our *Five Rules* prevent and correct insulin resistance, leptin resistance, adrenaline resistance, fatigue, and mood problems. They promote a metabolic balance that leads to relatively easy fat burning, even for those who have struggled with their weight.

If a person can violate these rules and still maintain a healthy weight and good energy level, they are fortunate and blessed with good genetics. However, sooner or later they will not be able to eat in violation of the *Five Rules* and get away with it.

If a person tries to follow the *Five Rules* and is not able to, they need to work themselves into a better level of "eating fitness." It is workable to begin implementing some of them, and as there is improvement, keep working on all of them.

Even though there is tremendous biochemical individuality, the *Five Rules* are of fundamental importance to virtually everyone. This is because the rules are based on survival, and they facilitate correct signals in the body relating to survival. The *Five Rules* address the subconscious brain at a core level, a much more powerful principle than conscious-level individuality. The *Five Rules* are the essence of mastering leptin from a dietary point of view.

Eating in such a way as to not confuse basic communication signals in the body relating to survival is the single most important point about how to eat. If such principles are violated, it will minimally feel like rowing a boat upstream. More commonly, it feels like health is slipping away.

Following the *Five Rules* is the foundation of a healthy eating lifestyle that facilitates energy needs and helps keep the body efficiently metabolizing calories throughout life, including the accessing of fat-burning mode for the purpose of healthy weight loss. These simple eating rules are the keys to growing older healthfully. They form the foundation of being a competent Health Asset Manager.™

19

Taking Steps to Conquer Stress Eating

*L*ook around. How many things just have to get done? How many projects are on the backlogged "to do" list? How many demands are there today or this week? Many of these demands are responsibilities essential to living, such as working and raising children. There seems to be no end to how energy can be spent. Are the demands of life in any reasonable state of balance in terms of ability to recover? When can time be made for oneself?

Most individuals with leptin resistance have trouble with the balance of demands in their life compared to recovery, relaxation, fun, and enjoyment.

In terms of food, the fastest way to leptin resistance is to overeat. In terms of exercise, the fastest way to leptin resistance is to do none. In terms of lifestyle, the fastest way to leptin resistance is to stress out. When the "solution" to stress is eating, there is double trouble.

STRESS FUELS ADRENALINE EXCESS

Stress generates an adrenaline response to meet the demands of the stress. This is a survival trait to be able to deal with emergencies. In today's world, we have ongoing stress that is generally not life threatening. This leads to excessive adrenaline production on a regular basis due to the demands and pressures in life.

Excess adrenaline is behaviorally manifested in different ways. Some feel anxiety or fear; others feel anger, irritation, and frustration. Some express these feelings; others internalize them. Regardless of how the excess adrenaline is manifested, the bottom line is that there is too much of it.

FALSE ALARM

Normally, the hypothalamus gland, the 911 control center in the brain, signals fat cells to release energy by sending an adrenaline message to them. This is a normal survival mechanism wherein adrenaline is associated with an increased energy need, and increased fuel is supplied to meet the emergency demand. This method of survival is certainly handy when confronted by saber-toothed tigers.

However, what happens when the body cries wolf? Maybe it does not seem like the stressors in life are like "crying wolf," but from a genetic survival point of view, the great majority of today's stressors are in the "crying-wolf" category. In essence, the survival instincts to deal with major stress are activated by relatively trivial issues. At first, the body behaves according to the genetic program. After a while, the body realizes there is a false alarm.

The fat cells are no longer going to listen to the "crying-wolf" adrenaline release. The fat cells develop adrenaline resistance due to excess trivial stress, in turn causing the fat cells to become metabolically numb and slow down. Sluggish fat cells easily expand causing weight gain.

Adrenaline resistance is one-third of the key triad of weight gain issues, along with insulin resistance and leptin resistance. Once one of these three is in motion, the other two follow. True enough, people may overeat in response to stress. However, the main reason they gain weight from stress is because of adrenaline resistance.

STRESS CHANGES ENERGY NEEDS

Stress is the wildcard that wreaks havoc with fuel regulation. Stress comes in many sizes and shapes. There can be major stressors such as accidents, surgery, chronic illness, or loss of a loved one. There can be emotional stressors such as conflict or other relationship issues that involve bad feelings.

There can be physical stressors such as living with pain, not getting enough sleep, physically demanding work, a flu bug, or intense exercise. There can be acute intense stressors such as a large argument or unexpected change.

These various demands and challenges of life, regardless of their size and shape, are intimately connected with fuel regulation systems in the body. The reason for this is easy to understand. When there is an increased demand on the body, there is an increased need for fuel.

Too much stress not only offsets schedules and routines, it can offset the underlying fuel balance in the body. This causes food cravings, energy fluctuations, and fatigue. This is a fast track to weight gain or causes disruption of a good weight-loss routine.

ONGOING STRESS

Managing acute or short-term stress is difficult enough, but what happens when stress is ongoing for a number of years?

The hormones released under stress are adrenaline and cortisol. Adrenaline is released by the nervous system; it is also secreted by the inside part of the adrenal glands called the adrenal medulla. Cortisol is secreted by the outside part of the adrenal glands called the adrenal cortex.

Adrenaline and cortisol are friendly with glucagon but not as compatible with insulin. Since insulin works with food to help store it, it is not a good hormone to help make extra energy on demand. Conversely, glucagon is the hormone that synthesizes fuel from storage and helps protein and fatty acids to be burned for fuel. This makes sense that adrenaline, cortisol, and glucagon all work together to produce more energy in response to increasing demands, especially stress.

In the absence of stress, glucagon does its basic role of maintaining blood sugar between meals and setting the stage for consistent blood-sugar support during sleep. It is much easier to maintain proper blood sugar during sleep if glucagon is not also having its volume turned up by adrenaline and cortisol.

In the presence of stress, the release of adrenaline and cortisol signal the liver to dramatically increase the supply of blood sugar. In essence, there is a synergistic effect between glucagon, adrenaline, and cortisol. The liver responds to this combined hormone stimulus by making fuel from stored glycogen and by synthesizing fuel from protein. Fatty acids may also be used if the stress is prolonged.

On the one hand, this might sound like a great way to lose weight; unfortunately, stress hormones break down the protein of the body structure before they burn fatty acids for fuel. Stress-induced weight loss is debilitating to heath due to the loss of physical fitness; the physical feeling of wear and tear is obvious.

STRESS EATING

Stress causes a rise in blood sugar; this is a hyperglycemic state. This means there is a higher than normal amount of blood sugar so that a person can either run away or go into battle. Genetically, this was for fight or flight purposes. This hyperglycemic response activates many subconscious behavior patterns associated with survival.

These patterns are not necessarily rational. Hyperglycemia drives violent and aggressive behavior. It also causes anxiety and fear, and in the case of children, causes irrational and emotional outbursts and odd social behavior such as ADHD. If there is a large amount of it going on before bed, a person will not be able to get to sleep, stay asleep very long, or sleep restfully.

Hyperglycemia causes the body to run hot. The engines are hyper aroused, as if prepared for battle, whether real or imagined. One way to cool off a hot hyperglycemic reaction is to eat food. The higher the concentration of calories, the faster the stress reaction will cool off.

The reason this works is because eating food causes a rise in insulin. The fastest way to raise insulin is to eat fats and carbohydrates in combination. The rise in insulin causes a depression of glucagon, turning off the liver's ability to make excess sugar. This settles down the hyperglycemic reaction to stress, sometimes in a matter of minutes. When stress is more intense or has gone on for a long time and the hyperglycemia is more severe, then dense fatty/salty junk foods sound better than sweets.

This is why people stress eat; it is how excess food becomes an individual's best friend. It is a temporary solution to turning off unpleasant feelings. It has a short-term "workability" with major adverse, long-term consequences. Regular stress eating is a fast track to leptin, insulin, and adrenaline resistance.

STRESS WHEN ALREADY FED

Let us say that something stressful happens after eating. In this case, insulin is already the dominant hormone in the system. The release of stress hormones upsets the digestive system, as they reduce peristaltic motion and take blood away from the digestive tract.

Additionally, insulin response is blunted by the stress hormones causing improper refueling. The liver does not want to store energy under stress; it wants to synthesize energy.

Therefore, stress in a fed state causes liver confusion and indigestion. This destabilizes energy and results in energy dropping either immediately, if stress tolerance is not good, or in several hours, causing food cravings between meals due to low-blood sugar.

FIND ALTERNATIVES TO STRESS EATING

Instead of eating when there is a stress feeling in the body, do something physically active. Go for a walk, do some jumping jacks, briskly climb up and down the stairs ten times. This has the effect of putting the high blood sugar to use, at which point the craving for food will cease.

The more stress a person has as part of their life, the greater the importance for consistent relaxing exercise or activities to remain in balance. This helps build up the relaxed reserves of the nervous system so there is more tolerance for stress. Just getting in a good rhythm with the *Five Rules* can make a big difference in terms of improved stress tolerance and less likelihood to embark on stress eating.

SUMMARY

Stress is one main factor that deregulates the natural balance of insulin and glucagon, setting the stage for leptin resistance. If these hormones are already out of balance from food issues, then stress simply makes matters worse.

Eating and exercising in a good rhythm and pattern are the basics to handle and tolerate stress more effectively. Building a good "savings account" of relaxed reserves is essential for any person with a physically or emotionally demanding life.

In order to grow older with health intact, good eating patterns and stress management are essential components that exist along with proper blood-sugar control and healthy immunity.[97]

Finding comfort and pleasure in alternatives to stress eating, such as enjoyable walks, is an important issue for individuals prone to this behavior.

20

Is Caffeine Good or Bad?

*C*affeine is one of the most widely consumed and addictive substances in the world. It serves as an example of how a substance can be beneficial or harmful, depending on the person consuming it and their existing health situation.

The most basic view of caffeine is as a metabolic stimulant. It works by increasing sympathetic nervous system activity that in turn increases metabolic rate.[98] The ability of caffeine to increase metabolic rate is the opposite of the slow and "perceived starvation" metabolism of the typical overweight person, thus it has been incorporated into various weight-loss plans.[99,100]

Caffeine has been found to increase the rate of fat burning in the liver, enhancing the burning of fat for fuel.[101,102] It has been hypothesized that caffeine, via its increase in sympathetic nerve activity, can help reduce abdominal weight gain, the type of fat most associated with cardiovascular disease.[103]

Caffeine may even help protect the liver from damage.[104] Caffeine consumption reduces the risk of gallstones by helping the gall bladder contract and thus move along its contents more efficiently.[105] This is the same reason coffee enemas have been in use for over 100 years. Caffeine also helps the bowels move along promoting a better elimination and rate of overall toxin clearance.[106] When caffeine works in a friendly manner in the body, it helps to depress leptin.[107,108]

It was recently reported in the *Lancet* that individuals drinking seven cups of coffee per day had one-half the chance of developing type II diabetes compared to individuals who had two or fewer cups of coffee per day.[109] This study of Dutch coffee drinkers did not compare coffee drinkers to healthy non-coffee drinkers; thus, while this study made national media headlines, it is misleading.

Navy Seals, intentionally sleep deprived and placed under a variety of intense physical stress, had significantly better cognitive function and performance with the assistance of 200 mg of caffeine.[110] It is safe to assume that due to the needed level of physical fitness, most Navy Seals do not suffer from leptin resistance. This study shows that individuals in good physical fitness may benefit from caffeine stimulation when under stress. This is a short-term response to caffeine stimulation.

The cognitive effects of caffeine seem most prominent in individuals who are deprived of caffeine and then consume some. These improvements tend to be lost with regular caffeine consumption.[111]

In a rather interesting experiment, researchers tested the accuracy of timing perception in individuals who consumed no caffeine, less than 135 mg a day, and more than 135 mg a day. The moderate caffeine consumption group had the best timing perception. Higher caffeine consumption or no caffeine consumption did not score as well.[112] Since body rhythms are a matter of proper timing and being in sync, this study provided evidence that a moderate amount of caffeine may be helpful for some individuals in achieving natural balance. Whether caffeine actually has this effect depends largely on the amount consumed and the existing health of the individual.

CAFFEINE PROBLEMS

Individuals with eating disorders are known for their over consumption of caffeine and other metabolic stimulants such as nicotine.[113,114] Caffeine excess can lead to very serious health problems in these individuals, including psychosis[115] and heart attack.[116] Individuals with eating disorders attempt various strategies to suppress leptin out of existence so that no weight gain is possible, then they get stuck in the problem and can't get out.

Caffeine can be used as a substance to facilitate this misguided behavior, an example of too much metabolic stimulation in an individual who is already malnourished. Such individuals frequently live on diet soda and cigarettes as their primary "nutrient" intake.

The other side of the coin is the person who is over nourished, even though their body may think it is starving. While consuming caffeine can potentially help such a person, this is frequently not the case. For example, instead of getting improved bowel function, such individuals simply get heartburn or a sore stomach from consuming caffeine, especially when they exceed a small amount.

Even in healthy individuals, caffeine can tilt metabolism in a manner that begins to induce insulin resistance.[117] As a healthy person begins to run on stimulants, the natural balance in the insulin system is disrupted. Every indÿividual has a different tolerance level for this shift, meaning that some individuals are able to consume more caffeine than others.

However, at some point, over-stimulation with caffeine begins to create insulin resistance. Once insulin resistance occurs, leptin resistance and adrenaline resistance are close behind. When a person who consumes caffeine is gaining extra weight, this fact is impossible to deny. At this point, caffeine has crossed the line.

In our experience in observing overweight individuals who consume caffeine, it is common that caffeine moves leptin timing too early. Instead of leptin hitting its highest level during sleep, this timing is moved forward. This results in excess cravings for carbohydrates between meals, overeating at night, and/or poor quality sleep. In essence it causes an individual to violate the two most important rules of eating properly.

By reducing caffeine intake, especially morning caffeine, this adverse effect of food cravings later in the day can be avoided and a person can stay in better balance. The bottom line is a person with obvious leptin resistance should seek to avoid excess caffeine consumption. Reduce consumption to a point that does not induce poor eating patterns.

Some individuals may need to eliminate caffeine in order to wake up their sluggish fat cells that are adrenaline resistant.

If caffeine raises blood pressure, contributes to weight gain around the middle, and/or there is great trouble following our *Five Rules*, then it can be assumed that caffeine intake is excessive. This is because excess sympathetic nerve stimulation causes a numbing effect on fat cells in the abdominal area leading to excess weight gain around the middle. In such situations caffeine is making adrenaline resistance worse.

The excessive amount also has a stimulating effect on the kidneys leading to high blood pressure and over-reactions to stress.[118] Therefore, the over-caffeinated individual is irritable, hyper, prone to high blood pressure, has trouble sleeping, has insulin resistance, and is gaining weight around the middle. Such individuals are also fatigued and think they must have caffeine for energy stimulation.

A person who is leptin resistant may already have these problems even though they do not consume any caffeine. Caffeine consumption may simply make existing problems worse.

Caffeine issues are complicated with a coffee shop on every corner. Many drinks ordered in these shops contain excess sugar and fat calories along with the caffeine. When such drinks are consumed between meals, they count as a snack, directly unbalancing the *Five Rules*. This is also true for the person consuming excess sugar or nerve-irritant artificial sweeteners in their excess soft-drink consumption.

Too much caffeine has the same effect as too much leptin; it simply causes a breakdown in normal communication and natural balance.

SUMMARY

If a person has a moderate amount of caffeine, sleeps well at night, sticks with the eating pattern of the *Five Rules*, has normal blood pressure, maintains an optimistic mood, and is losing weight or maintaining optimum weight, then caffeine may actually work towards improved health and metabolic fitness. At least it is not noticeably detracting from health.

The problem for most individuals who are leptin resistant is that they are prone to compulsive or addictive consumption patterns, easily leading to excess intake of caffeine, therefore, wiping out any benefit they may have had.

Individuals with a history of weight issues, leptin resistance, and any type of drug/alcohol abuse need to be quite wary of falling into the trap of excess caffeine consumption. Any person who "has to have" caffeine every day is on the edge of, if not already in, a significant problem with energy and metabolism.

21

Brain Cravings

*W*hen all is said and done, a person will eat when they are hungry. Hunger sets in motion powerful subconscious survival instincts. The key issue is whether or not the hunger signal the person is experiencing is a proper hunger signal or one that is misguided. The abnormal hunger signal leads to excess weight gain and serious health problems as the years go by.

The issue of leptin resistance is the key factor that sets the stage for a truly misguided hunger signal as the brain cannot properly sense the amount of fuel stored in fat, therefore, enforcing a hunger signal. This keeps sending the eaten food into fat storage.

Insulin resistance and adrenaline resistance work together with leptin resistance to lock in eating patterns that are erratic. Individuals with these issues lack stress tolerance and try to use food to cool off or settle down emotional feelings. This results in the emotional eater who locks in the problems of leptin, insulin, and adrenaline resistance.

In virtually all situations of inappropriate eating due to a faulty hunger signal, a person feels better for a few minutes or a few hours after eating. However, there is no stability in their daily energy, mood, eating patterns, or sleep patterns. Any benefit from the improperly ingested food is easily offset by the consequences to energy level, weight gain, and overall natural balance.

We are learning more and more about the science behind food cravings. It may help one to combat food cravings if such science is more thoroughly understood. However, the bottom line is an issue of staying in natural balance. The better a person can do this, the fewer improper hunger signals they will experience.

NEUROPEPTIDE Y

The hypothalamus gland in the brain is the subconscious command and control center for the entire body. It is the part of the brain that senses the amount of leptin on hand. When it senses the correct amount of leptin, it means there is plenty of fuel in storage so it turns off appetite and enables a faster metabolism.

If there is truly a lack of food or if there is leptin resistance, then the hypothalamus will keep hunger signals elevated in an effort to motivate the gathering of more food.

Neuropeptide Y (NPY) is the key hunger signal in the brain. This signal must be turned off in order to feel satisfied. If this signal stays elevated, then eating continues. (Figure 10)

Leptin and NPY are opposites. As leptin levels rise inside the brain, NPY levels fall. Unfortunately, when there is leptin resistance, leptin does not enter the brain at the proper rate. NPY levels stay high causing an individual to eat more than they need before the brain gets the message that they are full.

DOPAMINE AND NEUROPEPTIDE Y

As we have pointed out, leptin is closely related to sympathetic nerve function. The primary neurotransmitter relating to leptin is dopamine. Dopamine is involved with reward behavior. The fastest way to increase dopamine is to eat fat; in turn this raises leptin and shuts off NPY.

This makes the person feel rewarded on a subconscious basis; they feel satisfied. The primary protein needed to make dopamine is the amino acid tyrosine, found in animal proteins and cheese. Therefore, high tyrosine and high-fat foods, such as a steak dinner, pizza with meat, and high-calorie Mexican food, are foods that individuals may turn to so that the dopamine-reward system in the brain feels satisfied. Individuals who crave high-fat proteins generally crave energy.

Food Cravings

Figure 10

Stress places demands on the nervous system. When stress is not managed well or when stress is too great, then food cravings will intensify. When a person eats in response to stress, it sets the stage or locks in the problems of leptin resistance, insulin resistance, and adrenaline resistance.

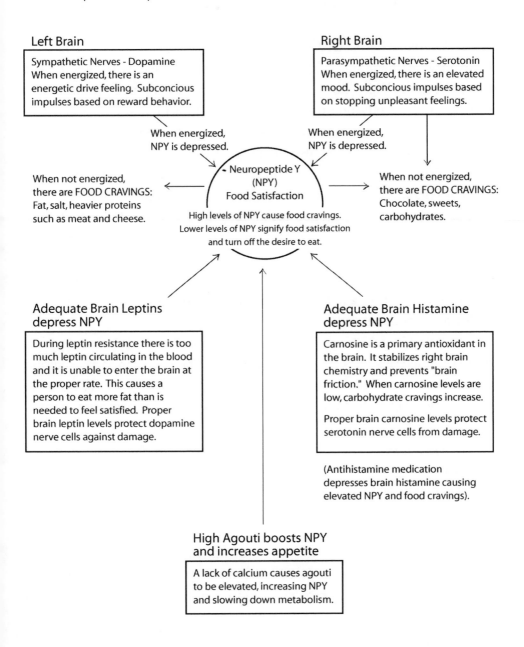

Left Brain

Sympathetic Nerves - Dopamine
When energized, there is an energetic drive feeling. Subconcious impulses based on reward behavior.

Right Brain

Parasympathetic Nerves - Serotonin
When energized, there is an elevated mood. Subconcious impulses based on stopping unpleasant feelings.

When energized, NPY is depressed.

When energized, NPY is depressed.

Neuropeptide Y (NPY)
Food Satisfaction

High levels of NPY cause food cravings.
Lower levels of NPY signify food satisfaction and turn off the desire to eat.

When not energized, there are FOOD CRAVINGS: Fat, salt, heavier proteins such as meat and cheese.

When not energized, there are FOOD CRAVINGS: Chocolate, sweets, carbohydrates.

Adequate Brain Leptins depress NPY

During leptin resistance there is too much leptin circulating in the blood and it is unable to enter the brain at the proper rate. This causes a person to eat more fat than is needed to feel satisfied. Proper brain leptin levels protect dopamine nerve cells against damage.

Adequate Brain Histamine depress NPY

Carnosine is a primary antioxidant in the brain. It stabilizes right brain chemistry and prevents "brain friction." When carnosine levels are low, carbohydrate cravings increase.

Proper brain carnosine levels protect serotonin nerve cells from damage.

(Antihistamine medication depresses brain histamine causing elevated NPY and food cravings).

High Agouti boosts NPY and increases appetite

A lack of calcium causes agouti to be elevated, increasing NPY and slowing down metabolism.

Such a craving may be based on an actual need, as in the case of an active person who is maintaining proper body weight. It may also be based on a faulty "need," as in the case of a leptin-resistant individual who seemingly must eat this type of food to feel satisfied but then it is converted to an expanding waistline. A person with leptin resistance eats more fat to get the satisfied feeling than is needed. This leads to eating too many calories.

SEROTONIN AND NEUROPEPTIDE Y

The parasympathetic side of the nervous system is fueled by the neurotransmitter serotonin. This side of the nervous system has no direct connection to leptin at all.[119] It relies on tryptophan, an amino acid, and higher carbohydrate intake in order to increase the serotonin production.

A higher serotonin level also depresses NPY. This results in a satisfied feeling. While there is no direct connection between leptin and serotonin in terms of regulating each other, they share a common effect on NPY.

The most famous serotonin-raising food is chocolate. Individuals who crave carbohydrates generally try to improve their mood, especially to create a relaxed feeling.[120]

On a subconscious basis, the right brain tries to avoid pain. Therefore, as serotonin levels drop, a person craves carbohydrates in an effort to turn off unpleasant emotional feelings.

Depressed individuals crave more carbohydrates in an effort to raise their low serotonin levels.[121] A far better choice would be to do a moderate aerobic exercise such as walking. Mood fluctuations prior to the menstrual cycle can cause powerful carbohydrate cravings for the same reason, depressed serotonin.[122]

The last thing a person needs when they are in a good eating pattern is too much stress that induces cravings for food to satisfy energy or mood needs. Eating to make one's head feel better may work in the short run, but it is a fast path to frequent eating and overeating, behavior that is sure to induce leptin resistance and weight gain.

If a person knows they will have a demanding day, it is better to eat a large breakfast or lunch as opposed to having their energy crash and get into craving patterns that cause problems. Once leptin resistance sets in, hunger signals are more likely to be incorrect, leading to an inability to lose weight and a tendency to progressively gain weight.

HISTAMINE AND NEUROPEPTIDE Y

There is a new wave of information relating to brain histamine and food cravings. Higher neuronal histamine in the hypothalamus gland of the brain depresses appetite.[123] The action of brain histamine is synergistic with the action of leptin to depress appetite in the hypothalamus gland of the brain.[124] The working hypothesis in this emerging research is that higher histamine depresses NPY.[125] This also explains why antihistamine medication and antipsychotic medication with antihistamine effects cause weight gain.

Ongoing brain histamine research over the last 15 years has demonstrated that a proper amount of brain histamine not only helps control excess appetite, it is essential for the brain to feel properly awake.[126]

The nutritional supplement carnosine is a naturally occurring histidine peptide, highly concentrated in the brain, muscles, and heart. New research shows that carnosine is a primary antioxidant in the brain.[127,128] It offers considerable protection from changes in brain structure that lead to dementia,[129] and it is being considered a novel way to stop changes in the brain that lead to Alzheimer's disease.[130]

Carnosine is a major part of the foundation of the relaxed reserves in the brain.[131] When carnosine levels are proper, the brain can tolerate stress and stimulation. When carnosine levels are lacking, stress induces damage to brain cells and leaves the nerves in an excess adrenaline state that contributes to high blood pressure due to a lack of ability to tolerate stress.

In a groundbreaking study, carnosine stopped the effects of excess adrenaline on the kidneys leading researchers to conclude that carnosine may offset the obesity-associated hypertensive effect of leptin.[132]

Carnosine levels in the brain are directly associated with protecting the brain from damage. Carnosine also helps appetite control, generates a relaxed and awake feeling, and has an ability to reduce adrenaline and leptin resistance.

LOW CALCIUM CAUSES FOOD CRAVINGS

The issue of calcium and weight loss is another emerging finding related to genes and fat cells. Calcium has a direct influence on a brain signal called agouti. Agouti is a best friend of NPY, acting to stimulate food intake while slowing down metabolism.[133] In fact, it is known that this combination of high NPY and agouti block thyroid function, even though common thyroid lab tests appear normal.[134]

Agouti is one of many brain signals involved with promoting appetite. In our genetic evolution it was common to not have enough food. Thus, as we evolved we developed numerous signals to help the ingestion of food and very few to turn off appetite. This may have been handy many years ago, but it is extra genetic baggage that we do not have a great deal of use for now.

Agouti is a gene signal that amplifies the production of leptin from fat cells, and it blocks the ability of the hypothalamus gland to sense leptin in the brain, thus helping to promote the leptin resistance problem.[135] The net result of this problem is to increase fat storage and inhibit fat breakdown.[136] The agouti gene is regulated by calcium intake.[137] Extra calcium intake can cool off this agouti gene and thereby remove a stressor that enhances the production of excessive leptin and reinforces higher levels of NPY causing food cravings.

Furthermore, too much agouti causes a person to gain weight eating the same amount of food they could previously eat, because it slows down metabolism.[138] A higher level of calcium intake improves thyroid function and metabolism by lowering agouti.

Higher calcium levels also help to settle down excess production of adrenaline. It does this by relaxing the smooth muscles of the circulatory system, thereby helping to bring down high blood pressure. The calcium imbalance that contributes to high blood pressure is the same type of calcium imbalance that leads to obesity.[139] This imbalance is made worse with excess salt consumption and a lack of water.

To help weight loss, calcium is only going to work during times when a person is not overeating. If there are excess calories being consumed, the body is simply forced to store them as fat. The combination of appropriate dietary restriction and increased calcium intake has the best weight-loss effects.[140]

SUNSHINE REDUCES CRAVINGS

Americans are constantly being told to stay out of the sun. This results in a reduction of vitamin D, a fat-soluble nutrient. A recent scientific study shows that vitamin D is a powerful inhibitor of leptin secretion from white adipose tissue.[141] When one does not get enough sun, there is a higher risk of leptin excess leading to leptin resistance.

This takes its toll every winter in the northern states, where shorter and colder days mean less sun exposure. This does not help the tendency to over-eat, especially at the holidays, locking in a leptin-resistant pattern the rest of the winter.

Additionally, vitamin D is an important cofactor in calcium absorption. Thus, not only is the lack of vitamin D a specific problem that improperly increases leptin, it also decreases calcium uptake which predisposes a person to a higher than normal level of agouti. This in turn causes higher levels of neuropeptide Y and food cravings.

EATING TOO MUCH BECAUSE YOU ARE NOT EATING ENOUGH?

All of this information tells us that feeling satisfied from food is a complex issue. If we have strict rules that prevent eating fat or carbohydrates, we could easily get into a situation of elevated neuropeptide Y that does not shut off.

For example, a person attempting to eat a high-fat and high-protein diet who needs to raise serotonin will end up overeating fat because they cannot tell when they are full. Such diets are touted as a way to help prevent insulin resistance, as insulin is secreted primarily based on the amount of carbohydrates in a meal. However, when fat is eaten, it stimulates the intestinal tract to release a compound called gastric inhibitory peptide that causes insulin to rise higher.[142]

While not enough gastric inhibitory peptide can be a problem in making insulin, it is found that excess stimulation of gastric inhibitory peptide due to high-fat consumption can induce insulin resistance![143] This means that high-fat diets that are not supposed to cause insulin resistance are just as capable of inducing the same problem through a different mechanism.

Conversely, a person on a low-fat diet can easily eat too many carbohydrates because the dopamine-reward system is not satisfied, and the person does not feel like they have any sustainable energy or ability to focus.

In both cases, the individuals become overweight or stay overweight because they are eating too much, even though they think they are avoiding the "evils" of saturated fat or too many carbohydrates. If they had learned to eat an appropriate amount of saturated fat or carbohydrates, their cravings would turn off, their metabolism would run more efficiently, and they would not overeat in an effort to feel satisfied by eating extra food that is not satisfying.

A simplistic guideline about how much fat or carbohydrates a person should eat so they do not crave food is not possible because this is different for every person. Issues such as personality type, physical demands, emotional demands, sleep status, and many other topics factor into what is correct for any individual. However, if a person does not learn this information and how it applies to them, they can easily overeat because they are trying not to eat a particular type of food.

DO YOU HAVE A MISGUIDED SWEET TOOTH?

Interestingly, it has been proven that leptin influences the taste system. Properly functioning leptin enables a person to not crave sweets. There are leptin receptors on taste buds. When leptin communicates to taste buds, then the craving for sweet tastes is reduced.[144] If a person has leptin resistance, then the taste buds do not get the message, and over consumption of carbohydrates and sweets is likely.

A person without eating problems can induce them by trying to follow dietary advice that makes them feel unsatisfied. A few pieces of cheese can make the leptin-dopamine system feel good, preventing excess carbohydrate consumption. A few bites of chocolate can make the serotonin-satiety center feel good, preventing continued eating of other food.

Generally for more serious problems, an entire program needs to be implemented. This includes exercise, stress management, lifestyle modification, and appropriate use of nutritional supplementation. This heads towards the goal of being able to eat in a normal rhythm and pattern and to be satisfied on a moderate amount of food.

Even healthy people should be wary of a diet that is too low in fat or too low in carbohydrates as these diets can induce overeating by failing to produce proper feelings of being satisfied following a meal.

SUMMARY

The bottom line of any meal is that a person must feel satisfied or they keep eating. Feeling satisfied is a more complex event than one may imagine. It is especially hard to feel satisfied when there is a major problem with leptin resistance.

As one follows our *Five Rules*, leptin resistance decreases, and it is easier to feel satisfied on a moderate amount of food, especially less sweet food. Also, as physical fitness improves, food cravings decrease. Therefore, if a person can use their willpower for a few days and follow our eating guidelines, they begin to get leptin resistance under control, and it is easier to not crave meals that are high in carbohydrate and fat.

Stress is the wildcard variable that magnifies any weakness in a person's brain chemistry. If the weakness is on the dopamine side, cravings are for calorie-laden and salty foods. The subconscious goal is to have an energetic feeling of metabolic drive. If the weakness is on the serotonin side, cravings are for carbohydrates. The subconscious goal is to have a relaxed state of feeling or more pleasant mood.

When overall natural balance in a person's life is not good, then there is much less tolerance for stress. A person is likely to experience food cravings based on brain chemistry imbalance triggering stress eating, in turn causing a disruption in fuel utilization. This leads to leptin resistance, insulin resistance, and adrenaline resistance, a path of increased fatigue and bad moods no matter what is eaten.

22

Ghrelin, the Stomach's Cry for Food

*T*he gastrointestinal tract (GI tract) produces a variety of hormonal signals that communicate to the hypothalamus gland in the brain and affect hunger. These signals are part of normal appetite. When the body is out of balance, these signals cause inappropriate food cravings.

We have already described that the hypothalamus gland of the brain must be able to correctly perceive the true amount of leptin in order to regulate metabolism correctly. If there is leptin resistance, the hypothalamus gland does not sense the correct amount of leptin, and appetite stays higher than normal even though a person may be quite overweight.

Scientists have shown there are many diverse metabolic signals coming to bear on the hypothalamus gland, most of them seeking to stimulate appetite for one reason or another. It is believed that leptin plays the role of acting as a "brain toner" to enable the brain to properly respond and regulate these diverse signals.[145]

In addition to the hunger signals discussed in the previous chapter, many other appetite-related signals come from the GI tract itself. In this chapter, we will focus on a primary hunger signal coming from the stomach called ghrelin.

WHAT IS GHRELIN?
Ghrelin is a hormone produced in the stomach that says it is time to eat. The ghrelin hormone signal has a short-term effect lasting up to an hour. If a person does not eat when the hormone signal presents itself, then it goes away and appetite disappears. If there is too much ghrelin, then a person will overeat.

NPY and agouti stimulate the production of ghrelin, and ghrelin tells the pituitary gland how to influence metabolism.[146] This is rather amazing information. It means that the stomach is a major player in human behavior and metabolic rate, and that the brain must coordinate the stomach's input in order to have a harmonious situation.

This science reinforces the fact that solving stress eating is minimally a psychological issue and primarily an issue of achieving natural balance so that subconscious signals get along with each other. People can endlessly look for the reasons for overeating and beat themselves up for having such feeble willpower, when in fact this path of looking for solutions is likely to have minimal value.

Any person who chooses to view weight and obesity issues from a psychological perspective may find this hard to believe, but eating issues are primarily issues of hormone imbalance. Solutions that work are ones that help establish natural balance. To this end, managing stress more effectively is helpful, but root causes are programmed into genetic survival information relating to energy needs and controlled by subconscious signals that involve the brain and the entire digestive tract. Unless these issues are solved and natural balance is returned to these systems, craving patterns and eating problems will simply persist.

GHRELIN, INSULIN, AND LEPTIN

Ghrelin levels rise when the blood levels of leptin and glucose fall. High fat diets that cause a rise in leptin, depress ghrelin levels. Conversely, diets high in carbohydrates increase the production of ghrelin.[147] Ghrelin directly communicates to the brain to increase the production of NPY, the brain's main hunger signal.

In normal function, once the ghrelin signal is released, it will turn off for one of two reasons:

1) No food is eaten. The hormone can last up to an hour; after this time it goes away.
2) Food is eaten. The food itself, not insulin, turns off the production of ghrelin.[148]

Very importantly, a normal amount of ghrelin is essential for gastric motility, the forward movement of food through the digestive system, and the correct release of stomach acid to digest protein.[149] A proper amount of ghrelin is essential for the emptying of food from the stomach into the small intestine.[150]

In addition to primary ghrelin production in the stomach, it is also produced in the small intestine,[151] pancreas,[152] and thyroid.[153]

In a normal-weight individual, ghrelin rises before meals to signal hunger. Between meals, in healthy metabolic individuals, ghrelin and leptin rise together in the bloodstream throughout the day. They create a normal "tone," playing off each other to help maintain normal "appetite drive."[154]

Inside the brain, leptin and ghrelin act as metabolic opposites. Ghrelin helps NPY go up, thus stimulating the brain's desire to eat. Leptin makes NPY go down, thus allowing the brain to feel there is no longer any need to eat.[155]

GHRELIN IN OVERWEIGHT INDIVIDUALS

The difference between ghrelin levels in normal-weight individuals compared to overweight individuals is quite interesting. In overweight individuals, the usual amount of ghrelin before eating is lower than normal.[156]

In normal-weight individuals, ghrelin levels drop when food is ingested. In overweight individuals, ghrelin levels stay elevated after food is eaten, leading to excess consumption of food.[157] Overweight individuals have a blunted response to ghrelin working as it should.

Once again, it is an issue of efficiency. Ghrelin loses its normal rhythmic function in overweight individuals; it is an out-of-balance stomach hormone that adversely affects eating and behavior! Why does it do this? Leptin is too high. As soon as high leptin levels come down, ghrelin goes back into natural balance and normal appetite patterns of ghrelin reappear.[158]

The issue of leptin resistance causes the higher than normal blood levels of leptin, that in turn cause ghrelin to be released for an abnormally extended period of time during the meal, stimulating excess eating in order to feel full. This especially causes excess eating of carbohydrates. The fundamentals to lower leptin and normalize ghrelin are following our *Five Rules*.

A recent animal study shows that taking melatonin can decrease ghrelin levels by enhancing normal rhythmic function of leptin.[159]   Melatonin levels drop in individuals as they age and in the winter when days are shorter and there is less sunlight. Also, leptin levels generally rise as an individual ages. Now we know that this combination sets the stage for improper ghrelin timing, a key hormonal signal that fuels the subconscious overeating drive.

SUMMARY

Eating some carbohydrates is essential for normal ghrelin activity and production. The importance of this is further explained in Chapter 31 on growth hormone. At this time it is important to understand that carbohydrate cravings and eating excess carbohydrates are problems associated with ghrelin being released at the wrong time in relation to eating.

In overweight people there is not enough ghrelin before the meal and too much ghrelin after the individual starts eating, causing an improper signal to keep eating. This is a major reason why overweight people overeat; once they get started, they cannot stop until they have eaten too much food for their true energy need.

Furthermore, natural ghrelin release is essential for normal gastrointestinal flow and digestion. Thus, ghrelin issues cause the GI tract to become sluggish, resulting in indigestion and heartburn. As a person solves this issue by bringing leptin down, then ghrelin timing normalizes, excess carbohydrate cravings stop, and digestion improves.

23

Dangerous Weight Loss

*I*n 1997, it became obvious that the widely used weight-loss drug, fenfluramine, caused cardiovascular toxicity and heart-valve damage. The lesson to be learned from this catastrophe is that even though a drug can suppress appetite by manipulating the brain signals that control hunger, the consequence to the rest of the body can be quite damaging. The drug disrupted natural balance. Yes, it forced down the brain's level of NPY, but it did so at considerable expense.

Even though the drug was removed from the market due to its heart issues, a closer look at it shows that it caused four times the amount of serious episodes of major depression compared to overweight individuals not taking the medication.[160,161] This is due to the drug disrupting natural balance in the brain.

This book is about restoring natural balance everywhere in the body so that metabolism works correctly. This skill is the hallmark of the competent Health Asset Manager.™ If this lesson is not learned now, the unwitting public will be subjected to the next wave of weight-loss drugs, all attempting to regulate leptin and NPY in some way and throwing the body out of balance.

RATIONALIZING THE MEDICAL ROUTE

Health-care costs relating to obesity are skyrocketing. Disease in our society as a result of obesity is at epidemic levels. Society turns to the medical profession for a quick-fix answer.

Currently, the two medications approved for long-term weight loss are rather tame by comparison to fenfluramine and to what is waiting in the wings.

Orlistat is a fat-absorption reducing medication. The primary side effect is disruption of the GI tract. The GI tract must run smoothly and without symptoms in order for natural balance to be obtained; thus, the drug works against a primary goal of long-term weight management.

Three years of data regarding widespread Orlistat use has shown that the drug has only a slight ability to assist weight loss.[162] It has failed to demonstrate that it can reduce diabetes or heart disease. All a person has to do is get in some reasonable condition of natural balance and they will eat less fat. This result can be obtained without upsetting the GI tract and further disrupting natural balance.

The other current weight-loss drug is called sibutramine, a serotonin and norepinephrine transporter blocker. It works by interfering with the normal flow of neurotransmitters in the brain. It hopes to prop them up and have the side effect of depressing NPY. It does not act on NPY or any of the core signals or molecules in the subconscious brain that are under current intense research for the next weight-loss "miracle."

Whenever brain chemistry is manipulated, there are side effects. Medications that target appetite suppression by modulating NPY are likely to have adverse stimulant side effects. This means that adrenaline is extra hyped up and the heart bears the burden, as in an anxious prone nervous system.[163]

The most common reported side effects of sibutramine are dry mouth, constipation, insomnia, and an increase in heart rate and blood pressure that persist for as long as treatment is continued.[164] Those promoting these drugs rationalize that these disruptions of natural balance are not as bad as being overweight.

That view is likely to change as the cardiovascular distress picture becomes clearer with ongoing use. In November 2002, researchers from Germany quietly plead with the scientific community to more fully understand the adverse consequences of this medication to the cardiovascular system: "Our findings strongly suggest that current concepts regarding the action of sibutramine on the sympathetic nervous system should be reconsidered."[165]

Medications that affect the brain show side effects in areas other than cardiovascular risk. Researchers at Vanderbilt University proved that diet pill use before pregnancy or during pregnancy significantly increased the risk of leukemia in their children.[166] The risk was even greater if both parents took such stimulants.

The leukemia risk also included the use of antihistamines and allergy medication during pregnancy. This finding is not surprising either, as we pointed out the importance of brain histamine in maintaining natural balance in the nervous system in Chapter 21. Although this major side effect was recently discovered, rest assured that it will not be discussed with patients before putting them on stimulant diet pills. How long will it take health authorities to warn pregnant mothers or women who may become pregnant of increased risk for leukemia in their offspring if they take antihistamines or allergy medication while pregnant? Meanwhile, the quick-fix oriented public is continuing to pop sibutramine pills.

BROWN ADIPOSE TISSUE - A COMMON TARGET OF THE QUICK-FIX WEIGHT LOSS MENTALITY

Brown adipose tissue is different than white adipose tissue. Prior to the discovery of leptin in 1994, brown adipose tissue was the only one considered to have a major metabolic role. It is brown in color because it has a heavy blood supply and many nerves going to it. Inside brown adipose tissue fat cells, there are numerous and very large mitochondria, or cellular furnaces, for metabolizing fat.

These cells are different than all other metabolizing cells in the human body. Normally when cells burn calories, they create 65 percent energy and 35 percent heat. The brown adipose tissue cells make 100 percent heat. In other words, they completely burn and dispose of calories. They help keep the body warm; they are involved in the shiver response to cold as a fast way of heating up the body.

In theory, this is a great way to lose weight; turn up the stimulation of brown adipose tissue and simply dispose of extra calories by turning them into heat. Many weight-loss regimes and products have been targeted at stimulating brown adipose tissue into action. These plans use sympathetic nerve stimulants such as ephedra and caffeine. Beware of such programs!

Results over time will not be there as the body will slow down even further to compensate for the excess artificial stimulation. Eventually the fat cells become resistant to such stimulation, but the heart and kidneys do not. Over the long term, such stimulation efforts are at the expense of cardiovascular[167] and kidney health, and they can become quite dangerous. They also have the long-term result of making leptin resistance worse.

The real solution to weight loss is not in manipulating and artificially stimulating brown adipose tissue. The solution is in fixing the hormonal signals and other signals coming out of white adipose tissue. This is an entirely new view on the subject of weight management.

GASTRIC BYPASS INSANITY

A basic rule of natural balance is to keep all body parts whenever possible. If a body part is altered, then natural balance will be forever altered.

Gastric bypass surgery was once reserved for the morbidly obese. It is being promoted as a glamorous way to lose weight with various celebrities on covers of magazines and in the media. The frenzy is backed by a medical profession that is too eager to make money removing body parts. In fact, not only do they want part of the stomach, they want to take the gallbladder for "preventive purposes."[168]

Gastric bypass surgery is complicated and requires considerable skill. The most alarming adverse side effect is an inappropriate higher level of death, due mainly to blood clots in the lungs that occur even when precautions are taken prior to surgery to prevent them.[169]

If a person makes it past this initial risk factor, there is a 9.5 percent chance of developing a serious complication that requires more surgery.[170] These are not the annoying GI tract disturbances that are also common, they are major ones.

Nevertheless, a certain number of individuals are willing to take these risks in an effort to be thinner and reduce other types of risks.

Unfortunately, this is a situation where the long-term risks of doing the surgery are just as bad as the health risks of being overweight, they are just different.

It is coming to light that individuals with gastric bypass surgery need to contend with the issue that they are likely to develop serious metabolic bone disease as they grow older. This is a well-documented side effect of this surgery.[171] In the past, it was thought that this side effect was due to malabsorption of food or eating too little or both.

New science shows a different cause; the surgery is ruining metabolism in the body. How is this possible?

The surgery reduces the amount of functional stomach. As stated in the previous chapter, the stomach makes a hormone called ghrelin, a key hormone that stimulates hunger and leads to overeating in overweight individuals.

As it turns out, gastric bypass dramatically lowers the levels of ghrelin because there are fewer stomach cells that can make it. This is permanent. A person might think this is good because they will not be hungry as often.

However, once the surgery is complete there is no normal ghrelin response to food.[172] This is quite different than a normal-weight person's correct and healthy ghrelin function. Gastric bypass surgery permanently destroys normal ghrelin function and rhythm.

This one finding is enough to call a halt to such surgeries. Why? Because ghrelin is the key signal in the body that enables the proper release of growth hormone.[173] Ghrelin is a major discovery in the growth hormone field. Without proper ghrelin function, numerous parameters of aging worsen as the body cannot correctly repair itself. One side effect that is already noticed is the bone-disease issue; a finding that has been confirmed by animal studies showing that low ghrelin suppresses bone mineralization.[174]

SUMMARY

There are no quick fixes for weight loss. Due to the severity of problems in our society, there is considerable research money being poured into finding drugs or surgeries to help individuals lose weight.

Since there will be adverse effects from such drugs and surgeries, the companies making the drugs or the health professionals involved use the age-old marketing ploy that the benefits outweigh the risks. Once the government agrees, then the quick-fix and frustrated dieters jump on board. Years later, the adverse effects accumulate.

The widespread promotion of gastric bypass surgery is a new low. The economic forces behind it promote its "safety," downplaying its serious risks and problems with a marketing campaign appealing to thinner America.

There is only one safe and healthy way to lose weight and maintain quality of health. That is to implement a comprehensive approach to achieving and maintaining natural balance. All quick-fix weight-loss solutions are detrimental to natural balance.

The health risks associated with obesity are serious. Taking proactive steps on a consistent basis is essential. There are no shortcuts. There are healthy solutions.

24

The Foundation of Natural Balance

*O*ur five key dietary rules to mastering leptin form the foundation of a lifestyle and dietary pattern that establish natural balance. There are no shortcuts. These are not rules a person follows for a few months and then discards. These are the core rules for building stable natural rhythms in the human body that help a person efficiently burn calories and make energy.

A person following our *Five Rules* does not feel like they are on a diet. They do not feel deprived. Their significantly improved energy is obvious. It is also obvious when they revert to old ways and get too far off track. The fatigue, cravings, and other health issues are reminders of the wrong way of doing things.

It is incredibly important for individuals to establish for themselves proper dietary habits. Our *Five Rules* offer a blueprint on how to do this. They are not set in concrete. They are functional rules that have scientific basis.

Proper eating patterns and consequent energy production from food set the tone for other rhythms in the body. This enables an individual to have much greater potential to deal with any type of stress or demand and not get worn down.

Our *Five Rules* are the secret to maximizing the energy that can be extracted from food. When this ability declines then food too easily turns to stored fat instead of energy.

Some individuals struggle with this their whole lives. Others have a turning point, such as the start of puberty, going off to college, or having children. These turning points tend to flare up problems that may not have previously been significant. Maybe a person can violate the *Five Rules* and seem to get away with it. This only means that their metabolism is strong enough to tolerate the abuse. Sooner or later, it will catch up.

Individuals entering their forties know that their body just does not respond the way it did when they were younger. Now the *Five Rules* are mandatory. Violating them leads to slow and progressive weight gain and a whole host of other issues associated with aging.

In order to stay on track with the *Five Rules,* a person must understand cravings and what they mean. They must understand how to get back on track if they get off track. Problems with metabolism tend to progress towards obesity.

The *Five Rules* are the foundation of the true path to attain and maintain optimum body weight. Implementing them in one's life requires skill. The reward of doing so is an improved and ongoing quality of health.

PART 3

Solving the Hormone Puzzle

25

Timing, Inflammation, and Aging

*T*iming is everything. Our bodies are either regulated by a harmonic symphony, a heavy metal tune, or somewhere in between. Biological rhythms are the guiding force of human metabolism and natural balance. They are the essence underlying communication in the body. A person either feels in sync or out of balance.

Whenever extra demands are placed upon a person, they could potentially push the individual out of rhythm. A fundamental principle of the human body is that no matter what type of demand is placed on it, it tries to compensate and maintain natural balance.

Hormones are important communication signals in the body that seek to coordinate the body's ability to stay in sync and meet the extra demands or pressures. As a person begins to have problems, the body is thrown out of sync, and timing is off.

Poorly timed communication occurs in hormonal systems. This sets in motion a path of wear and tear. This out-of-rhythm situation generates friction; cellular function no longer clicks along in the proper way. Such friction causes inflammation that is excessive and inappropriate. This is not just an ache or a pain. This is inflammation happening at a cellular level throughout the body.

This cellular friction or inflammation is the primary cause of heart disease, both in terms of the progressive deterioration of the circulatory system over time and as a causative factor in a heart attack.[175,176,177,178] The problems of inflammation and cardiovascular risk are significantly elevated in the insulin-resistant and leptin-resistant condition.[179] The problems of inflammation extend to many aspects of disease risk, a fact that is being announced loud and clear to the American public.[180]

Slowing the aging process is related to having a good rhythmic base of natural balance and an ability to bounce back and manage stress so as to maintain the in-sync feeling.

KEEPING TIME AND ESTABLISHING ENERGY

The central biological clock that governs rhythms is called the suprachiasmatic nucleus (SCN), found in the hypothalamus gland of the brain. It is the primary timekeeper for all of the rhythms in the human body, much like the conductor in an orchestra. It seeks to synchronize the body through various internal functions, such as hormonal patterns and body heat. It adapts regulation to external cues, such as light. It may change the musical composition at a moment's notice based on some type of stress or demand. Each orchestra member, those being a body part or a cell, must also keep time and play on cue.

The hypothalamus gland sends out the rhythmic signal that sets the 24-hour leptin pattern, thus permitting energy to be used by other hormonal systems and body organs. When leptin works correctly, the 24-hour rhythm follows, as in an orchestra member following the conductor. There is a degree of tiredness or fatigue that is not proper when leptin and the hypothalamus are out of sync. Such a lack of energy is frequently the first symptom of a problem.

The conductor must figure out what musical composition can be played based on the energy required to perform the composition. In order to figure this out, the conductor must perceive the level of leptin signifying the amount of fuel on hand. Once determined, the conductor will set the pace and energy expenditure of the orchestra as a whole. Leptin has a powerful influence on metabolic rate and the feeling of good energy at the most fundamental level.

AGING AFFECTS RHYTHMS

As a person ages, the biological clock system begins to lose its ability to keep time, resulting in a direct deterioration in the quality of health. There are several changes that occur. All changes result in a lowered quality of communication taking place in the body with a concurrent increase in inflammation due to the friction caused by the inefficiency.

One change is that the rhythms lose their ability to hit a peak, such as the singer who can no longer hit the high notes. This causes the rhythm to "flatten out" resulting in the inability to get the job done with the same quality. The singer can still sing; it just does not sound as good as before.

Another change is overall timing. The conductor of the orchestra sends signals prematurely, causing instruments to be played at the wrong time. It does not sound good, and it does not feel in sync. The general trend of aging is that the timing moves forward in the wrong direction. This is evident in wake/sleep patterns wherein a person goes to bed earlier and wakes up earlier, a sign that the body is losing proper timing.

Timing problems are combined with the problem stated above wherein the "peak" sleep rhythms do not occur properly, meaning a person does not get into a deep sleep correctly. Therefore, sleep occurs at the wrong time, and it is a poor-quality sleep. This interferes with the ability to repair and maintain the health and well being of the body.

These issues of timing and quality apply to all hormonal systems and body rhythms, not just sleep patterns.

Another problem with rhythms is that the members of the orchestra do not follow the conductor well. The conductor may be furiously signaling a whole section of the orchestra to play, like the liver section or the immune section, and they simply do not respond well. They have become resistant to their directions. The problem is not all in the central clock in the brain; it also occurs in areas of the body that receive the messages.

This is complicated by the fact that various body organs do not communicate well with each other. There is a breakdown in messages occurring between the pancreas and liver. This makes the job of conducting even more frustrating, as group members are not working together.

A TRIAD OF PROBLEMS

These breakdowns in communication are the essence of leptin resistance, insulin resistance, and adrenaline resistance. Such miscommunication causes internal friction and wear and tear, leading to inflammation and accelerated aging.

Leptin resistance, insulin resistance, and adrenaline resistance are the key triad of problems that lock in hormone imbalance. The "glue" that keeps them locked in is the pro-inflammatory signals, TNFa (tumor necrosis factor alpha) and IL-6 (interleukin 6). These are the primary immune signals that no longer work properly when a person is in a wear and tear trend. They become the primary source for generating the inflammation that leads to poor health and disease.

Insulin stimulates white adipose tissue to make TNFa.[181] As higher levels of insulin occur during insulin resistance, higher levels of pro-inflammatory TNFa tend to match the exaggerated insulin level.[182] TNFa can directly induce insulin resistance.[183]

TNFa also sends disturbing e-mails to the adrenaline receptors inside fat cells, telling them not to work, thus inducing the white adipose tissue resistance to adrenaline.[184] TNFa sends e-mails to its pro-inflammatory friend, IL-6, telling it to get into high gear.[185] IL-6 gets the liver all worked up and then C reactive protein levels increase, a key measure of cardiovascular risk.[186]

IL-6 also tells the digestive system not to move,[187] thus causing heartburn and indigestion. This is why many individuals in a wear and tear trend have heartburn, reflux problems, and/or sluggish bowels.

Furthermore, platelets in the blood, the cells that stick together in order to form a clot, have leptin receptors on them. The effect of high leptin on platelets is to induce them to stick together too much. This dramatically increases the risk for excessive clot formation,[188] and thus an occlusion in the circulation that can cause a heart attack or stroke.

A common theme in Part 3 of the book is showing how excess inflammation becomes the cause of a variety of health problems. We explain how this issue relates to every major hormone and to numerous diseases. Once a person understands this information, it is no longer a mystery why there is disease; it is only an issue of how to solve the problem.

BASIC RHYTHM MANAGEMENT IS PART OF THE SOLUTION

By keeping our bodies in better biological rhythm, we have more tolerance for stress. Having some level of consistency with our daily behavior and routines can help. This is a form of anti-aging exercise for body rhythms. Scientists have proven that regular behavioral rhythms are conducive to good health and well being.[189] Establishing routine eating times, sleep times, exercise times, and other life-related timing under our control can have a powerful influence on health.

Many of the hormones work in harmony or disharmony with one another. It is not possible to isolate one from the others; they must all be considered members of the orchestra. They either sound good and make beautiful music or they do not.

In the context of metabolism and food, eating a meal causes insulin to rise. This is the short-term response to the food. There is also an underlying health issue in the insulin system, one that is part of the overall health trend of the body. This is a longer-term pattern, one that reflects the function of insulin in relation to other hormones and body organs on a week-in and week-out basis, independent of a single meal.[190]

Insulin resistance is an issue of this long-term pattern, as it is a series of ongoing abuse that leads to the problem. This is involved with progressive leptin resistance and adrenaline resistance.

Hormones are powerful controlling signals in the body. When they work in harmony, they play like a well-rehearsed orchestra. Everything goes according to plan; timing is perfect; harmony and natural balance are the result.

SUMMARY

Good eating, exercising, and sleeping patterns form the basis for consistency that sets healthy biological rhythms. These are steps we can take to directly affect how our own hormones work towards the goal of keeping everything in natural balance.

The tendency of the aging process is losing quality and timing in hormonal communication systems. Once this happens, an inflammatory path of wear and tear sets in. If it is not resolved, this path heads for increased risk of disease and accelerated aging.

Leptin is the most powerful hormone in the human body. When it works properly, it smoothly interacts with other hormones. When there are health issues, there is friction and disharmony between leptin and other hormones. Timing is off. Rhythms are erratic. Resistance to hearing the hormonal phone call is common. An individual simply feels out of sync.

In the first two sections of this book, we have focused on the hormones leptin, insulin, glucagon, and adrenaline. We have discussed dietary steps an individual can take to reduce stress and friction in hormonal systems.

In this third section of the book, we explain how leptin relates to other hormones including cortisol, growth hormone, thyroid hormones, and sex hormones.

Once there is a comprehensive picture of how hormones work in relationship to each person on an individual basis, then one can take steps to effectively manage them so that they can work together in sync.

26

Stress and a Fat Stomach

*H*ow much stress can a person handle on a day-to-day basis before it takes its toll on health? Every person has a different ability to tolerate, adapt to, and manage stress. At the point stress throws the body out of rhythm, it sets the stage for problems with metabolism, food, weight gain, and poor health.

On an emotional level, such stress feels too out of control and uncomfortable. On a physical level, there is wear and tear. The first sign of this wear and tear is fatigue that is not normal. The person no longer pops out of bed in the morning. It is harder to get going or keep going. There is less tolerance for stress because the brain does not have the same energy to deal with issues. As time goes along, one of the undeniable physical issues accompanying this inflammatory wear and tear is weight gain around the middle.

Stress complicates the whole picture of fuel utilization, biological rhythms, and hormones. Stress implies that there is an increased pressure or burden, and therefore, an increased need for fuel. Stress can come from external pressures. These include emotional and physical demands as well as not sleeping enough or poor quality sleep. It also comes from internal demands such as the energy needed to run a menstrual cycle or to fight an infection. Many times there is a combination of external and internal stressors.

Many individuals are already out of sync from wear and tear in their lives. What happens when they get under additional stress? The already inefficient and inflamed body may get overworked and overloaded. If it is unable to meet the demands of the extra burden, a major health turning point occurs.

Sometimes this happens as progressive wear and tear catches up with a person over the years. Other times, there is a major event or series of events that trigger the stress overload. Once this happens, it is the same as a major thunderstorm that knocks out power and downs power lines. This magnifies the degree of communication problems in the body, as the structural integrity of the nervous system and hormonal systems are not functionally up to par.

ADAPTING TO STRESS

If life never had any variables and clicked along at a predictable and monotonous pace, there would be no such thing as stress. Life would also be quite boring. To the contrary, a great deal of human evolution involved adapting to or overcoming significant threats to survival.

The key hormone that orchestrates the ability to respond to stress is cortisol, produced by the adrenal cortex. In terms of general nonstressed function, cortisol is highest in the morning acting as a cellular activator to "turn on the light switches" in all cells to wake up and get going for the day.

Morning fatigue or taking a long time to feel energized are common signs that cortisol is in a poor condition. For example, we know that leptin levels must be low for proper cortisol release in the morning. Thus, if a leptin-resistant person overeats at night, their leptin level stays higher during sleep. It will also be too high in the morning, thus blunting the proper time for the release of cortisol.[191] This makes a person feel tired and out of balance in the morning.

In fact, once leptin resistance takes hold, the problem gets worse because the normal 24-hour rhythm pattern of leptin is chronically blunted, leading to a 4-8 hour delay in proper leptin timing and insulin function. This leptin problem forces normal daily cortisol release to happen at the improper time, thus resulting in fatigue and throwing the entire body out of natural rhythm.[192] This is why a person with leptin resistance has some abnormal level of fatigue, tiredness, or stress intolerance.

Cortisol is secreted in higher amounts under stress. This helps the liver get into action to synthesize blood glucose at a higher rate to meet the need. It is part of the adaptive system of the human body. Think of it as a rubber band stretching. After the stress is over, the rubber band returns to its normal position. This indicates good stress tolerance.

Under the wear and tear of stress, the rubber band does not bounce back properly. A person feels this in an energy level that has increasing periods of fatigue. There is a feeling of physical wear and tear. Moods are noticeably affected; there is a short temper and ongoing negative feelings such as agitation, sadness, apathy, or even depression. This type of wear and tear causes the body to lose biological rhythms associated with stress tolerance and fuel regulation. A common consequence of this problem is gaining fat around the middle.

LEPTIN AND THE STRESS RESPONSE

We have mentioned that leptin is essential for survival. One key to its operation is managing the body during periods of low food supply and helping the body replenish itself once the period of food deprivation is over.

Leptin also is involved with the short-term energy needs relating to stress. However, leptin is an integral part of the stress response and is released on purpose when inflammation occurs.[193] The body must initiate a change of normal operation in order to deal with the stressful irritant. Leptin is a key part of this healthy reaction.

Leptin initiates a wide variety of changes:

1) Leptin enables blood vessels to enter tissue that does not normally contain them, thus enabling a temporary communication and transport system to an area of the body that has been irritated or injured.

2) Leptin stimulates the production of red blood cells. This is essential if there is a wound that causes blood loss.

3) Leptin stimulates the production of white blood cells so that an immune response can be effectively mounted against any pathogens that have entered.

4) Leptin stimulates macrophages, immune cells that help clean up debris. Leptin also turns up the signals in macrophages, including highly pro-inflammatory signals such as TNFa and IL-6, to help orchestrate the inflammatory response to stress. This is the normal and appropriate use of these inflammatory signals to help deal with an acute challenge.

The net result of this activity is proper wound healing or healing stressful trauma in the body wherever it may be. This is essential for survival. It is part of the body's perfect defense system. Several scientific papers explain the role of leptin in this capacity.[194,195]

Why would the body utilize a hormone secreted by fat cells to help regulate the inflammatory response to stress? So that it may enable the body to have enough energy to deal with stress without having to digest food.

Digesting food requires a tremendous amount of energy. If energy is needed for an emergency, then eating food forces energy to be used for the purpose of digestion. This is why a person loses their appetite when they get sick. It is why animals do not eat when they are stressed. It is why some humans lose their appetite when they are stressed. Those who eat in response to stress have serious leptin resistance.

There must be a supply of energy to deal with stress. The body already has a hormonal signal that it uses to manage the longer-term issue of the available fuel supply; it is called leptin. Therefore, when there is plenty of fat in storage, leptin levels are higher and signal the brain not to eat anymore. This is what leptin does unless a person has leptin resistance.

When stress causes an inflammatory emergency, the rise in leptin tells the body not to eat. This is essential for a proper immune response to the emergency.[196] If the stress is dealt with in a shorter period of time, that is great. If not, the body uses the energy in fat cells to fuel the stress response until the problem is brought under control.[197]

If a person is at a normal body weight and in good natural rhythm, then leptin works as designed. Leptin will be a friend in the process of having a perfectly working stress response.

LEPTIN RESISTANCE AND INFLAMMATION

Leptin resistance is the situation of having too much leptin already in the blood. It is the most common issue in any person who is overweight. There are two situations where leptin is higher. One is a natural response to stressful inflammation and the other is leptin resistance. Are they the same? No.

Leptin levels rise during stressful inflammation, but there is a 50-50 ratio of free leptin to bound leptin. Half the leptin is biologically active. In leptin resistance, only 10 percent of the leptin is biologically active.[198]

It has recently been proposed that obesity is an inflammatory condition. Overweight children and adults have elevated levels of C reactive protein, IL-

6, and TNFa, all markers of inflammation.[199] Normally, these signals rise when the body mounts a stress response for a given purpose.

In overweight individuals, these markers are stuck at higher levels due to the generation of these immune signals on a chronic basis from the extra pounds of fat. Remember, 30 percent of cells in white adipose tissue are immune cells. Overweight individuals have more than a normal amount of TNFa because of the amount of fat they have on hand.[200] The rise in TNFa is the actual cause of signals that generate excess inflammation for the rest of the body.[201]

Scientists are just beginning to comprehend the dramatic and far-reaching nature of this information. For example, the inflammation generated by TNFa is understood to be a cause of diabetic retinopathy, which the scientific report calls a "newly recognized inflammatory disease."[202]

CORTISOL AND LEPTIN

Cortisol and leptin generally communicate in a reciprocal manner, as one rises the other tends to fall. In nonstressed situations, both cortisol and leptin follow a 24-hour rhythm. The peak level of leptin is between midnight and 2 a.m.

Leptin is mostly an anabolic hormone; correct and properly communicating leptin levels during sleep are essential for repair of the human body. The peak cortisol level is 6 a.m.; it is the primary get-up and go hormone. In a healthy individual, the two hormones have a "communication tone" between each other that is fundamental to natural balance, enabling an individual to respond to stress, deal with stress, and recover from stress.

We know that cortisol is not in control of leptin. Mice that have had their adrenal glands removed still have a normal 24-hour leptin pattern. However, cortisol can influence leptin under stress. Cortisol acts to turn up the volume of leptin activity in fat cells.[203] This is a genetic response wherein the body needs more energy to deal with stress and needs the help of leptin to orchestrate the healing response to stress, including the appropriate inflammatory changes that need to take place so that healing can occur.

When this normal reaction to stress becomes unbalanced and natural rhythm is lost, then the same hormones that are needed to combat stress begin to miscommunicate. Cortisol still stimulates leptin production, but the condition of leptin resistance develops. For example, in Cushing's syndrome and other metabolic conditions like Cushing's, there is a chronic overproduction of cortisol. Such patients have markedly elevated levels of leptin, yet the leptin activity inside of fat cells is blunted.[204]

The combination of excess cortisol from stress and leptin resistance blunts the metabolic activity of abdominal fat cells. [205] This is a serious issue, not just unpleasant fat. Abdominal obesity is a primary indicator that there are disruptions between cortisol, leptin, and neuropeptide Y. Remember that elevated NPY causes a person to be hungry all the time. Scientists have proven that these hormone imbalances are the actual cause of diseases and mortality associated with the extra abdominal fat.[206]

THE TRUE CAUSE OF STRESS EATING

Yes, a person can seek to manage psychological factors that relate to stress. Anything a person can do as a life strategy to feel more in control will help them release less cortisol in response to their personal perception of stress.

However, stress eating is not a psychological issue; it is an issue of disrupted natural balance. It is a key sign that the body is out of rhythm and unable to properly tolerate the perceived demands. It does not matter if the stress is a current issue or a past trauma.

Stress induces overeating only when stress is followed by excessive cortisol release. When this issue is ongoing, there is excess cortisol, leptin resistance, and weight gain around the middle.[207] As mentioned above, this is combined with elevated NPY. Thus, the person has a constant hunger signal locked in place.

ELIMINATE ABDOMINAL FAT TO STOP DISEASE

Scientists have proven in animals that when this extra abdominal fat is removed, insulin resistance, diabetes risk, and the diseases related to these hormone imbalances are significantly reduced or eliminated.[208] How to do this is discussed in the next chapter.

SUMMARY

Good health and proper weight management establish and maintain healthy rhythms. It is important to have a core rhythmic lifestyle pattern in place, especially so there is more ability to tolerate a stressful demand when it happens. This prevents excess cortisol from stress.

If a person does not have a good rhythmic base, then stress can throw the entire system out of whack in a matter of days, leading to vicious patterns of weight gain, poor energy, and many other potential health issues. This sets up a problem of internal friction and ongoing excess inflammation, in turn setting the stage for disease risk.

A person does not need elaborate testing to realize there is an issue wherein stress leads to increased risk of serious health problems. Emotionally, it feels like too much is out of control. The longer a person feels this way, the more likely they are to be in a state of excess cortisol production.

Physically, it feels like accelerated wear and tear and a poor energy level. This is because cortisol acts by breaking down body tissue to make energy. When there has been too much cortisol secretion, it is physically wearing over time. A person with this cortisol excess problem is prone to stress eating, a behavior that is driven by out-of-balance hormones.

Eventually, these emotional and physical trends result in weight gain around the midsection. Over time, the metabolic strain of stress results in a true physical problem that is reflective of a much higher risk for disease.

27

Solving Weight Gain
Around the Midsection

*T*he key to understanding weight loss is getting leptin to work properly. Properly working leptin permits fat burning to occur. It is the hormone that controls the rate of fat burning in the liver, muscles, pancreas, and heart.[209]

Normal metabolism of fat and carbohydrate must be restored in order for weight to be lost correctly. In leptin resistance, there is a slowdown of fat metabolism in the liver. This leads to an accumulation of stored fat, since the fat cannot be burned as fuel. Normal-weight individuals do not have this problem.[210]

Furthermore, once fat utilization is disturbed, carbohydrates also turn into fat. This means that insulin resistance is a consequence of leptin resistance.[211] As long as leptin resistance is present, carbohydrates are likely to turn into fat because of the inability to burn fat.

Once a person is overweight, they have factors working against them that a normal-weight individual does not have. The calories contained in the same exact food are metabolized differently in an overweight person compared to a normal-weight person. The unfortunate tendency is for the overweight person to convert the food into stored fat.

This is an area where extra nutritional support can balance the playing field, giving the overweight person a significant boost in the ability to metabolize fat.

NUTRIENTS TO SUPPORT OPTIMUM HEALTH

This brings up an important issue about what we seek to accomplish with nutrition. We try to restore healthy structure and function to the body. We work to restore communication in the body so that it has the ability to establish and maintain proper biological rhythms. We may also need a plan to offset the stressful demands in our lives.

The new Daily Values for vitamins and minerals, formerly referred to as Minimum Daily Requirements, evolved based on the discovery of essential nutrients that when lacking caused nutritional deficiency diseases. A lack of Vitamin C causes scurvy, a lack of Vitamin D causes rickets, a lack of B12 or iron causes anemia, and so on. These stone-age concepts of nutrient needs serve a purpose, but they are woefully lacking when it comes to the general health needs of individuals.

For example, an individual may have 100 percent of what the government thinks is needed for health and still have a raging case of leptin resistance. Excess cortisol from stress makes the problem worse, and the individual gains weight around the middle. The problem is that what the government thinks an individual needs to prevent the old-time nutritional diseases has nothing to do with how that person tolerates stress and utilizes calories.

Let us define "need" in a relevant way. If we agree that leptin resistance, insulin resistance, adrenaline resistance, and cortisol excess are not good for health, then a main goal is to have no problems with these issues. Whatever a person must do to accomplish this becomes a minimum daily need.

One indicator that such a need is met is that the individual has a better tolerance for stress, and their midsection shrinks or stays flat while their muscle energy and drive in life is good. This is not complex; either a person feels this way or they do not.

There are shades of gray, wherein a person slips into a pattern of wear and tear or they may be gradually improving. It is important to look at the weekly and monthly trends as these tell how well a person is doing over time.

A person can do more than is minimally needed just to be on the safe side or for prevention, but that is a matter of personal choice. A true need is to resolve issues with leptin resistance, insulin resistance, adrenaline resistance, and cortisol excess. This not only helps one attain and maintain proper body weight, it reduces the risk for the diseases of aging.

EVERY PERSON IS DIFFERENT

There are many factors that come to bear on this issue besides vitamins and minerals. Food, stress, and sleep are of major importance. If a person eats well, exercises, effectively manages stress, gets adequate sleep, and has no signs of leptin resistance, insulin resistance, or adrenaline resistance, then they have achieved the goal. They are in excellent natural balance.

The great majority of people, especially those over the age of 30, have a difficult time getting in a state of natural balance simply by eating well, exercising, and making an effort to get adequate sleep. Certainly, improvement is experienced by making positive changes in these areas, but the goal of being in balance may be difficult to attain or maintain.

There are varying states of difficulty. There can be a moderate case of being 5-10 pounds overweight and feeling more sluggish than normal. A person can be stuck in a more significant problem of progressive weight gain, yo-yo dieting, or the inability to lose significant extra weight. A person needs help to get back on track and to stay on track.

Extra nutrient support can help make this possible by getting the person out of a health rut and heading in the right direction. This is a relevant use of nutritional support. If the person uses extra support and gets on track, there is a positive outcome that is relevant to healthy function and structure. In our way of thinking, this is the true minimum daily requirement.

Once a person is back on track and doing well, they may not need as much nutrient support to stay that way. Thus, two issues arise:

1) What does a person have to do to get on track and get back in rhythm?
2) What does a person have to do to stay on track once they are in a stable pattern?

Do not expect the government to issue guidelines to help people understand nutritional needs in this context. The government has a history of being 10-20 years behind the times.

For many years, the major medical journals have been anti-vitamin. Faced with overwhelming evidence of the health benefits of nutritional supplement support, they are changing their tune.

In a rather astounding recent article published in the *Journal of the American Medical Association,* it stated, "It appears prudent for all adults to take vitamin supplements."[212] The surprising aspect of this article is that this is mainstream medicine telling the world that even basic vitamins and antioxidants can prevent serious disease.

Leptin-resistance issues are clear; one either has them or they do not. If someone has leptin resistance-issues, they age faster, and their health deteriorates quicker than necessary. Something can be done and should be done while there is time. These are factors that help define minimum daily nutritional needs for any individual.

ESSENTIAL FATTY ACIDS AND LEPTIN RESISTANCE

Thirty percent of the cells in white adipose tissue are immune cells that produce the pro-inflammatory signals TNFa and IL-6. It is ongoing stress 24 hours a day, 7 days a week.

Not only do overweight individuals have to deal with the stress of life, they have to deal with the stress of highly inflammatory immune signals being generated by the extra pounds of fat they carry.

Changing the type of fat in the diet can change these inflammatory signals and help stop leptin resistance.

Long-chain omega 3 oils, such as fish oil, can reduce the output of TNFa and IL-6 from white adipose tissue.[213,214] Individuals in inflammatory states, such as arthritis, can have their inflammation signals, including TNFa, reduced by as much as 90 percent by fish oils.[215] By helping to reduce these pro-inflammatory signals, the stranglehold leptin resistance has on a person can be changed so that willpower can start to take charge.

Fish oils are also proven to reduce insulin resistance.[216] Fish oil has a direct bearing on enhancing glucose utilization,[217] including the ability of muscles to use and store glucose.[218] In order to get rid of leptin resistance, glucose metabolism must work properly. This is why extremely low and no-carbohydrate diets do not work in the long run.

It is essential to restore glucose utilization in order to stop excess leptin production.[219] Therefore, fish oils, with their ability to enhance glucose utilization, are one of the many unique nutritional supplements that can have a significant impact on returning natural and normal energy balance to a person who is otherwise stuck in an extremely bad rut.

In a recent study, fish oil and an oil called GLA demonstrated the ability to reduce pro-inflammatory immune cell activity by up to 65 percent within four weeks.[220] Flax oil, another oil rich in omega 3 fatty acids, has also shown to reduce these pro-inflammatory messengers, leading researches to recommend flax oil for the prevention of high-cholesterol induced heart attacks and strokes.[221] We frequently recommend combination capsules of fish oil, flax oil, and borage oil (containing GLA) to fortify the diet.

Three to nine grams of these oils added to the diet change the excessive inflammatory problems generated by the extra pounds of fat. This is a form of stress management for fat cells, helping to cool them off so they stop generating aches and pains for the rest of the body, as well as locking in conditions of hormone imbalance.

Omega 3 oils were in much higher amounts in our diets when animals were free-range and they grazed on grass. This caused their fat to have much higher levels of omega 3 oils. Today, other than eating deep-sea fish such as salmon or tuna, it is difficult to obtain the needed amount of omega 3 oil in the diet. We end up eating too many pro-inflammatory fats without a natural amount of anti-inflammatory fat to keep things in natural balance. This tilts the scale towards inflammation and leptin resistance.

In overweight individuals, extra amounts of these oils become a minimum daily requirement to offset the extra pro-inflammatory immune signals coming from the extra pounds of fat. This serves as a basic example of an increased daily requirement for nutrient intake. The minimum daily requirement relates specifically to how many pounds of extra fat the body has on hand.

PANTETHINE: THE METABOLIZER OF EXTRA FATS

Pantethine is a special form of vitamin B5, pantothenic acid. It is a coenzyme form of the vitamin, meaning it is exactly the form naturally used in metabolism. It is extremely biologically active, much more so than plain vitamin B5. If we think of fats in the body as a long train, pantethine acts like the locomotive, hauling and transporting fat into metabolic action. No other nutrient is as effective as pantethine.

Pantethine can lower LDL cholesterol,[222,223] raise HDL cholesterol,[224,225] lower triglycerides,[226,227] and make blood less sticky.[228] Unlike drugs, these cardiovascular risk-reducing features are accomplished by restoring normal metabolism of fat without any adverse side effects, thus promoting the restoration of natural balance. This includes naturally stimulating the breakdown of stored fat in white adipose tissue.[229]

In a recent study with 16 individuals who had fatty-liver disease and high triglycerides, each was given 600 mg of pantethine a day for six months or longer. At the end of the study, nine of them no longer had fatty-liver disease. Furthermore, CT scans of their abdominal areas showed significantly reduced visceral fat (abdominal fat), the type of fat around important body organs that is the largest concern for fat-associated serious disease.[230]

This study is important because it proves this nutrient helps metabolize the type of fat, abdominal fat, that is most associated with the onset of disease. It changes the problem of excess cortisol and leptin resistance.

A 20-year scientific track record of the safe use of pantethine, even in patients with diabetes and kidney failure, demonstrates the power of this natural way to improve fat metabolism. A case can be made, from a healthy function point of view, that this nutrient is essential in higher amounts (600-900 mg a day), amounts that far exceed what an individual could get from the diet, for the safe and natural reduction of abdominal fat.

CALCIUM, A NEW SOLUTION FOR STOMACH FAT

In Chapter 21, we mentioned the importance of calcium in controlling agouti, a gene signal in the brain that helps bolster neuropeptide Y. NPY makes a person hungry while at the same time blocks the brain's perception of leptin, thus locking in leptin resistance. In the previous chapter, we pointed out how excess cortisol, leptin resistance, and elevated NPY are locked into a metabolic pattern in the stressed-out, overweight individual, placing them at high risk for stress eating.

As it turns out, agouti and NPY gang up on the body to cause excess food cravings and eating. Excess agouti is directly related to the accumulation of excess abdominal fat.[231] The more overweight a person is, the higher the agouti.

It is easy to cool off the agouti gene. To do this, a person needs to take enough high-quality calcium. This may require calcium ranging from 2,000 mg to 3,000 mg a day. When the right amount is reached, many cravings for food stop, energy is noticeably improved, and there is weight loss around the midsection.

In our clinical experience, we have had the best results using calcium AEP and coral calcium to accomplish this result.

SUMMARY

Freeing the body of extra abdominal fat is essential to reducing the risk for disease and slowing the rate of aging. When a person gains weight around the middle, it signifies that many issues relating to hormones are going in the wrong direction and that natural balance is disrupted.

If a person is able to eat better and exercise, thereby losing weight, then that is all that is needed to return the body to natural balance.

This issue becomes progressively more difficult to solve when ongoing stress and poor eating habits have set up problems with cortisol, leptin, insulin, NPY, and agouti. These problems tend to lock each other into place and get progressively worse as time goes by.

It is proven that various nutrient supplements can help the body regain better control of fat metabolism and reduce the inflammation coming from fat cells. At the forefront of nutrients in this category are essential fatty acids, pantethine, and calcium.

The science is overwhelmingly clear that these nutrients are safe and effective to help restore natural balance in fat metabolism. From a functional point of view for many overweight individuals, this type of nutrient support is essential to overall health and well being.

For many others, this information is of value to help make weight loss easier or to prevent weight gain from stress. It can be used as part of a health maintenance and anti-aging approach to help metabolism run more efficiently.

28

Resolving Eating Disorders

*P*eople are constantly bombarded by advertising images promoting ultra-thin as desirable. In an effort to achieve this thin state, one attempted solution is to eat little food.

Frequently, this involves younger women trying to attain or maintain their idea of a proper body image. Their fears of food are reinforced by their observation that when they eat more they gain weight. Quite often, they look at their overweight parents and do not want to turn out that way.

Individuals heading down this path can easily get into a metabolic pattern they cannot get out of, resulting in a clinically definable eating disorder. The essence of this disorder is that starvation metabolism becomes locked into place, and the individual cannot get out of the problem.

MILLIONS OF BORDERLINE EATING DISORDERS

Millions of Americans who think they do not have eating disorders are headed down this path. This is partly because the public-health officials in charge of dietary advice have been preaching low-calorie and low-saturated fat diets to the general public for years.

The public has become brainwashed into thinking this type of diet is heart healthy as well as the best way to lose weight. Since it is a general public recommendation, many women who try to be healthy and stay slim employ this method of eating to watch their weight. This is a quick way to enter starvation metabolism.

Starvation metabolism comes in degrees of severity. Those most likely to encounter this low-leptin problem are:

1) People who significantly reduce calories on a diet.
2) Young women trying to be thin.
3) Middle-aged women trying to stop progressive weight gain or maintain a too thin body appearance.
4) Athletes with demanding energy output. Female gymnasts are particularly at risk.
5) People with stress induced lack of appetite that causes fatigue, muscle wasting, and weight loss.
6) Elderly individuals whose appetite and health are sliding.
7) Individuals suffering from chronic or serious illness.

THE SIGNS OF EATING DISORDERS

There are many shades of gray between optimum health and a clinically definable eating disorder. A clinical disorder is characterized by the pervasiveness of the starvation metabolism. In some cases, this is caused by a disease process such as cancer or the wasting away associated with advanced aging. In other cases it is by choice, in an effort to lose weight or stay slim.

The hallmark of the starvation metabolism is a low-leptin situation. Since leptin permits a healthy metabolic rate to take place, a low-leptin starvation metabolism forces the body to run slowly, as if in a hibernation mode.

Forcing a hibernation metabolic rate onto an individual can have devastating metabolic effects. For example, young female gymnasts are known to have a low-leptin problem. This has a profound effect on their estrogen levels, normal female development, hormonal function, and bones. By comparison, elite male gymnasts do not have the same type of problems.[232] Having enough leptin is important to women.

In less obvious low-leptin situations, it is still fairly easy to observe if there is a problem. This is because there is not enough energy for the body to work properly. Body needs that are energy intense, such as the monthly hormonal pattern or the immune system, do not work properly.

Many young women are naturally thin because they have an efficient and highly functional metabolism. How does one tell the difference between such an individual and one heading down the path of an eating disorder?

This is relatively easy. There should be a normal appetite. Onset of menstruation should be at a normal age, and the menstrual cycle should run each month in a timely manner without symptoms. The individual should not catch colds easily and should get over bugs readily if they do get ill. Mood should be good with no proneness to irritability and depression. Posture should be excellent with no slumping shoulders or evidence of scoliosis. If a young lady is trim and has no issues with any topic in this paragraph, then she is generally eating enough.

Problems in this area range from slight malnutrition to full-fledged anorexia. Excessive exercise, whether done to keep ultra trim or as a result of competitive athletics, aggravates any issue in this category. This is because extra activity requires extra fuel. If a person does not eat enough, the body breaks down protein, fat, and bone to sustain energy needs. This can develop into a full-scale stress response and malnutrition syndrome that is quite serious.[233]

Many athletes fall into this problem by not eating enough fat to sustain their energy. They think that saturated fat will make them have too much body fat. However, the failure to take in adequate food results in adverse effects on performance, directly related to lacking leptin.[234]

Underweight individuals tend to be in low-leptin metabolic patterns, especially if they have any type of ongoing health issue. However, a person who is on a low-fat diet, in an effort to maintain a given weight or in an effort to lose weight, may also enter into a low-leptin metabolic condition.

Many middle-aged women gain weight and then employ starvation metabolism diet strategies in an effort to prevent gaining any more weight. This induces problems with fatigue, menstruation, hormones, and their immune systems. These problems are obvious. They normally blame their problems on the stress of raising children, working, and so on. These stress factors do indeed raise cortisol, stress-related factors that help to send them down the wrong health path. However, the diet strategy makes their health worse and locks in excess cortisol due to the wear and tear of the diet itself.

This person is not anorexic by clinical definition; they are anorexic-like in their metabolism because they live in a starvation metabolism. They can be in this metabolic pattern even though they are overweight or their general trend is to continue to gain weight. This can seriously speed wear and tear and accelerate aging, the exact opposite of what they were hoping to accomplish with their low-calorie diet.

We also have the middle-aged woman who tries to maintain a super thin appearance because she thinks it looks good. These individuals frequently run on stimulants such as diet soda, excess caffeine, and/or cigarettes. While these individuals may be thin, it is unhealthy as they are in a catabolic wasting pattern. Such individuals invariably have a variety of health complaints that are difficult to resolve because they do not have a normal metabolic energy capable of fixing their health problems. By the time they are in their fifties, they are likely to have serious bone-loss issues.

It is easy to observe by looking at the skin that there is accelerated catabolic wasting in such individuals. This is because the normal fat layer under the skin is weakened or broken down by this catabolic dieting strategy. This causes the skin to wrinkle much faster than normal. Many such individuals have already been to the plastic surgeon for face-lifts to help correct their sagging skin structure. However, the neck and the hands are two areas that can easily be observed that reflect this problem.

This catabolic break down of fat also causes cellulite. This is a main reason why a thin person or a person 5-10 pounds overweight has cellulite.

If a woman does not want to wrinkle or develop cellulite any faster than she needs to, the best way is to maintain a functional level of leptin that is proper for correct metabolic rate. This will not cause a breakdown in the fat layer under the skin at an accelerated rate. While a person with too low a supply of leptin may look thin, it is quite noticeable when this thin look is not a healthy look.

There are a number of unmistakable symptoms of the "middle-age" eating disorder. The individual tries, and possibly succeeds, in using incredible willpower to not eat, especially foods that they have been conditioned to believe are bad. If they are not governed by some fear of food or rule about fats in food, they will gladly indulge.

This is accompanied by abnormal fatigue and a feeling of wear and tear. Of course, if such an individual has a stressful life, then all factors of fatigue and wear and tear are made worse.

Such individuals do not have the energy to exercise, or when they make themselves exercise, they do not feel good. Even if they feel OK exercising, their response to exercise is not as good as it used to be prior to entering the wear and tear condition.

Sex hormones, whether in men or women, are not in normal balance and function; there are symptoms of one type or another. Women with this problem are prone to infertility and miscarriages. In this metabolic condition, a person is more prone to get sick, have constipation, or have sluggish bowels.

Every factor in these paragraphs is present, to a greater or lesser degree, in any individual heading down the path of starvation metabolism eating disorders. Remember, there are a thousand shades of gray. However, the metabolic trend and picture are clear, there is no hiding these symptoms.[235]

LEPTIN REGULATES HEALTHY METABOLIC RATE

People with symptoms of the anorexic-like starvation metabolism have one thing in common – too low leptin levels. Adequate leptin tells the brain there is adequate fuel on hand, thus metabolic activity in the body can function at an active metabolic rate. This is healthy, a condition whereby natural balance can occur.

Too little leptin tells the body it is starving; therefore, the brain turns down metabolic rate and function. The longer and more sustained the anorexic eating metabolism becomes, the greater the chance for chronically induced low-leptin levels. When a person gets stuck in low leptin over a period of time, it locks in a serious eating disorder with serious health consequences.[236]

Many problems of not enough leptin are similar to those of too much leptin. This is because leptin resistance means the leptin message does not get through to the brain. In leptin resistance, there is low leptin in the brain, high leptin in the circulation, and leptin resistance in the pancreas causing metabolic syndrome X. Excess cortisol combines with high circulating leptin to make a person fat in the stomach. This results in a condition of fatigue and increased risk of disease.

On the flip side of this picture, the clinical anorexic has low levels of leptin in the brain and low levels of leptin in the circulation. There is excess cortisol, a catabolic hormone, combined with low leptin. This combination forces body wasting to occur. There is also fatigue and increased risk of disease.

In the middle of these two is the leptin-resistant individual who keeps trying to employ the low-calorie diet to lose 10 pounds and can't do it. The dieting itself makes the person have anorexic-like wear and tear, yet the 5-10 pounds on the tummy will not budge.

The leptin-resistant state and the low-leptin anorexic state share these common features: low leptin in the brain, high cortisol in circulation, fatigue, increased risk of disease, and accelerated rate of aging.

Many individuals flip-flop between leptin resistance and low-leptin issues, the essence of yo-yo dieting. Many dieters hit a starvation metabolism brick wall long before they get to their goal weight. The longer they stay in this dangerous condition, the more body muscle and bone they lose, not fat.

Thus, we have the starvation dieter who has the metabolic profile and faulty immune response of an anorexic. This includes low-leptin induced depression,[237,238] muscle weakness that has been diagnosed as fibromyalgia, and loss of bone density, [239,240] yet they may be 50-100 pounds overweight!

Additionally, animals lacking leptin demonstrate that immune cells in their livers become overactive, generating inflammation that damages other healthy liver cells and leads to liver disease.[241]

Women who get stuck in the anorexic metabolic pattern begin to lose function of their hormonal cycle; this may show up as scanty or skipped cycles.[242] If the low-leptin problem is left unchecked, it can develop into infertility or a higher risk for miscarriage if there is a pregnancy.[243] This is a primary health issue for the low-leptin anorexic metabolism, and it is present as the hallmark of this situation regardless of the person's body weight. This is a serious health issue. These problems also occur in the leptin-resistant individual.

WHAT IS CACHEXIA?

Cachexia is a term given by the medical community to a disease process, such as cancer, that forces the body into an anorexic metabolism. Common anorexia is frequently encountered due to high stress, fears regarding food, or misconceptions about how to lose weight. Cachexia is the same physical problem as anorexia; it is simply caused by a different source, a disease that makes the body waste away.

Overcoming the cachexia problem is crucial to surviving cancer. High leptin sets the stage for cancer risk. Initially, high leptin may fan the flames of cancer and make it grow and spread. However, as the cancer takes root, courtesy of chronically elevated NF kappaB, it attacks body structure and destroys protein structures as well as white adipose tissue. As the white adipose tissue is destroyed by cancer, the leptin levels will drop quite low.

This problem of cachexia is responsible for 30 percent of the deaths in cancer situations.[244] It is fascinating to note that men with advanced prostate cancer seldom have cachexia. This is because they are treated with testosterone-blocking drugs, which in men have the net effect of increasing their leptin.[245] This same wasting-away issue and low-leptin levels have also been documented in patients with chronic obstructive pulmonary disease.[246] The main point here is that too little leptin during cancer or other chronic illness causes the body to accelerate the wasting-away problem, leading to serious life-threatening malnutrition.

IMMUNITY ISSUES, A SIGN OF MALNUTRITION

There is no simple way to think about leptin. Leptin is essential for survival. Too much leptin or too little leptin cause major health problems. A person must obtain a good understanding of natural balance and how to eat in relationship to the amount of energy they expend in order to maintain the right amount of leptin and optimum body weight so as to avoid major health issues. Low-fat diets are just as dangerous as high-fat diets. Somewhere in the middle is a healthy balance.

An important marker that helps define the right amount of food is a person's immune function. Individuals who are overweight frequently have impaired immune function.[247] Such problems may involve leptin resistance or may be due to a variety of other issues. Some overweight people have no problem with immune function.

On the other hand, the great majority of individuals with the anorexic-like starvation metabolism have a problem with immune function. A proper amount of leptin is essential to mount an efficient immune response. If the efficient immune response is not there, then the person is more prone to catching bugs and taking longer to recover. Such a person is also prone to a flare up of dormant viral infections, such as mouth sores.

One role of leptin is as an essential part of a proper response to inflammation and infection, key parts of the body's natural defense system.[248] Recent research proves that low leptin handicaps the immune response.[249,250,251] This issue is not open to interpretation. If a person is on the thin side or is attempting to restrict calories too much and is prone to catch bugs, struggles to get over a bug, or gets a breakout of mouth sores, leptin levels are too low and not enough food is consumed.

Low leptin causes the thymus gland to shrink, resulting in serious immune depression.[252] There is always the release of pro-inflammatory signals associated with inflammation and infection. It is interesting to note trends in various countries where food is in short supply and the focus is on immune dysfunction relating to malnutrition and immune depression.

AUTOIMMUNE DISEASE

Americans are mostly prone to overeating. As we pointed out, this leads to excess production of TNFa and IL-6 from the extra pounds of fat. The resting metabolic situation is already inappropriately hyper in terms of immune status. Researchers have identified excess leptin due to excess food consumption as a key factor behind the increase in autoimmune problems in affluent countries.[253]

This information sheds light on why some children may experience debilitating response to immunizations. A recent animal study shows that autoimmune nerve inflammation occurs as a result of immunizations given in the presence of excess leptin.[254] Baby girls have higher leptin than baby boys, placing them at higher risk. Any child that is overfed, overweight, or born to leptin-resistant parents is at a greater risk for such immunologic complications from immunizations.

This information also applies to leptin-resistant adults given flu shots. Once again, we find that public-health officials do not keep up with the current, available science and act on it in a proactive manner. Their focus seems to be on immunizing everyone, not on proving that immunizations are safe or figuring out who might be at risk for serious nerve damage from immunizations.

We learned in Chapter 8 that when there is low leptin in the brain, either due to generally low leptin or to leptin resistance, the brain is much more likely to experience nerve damage. In leptin resistance, the low leptin in the brain is combined with high leptin in the circulation, which overheats the immune system causing a high level of risk for autoimmune disease. This creates a metabolic risk profile of an overly hyped up immune system in the body and a brain more susceptible to damage. The fact that so many people are leptin resistant calls into question the safety of any broad-based immunization campaign. This information creates a link between the societal trend of increased obesity and the dramatic increase in autism in infants.

SOLUTIONS FOR EATING DISORDERS

In order to solve eating disorders, it is important to know that eating correctly does not promote excess weight gain. Understanding leptin explains why this is the case.

The next issue is to get the person to eat. Once eating occurs, the problem is likely to be improved. For example, getting young women with anorexia to eat restores their leptin levels and changes their bone metabolism so that they gain bone mass instead of lose it.[255]

In milder cases of eating disorders, whether in young women or adult dieters, it is simply a matter of explaining to them why diet-induced starvation metabolism does not work. This applies to underweight, normal weight, or overweight individuals.

In more serious situations of metabolic wasting, there are physical reasons why the person cannot eat. They are locked in a metabolic pattern where they have no appetite. They are nauseous, or when they eat they become nauseous. Even if they make themselves eat, they may not gain weight or energy.

This state of affairs is usually induced by major stress that resulted in unhealthy weight loss, purposely not eating and then getting stuck in the problem, or fighting cancer or some other chronic-wasting disease.

When such individuals agree that they should eat, the next issue is to get them to have an appetite so that they can eat and benefit from the food. This is not a psychological issue; it is a physical issue.

In our previous chapter, we pointed out how essential fatty acids, such as fish oil, borage oil, and flax oil, reduce excess leptin production by reducing the pro-inflammatory signals such as TNFa and IL-6. This causes a reduction in inflammatory immune signals coming from fat cells that lock in leptin-resistant overeating.

It is interesting to see that the same solution can work for individuals with low leptin, thus helping to solve eating disorders! In low-leptin states, the body is in a stressful wasting condition. There is excess cortisol fueling the wasting away of the body. This state of physical breakdown involves the excess production of TNFa and IL-6. However, this time, these highly inflammatory immune signals do not come from the excess fat, they come from the cortisol and/or disease fueled wasting process. They cause the loss of appetite.

A study was recently conducted with pancreatic cancer patients who were in a state of cachexia. Such problems are resistant to basic dietary therapy. The person is told to eat more food; however, in most cases, they do not have any appetite. Even if they do eat more, they do not gain weight. In this study, patients were given two grams of fish oil per day. Within three weeks, they had stopped wasting away and started gaining weight![256]

The researchers documented that the fish oils lowered inflammatory markers, such as IL-6, that fueled the catabolic process. This enabled the body to get out of high cortisol and highly inflammatory immune situations, thereby returning the body to a better state of natural balance. Once this is accomplished, the individual can eat food and gain weight.

Understanding this information, we began testing this principle on a variety of underweight individuals. Some had no appetite, and others had stress-induced weight loss. It generally required a dose of six, 1,200 mg of fatty acid mixture (400 mg fish oil, 400 mg borage oil, and 400 mg flax oil) to solve the problem. On this dose, appetite returned, body wasting stopped, and healthy weight gain occurred.

Another important nutrient in the recovery of the anorexic metabolic problem is zinc. A lack of zinc predisposes a person to anorexia in the first place.[257] A recent review of literature regarding zinc showed its extreme importance in helping recovery from anorexia.[258] It is proven that zinc supplementation is essential for the treatment of anorexia.[259]

Zinc is essential for hormone function of all types and hormone transport in the blood. It helps individuals that are stuck in an anorexic metabolic pattern. In can be helpful for moderate cases of anorexic metabolism, in terms of helping the body to run normally when more food is eaten. We recommend 25 mg – 75 mg of zinc per day to assist in restoring natural balance in any person prone to anorexia metabolic problems.

The other major issue in someone recovering from an eating disorder is the fear that they will gain too much weight once they start eating again. There is an element of truth in this concern, as leptin begins to rise as more food is eaten. This is normal and essential to replenish the malnourished condition.

If a person eats according to our *Five Rules* and moderately exercises as they regain weight, the leptin signal tends to be accurate; weight gain stops when they are properly nourished, and excess weight is not gained.

These are relatively simple solutions to what can otherwise be a very devastating issue.

In the case of the person who is 10 pounds overweight and losing energy on a low-calorie diet, they will tend to lose weight and cellulite by eating more and following the *Five Rules*. This is because they improve the efficiency of their body to use calories as well as prevent the catabolic wasting of anorexic-like starvation metabolism.

SUMMARY

Not having enough leptin can pose just as many health problems as having too much leptin. Bouncing around between high-leptin and low-leptin levels, as in the yo-yo dieter, is incredibly stressful to the body.

In order to avoid problems of leptin excess and lacking leptin, a person needs to adopt consistent eating and exercise patterns over the course of their lifetime, living in a state of leptin efficiency. This is a true commitment to healthy living, an important skill of the Health Asset Manager.™

29

Exercise to Solve Leptin Problems

*I*t is well known that exercise is an important part of any weight-loss program. This fact will not change. A lifestyle that places regular exercise as a priority is imperative. Hormones in the body do not work efficiently over time if there is no exercise, especially leptin.

Exercise conditions the fuel regulation systems in the body to work more efficiently. The better these fuel systems function, the less likely there are problems with weight.

EXERCISE, INSULIN RESISTANCE, AND LEPTIN

Exercise improves insulin resistance.[260] Exercise significantly enhances the ability of insulin to transport glucose into muscles so the calories can be used for energy.[261] When muscles are depleted of fuel, there is a demand to replenish the diminished supply.

The short-term positive effects of exercise on fuel utilization can last up to 48 hours. Minimally, a person needs to exercise 3-4 times a week. This allows for proper utilization of the foods that are eaten.

During the first 15-20 minutes of exercise, stored sugar in the muscles, called glycogen, is the primary fuel that is used. Even this small amount of exercise helps with insulin resistance, as the depletion of glycogen causes muscles to demand more fuel to go back into them. It has been conclusively proven that exercise helps lower insulin resistance.[262]

As exercise progresses beyond 20 minutes, glucose and free-fatty acids from the blood are the primary fuel. This is good because it helps clear stagnant calories out of circulating blood. During this time, the adrenal glands begin secreting higher levels of hormones, working with the liver to sustain energy for the exercise.

Individuals who are fatigued and have adrenal wear and tear cannot exercise longer than 15-20 minutes without having unpleasant symptoms. It is important to improve the adrenal reserves and improve liver fitness so that exercise can last 30-40 minutes and produce a pleasant relaxed feeling. This is the next step of strengthening the fuel regulation system. A positive response to exercise lasting 30-40 minutes has a beneficial effect on lowering insulin resistance and fatty buildup in the blood.[263]

After 40 minutes of exercise, fuel comes from a combination of stored liver glycogen and the breakdown of fatty acids from stored fat. The longer the exercise time, as long as the exercise is refreshing and not stressful to the cardiovascular system or physically exhausting, the more stored fat is broken down and burned.

When a person has insulin resistance, the liver does not efficiently store glucose as glycogen. It is difficult to exercise for longer than 40 minutes. This is due to the fact that fatty acids are most cleanly burned for fuel when some carbohydrate is present. If the liver cannot secrete glucose from its store of glycogen as it tries to burn fatty acids, excess numbers of ketones will form. Ketones are acid by-products of incompletely burned fats. This inefficiency to burn fatty acids causes hypoglycemia, a lack of energy, irritability, fatigue, and other issues.

A person recovering from wear and tear needs to find a balance in their exercise, seeking a refreshed response as a priority. Many times this means going at a slower pace than former ability, until overall health and energy reserves are built back up.

Exercise is necessary to repair fuel-regulation problems. As adrenal reserves and liver function improve, exercise will be possible for longer periods of time. A refreshing response to longer periods of exercise is important for solving insulin resistance, leptin resistance, and fuel-regulation issues. It may take some time for an individual to build up to this level of fitness; however, it is essential in order to achieve ideal body weight and to keep off the weight once it is lost.

Thankfully, as mentioned above, even 15 minutes of exercise begins to improve insulin resistance. As it gradually improves over time and the adrenals and liver get in better shape, then longer periods of refreshing exercise become possible.

In addition to the immediate benefits of aerobic exercise, it also lowers leptin when consistently done.[264] A consistent exercise program can improve leptin resistance and insulin resistance over time.[265] This fixes the long-term trend and rhythm, a true solution to insulin and leptin problems.

The problems of insulin resistance and leptin resistance are significantly improved when a person can exercise at a moderate pace for at least one hour, three times a week, and have a refreshing response to that exercise.

Such exercise is important for those with a problematic weight history. Even if beginning with only five minutes of exercise, it is essential to get started and stay with it.

THE RELAXATION RESERVES

In every person's nervous system, there is a natural balance between activation and relaxation. Activation is guided by the sympathetic nervous system. It leads to more assertive behavior and guides the basic stress response (fight or flight). Relaxation is controlled by the parasympathetic nervous system. It leads to a more easygoing and adaptive behavior. It acts as a savings account or "relaxation reserve" to help balance and tolerate the pressures of life without generating too much friction or internal wear and tear.

Leptin resistance disturbs natural balance in the nerves leading to excess sympathetic nerve activity with a loss of parasympathetic nerve tone. Leptin resistance, as well as an unbalanced lifestyle, uses up relaxation reserves. This causes the nerves to "run hot."

This frayed feeling in the nervous system generally accompanies leptin resistance. Eventually, this feeling turns into nerve pain that impacts the muscles, a problem referred to as fibromyalgia.

As relaxation reserves run low, there is constantly too much adrenaline active in the sympathetic nerves. Normally, white adipose tissue is metabolically stimulated by adrenaline. In this situation of excess adrenaline, the white adipose tissue fat cells become deaf to the adrenaline signal causing weight gain around the midsection. However, the heart and kidneys are irritated by this excess adrenaline.

Once this problem locks in, even on a generally nonstressed day, a person with leptin resistance induces excess adrenaline at night. This is because adrenaline rises in excess with leptin resistance, peaking as bedtime approaches.

This extra adrenaline is super activated by eating at night or by a stressful event at night. It can also be active at night simply due to the overall stress of the day.

It is quite common that a person with leptin resistance is prone to a racing, erratic, or unstable heart rate at night, especially when they lie down to go to bed. This may cause an excessive surge in blood pressure in the evening, disrupting sleep.

Most people understand how stress affects them on an emotional or relationship basis, as they are consciously aware of their feelings. If they had a stressful day, the heart symptoms mentioned above may be worse, especially at night. However, with leptin resistance, a person is prone to troubling heart rhythms regardless of how stressful the day may have been due to the excess irritating adrenaline that is in the circulation.

Rhythm disturbances in the heart can lead to ventricular fibrillation, the leading cause of unexpected cardiac death in industrialized nations. Many medications to control heart rhythms have simply failed to be of any value, causing increased cardiac mortality.[266]

Drugging the sympathetic nervous system into less aggressive function does little towards restoring sympathetic and parasympathetic natural balance. This should come as no surprise since drugs frequently do little to restore normal function. The risk for a cardiac event is proportionate to excess adrenaline relative to a loss of parasympathetic tone or balance.[267]

EXERCISE TO THE RESCUE

Aerobic exercise is the single best option for anyone who would like to reduce their risk of dying from sudden cardiac death due to heart-rate instability.[268]

Consistent aerobic exercise is the number-one physical act a person can do to correct leptin resistance. There is no shortcut. The biggest issue is consistency, rather than intensity. How fit one is must be taken into account in terms of how much exercise is done. One must get a relaxed response to the exercise, not exhaustion. It is important to do an amount of aerobic exercise so as to enhance the tone of the parasympathetic nervous system.

Even mild exercise, while watching the diet, has shown to improve parasympathetic tone and to reduce the effects of excess adrenaline.[269] In a study with mildly obese women who did not have high blood pressure, all of the women improved their heart-rate stability with exercise. At the same time, they lost weight, lowered cholesterol, lowered triglycerides, and improved insulin resistance issues. They improved the factors relating to leptin resistance, simply with consistent, moderate exercise and mild calorie restriction. The control group that did not exercise showed no improvement.

The reserves of parasympathetic nerve function act like oil in the engine of a car, keeping it from overheating. It is this parasympathetic tone that is the key aspect of natural balance in the nervous system, enabling the body to bounce back from stress and offset the potential wear of adrenaline output.[270] Without this natural balance, a person gets too wound up and too stressed. The degree of this problem is related to one's risk of dying from a heart attack.[271]

There is simply no question that exercise opens the door to recovery from leptin resistance by restoring parasympathetic tone to normal.[272] No drug can do this. The encouraging part about it for individuals who are not in good shape is that it is just a matter to get going and be consistent in order to have improvement.

Even mild or low-grade aerobics, such as walking, enhance parasympathetic tone in overweight individuals.[273] Walking 10,000 steps a day in one's course of activities can do this, plus reduce high blood pressure in hypertensive patients.[274] Study after study shows that mild aerobic exercise improves parasympathetic tone, thereby reducing excess adrenaline.[275,276,277]

GETTING ON TRACK

The better physically fit a person is, the easier it is to get back on track and recover from leptin resistance. If a person is fit enough to go out for a 30-minute jog, they can boost up the parasympathetic tone in a hurry. This can stop the binge eating and cravings of leptin resistance in one day. However, the program needs to be consistent, such as running at least three times a week, in order to maintain tone and build up the reserves in the nervous system.

If a person is not in this type of condition, they should not be dismayed. There is just a bit longer runway, but anyone can get to a point where leptin resistance can be controlled with mild and moderate, consistent exercise. As there is improvement, begin to do more if it is within physical capabilities. Always seek to obtain a relaxed and refreshing response to exercise, in order to replenish the parasympathetic tone in the nervous system. Doing too much too soon or exercising too vigorously will not be of any benefit.

A TRICK TO STAYING ON TRACK

It is quite common that the leptin resistant urge to eat will attack at night. It may come about even when one is fairly consistent and more or less on a good track. That overwhelming desire to eat starts. At first, it is ignored. Then it starts to take over. What should be done?

If there is enough willpower to overcome this urge to eat at night, congratulations. If not, the best thing to do is to get blood to flow to the head. Overweight individuals with food cravings have an exaggerated lack of blood in their conscious brain and an excess amount of blood overheating their subconscious brain fueling the drive to eat.

Instead of eating, vigorously exercise for a few minutes. Do some jumping jacks or push-ups or do weight-bearing exercises. Walk up and down the stairs ten times while taking deep breaths. Do something to stimulate circulation. Even go for a walk. Get blood to flow to the head to mechanically change the balance of power so that willpower is back in control; the craving will stop. Do not get in a wrestling match with the subconscious mind; it will most likely win.

Intense physical exercise can depress leptin on a short-term basis due to the increased demand for fuel to perform exercise. Furthermore, this reaction is felt over a period of hours, meaning that a good workout in the afternoon or evening can help prevent the nighttime desire to overeat. This lowering of leptin in response to resistance strength-training exercise has been demonstrated in athletes[278] as well as diabetics.[279] Short duration, intense exercise is a fantastic tool to bring leptin cravings under control.

BUILDING MUSCLE

As a person gains body fat, the internal appearance of muscle becomes more like a slice of bacon than a piece of lean beef. This accumulation of fat inside of the muscle is counterproductive to healthy function of insulin and leptin. As mentioned in the previous paragraph, there is a short-term improvement in leptin status from intense exercise. This is a different response than a resistance training program that converts muscle that looks like bacon back to a leaner and stronger appearance.

Recent scientific evidence shows that resistance training lowers body fat and leptin, and this reduction of body fat and leptin is the key that enables insulin to function correctly so that there is no insulin resistance in the muscles.[280]

A combination of aerobic exercise and resistance training in pre-menopausal women lowered their leptin and TNFa, in turn leading to a loss of all types of body fat.[281] These studies are important as they show that building strength over time helps restore leptin to normal levels, resulting in insulin-resistance problems resolved.

Strength training also creates a demand for fatty acids to be used by the muscles. This is because muscle tissue breaks down as a result of the exercise. This causes a higher demand of protein to repair the muscle and of fat to fuel energy supplies in the muscle.

When a person goes 5-6 hours without eating, the body begins breaking down triglycerides to use for fuel. Triglycerides are a combination of one glycerol, or sugar, and three fatty acids. As these fatty acids are liberated into the circulation, they must go somewhere useful. The muscles are the primary body tissue that uses fatty acids for fuel. The muscle breakdown that occurs during strength training may last 48 hours or longer, meaning that strength exercise three times a week keeps a constant demand for fatty acids to flow to the muscles.

If there is no muscle need for the fatty acids, the next time a person eats and insulin goes up, the fatty acids are packaged back up into triglycerides and sent back to storage. Thus, a person who eats properly but does not exercise may not get anywhere in terms of weight loss.

BODY HEAT AND EXERCISE

When cells throughout the body breathe correctly, energy is produced in an efficient manner. As glucose or fat are burned for fuel, energy is made (ATP) and heat is produced. Normal metabolism produces 65 percent energy and 35 percent heat. A person with the starvation metabolism problem conserves energy and does not produce adequate heat.

Body temperature is as important as light to help the body set biological rhythms. Scientists have demonstrated that proper body temperature is needed to activate certain parts of the brain that cause alertness during the day, and as bedtime approaches, heat signals other parts of the brain that promote sleep.[282] A shift in heat from the internal part of the body to the periphery signals the start of the sleep process.[283]

Furthermore, even middle-aged adults have already started moving this temperature rhythm earlier in time, indicating the onset of loss of temperature rhythm.[284] Body heat is now recognized as an important issue in setting the stage for proper sleep pattern and therefore, all other biological patterns.

This places new importance on exercise. Aerobic exercise increases body temperature; strength-training exercise increases muscle mass that in turn increases body temperature, even at rest. Proper production of heat can wake up the head, another benefit for individuals who make the wise choice to exercise regularly.

SUMMARY

There are six critically important reasons to exercise:

1) To improve the natural rhythm and pattern of fuel utilization in the body.
2) To increase the parasympathetic tone of the nervous system, building up the relaxed reserves.
3) To keep leptin food cravings and out-of-control behavior in check.
4) To enhance strength to more permanently stabilize leptin and insulin function.
5) To improve the muscle use of fatty acids so that weight loss is easier or optimum weight is more readily maintained.
6) To ensure adequate body heat, an important foundation for body rhythms and patterns.

The most important guiding principles of exercise are consistency and achieving a refreshed feeling from the activity. As fitness improves, the duration and intensity can be increased as long as consistency and the refreshed feeling are not sacrificed. As a person gains strength over time and can perform longer periods of aerobics, there is a consistent enhancement in fully solving the leptin problem. Exercising is a powerful tool for solving leptin issues.

30

Proper Sleep; a Key to Needed Repair

*Q*uality of sleep is another issue that must be well managed in order to solve leptin issues. In order to have quality of sleep, it is vital to maintain a steady supply of blood sugar during sleep. This enables one to dip into the reserves of fat while sleeping, an essential requirement for healthy weight loss. Sleep is prime fat-burning time, especially when there has been no eating after dinner.

Sleep enables the body to clean house and perform needed repairs. It is essential for recovery from wear and tear. The better the job one does of managing energy resources during the day, the better the quality of sleep at night. This is partly because there is less wear and tear to repair and partly because the body is in overall better rhythm.

The fastest way to disrupt sleep is to eat after dinner, eat too large a dinner, or eat dinner too late. This forces the body to digest food when it should be doing other functions such as fat burning and body repair. Also, as leptin resistance sets in, it causes higher amounts of adrenaline during sleep hours. This causes insomnia, light sleep, restless sleep, sleep apnea, and a general feeling of unrest.

There is no making up for a lack of sleep. A lack of sleep causes energy systems in the body to give out too easily. Even under little stress, a person who does not sleep enough finds it almost impossible to go 5-6 hours without eating. A person who is sleep deprived lacks tolerance for stress, leading to exaggerated hyperglycemic and eventual hypoglycemic responses to stress. Sleep-deprived individuals are irritable.

As a person has more demands in their life, it is imperative to keep exercise, eating, and sleep rhythms in a good pattern. A failure to do so results in a steady decline in the quality of sleep and daytime energy. Eventually this can lead to the problem called fibromyalgia, wherein sleep can be so poor that hardly any energy is possible the next day.

SLEEP AND FAT BURNING

Sleep is the most important time for burning fat. If the *Five Rules* are followed, there should be 11-12 hours of time between finishing the last meal of the day and eating breakfast. As the night progresses, more calories from fat are burned.

Ideally, as approaching sleep, one should be slightly hungry and tired. Avoid emotional stress before bed; this is the worst time to rev up the system with excess adrenaline. There should be an absence of hyperglycemic symptoms or hypoglycemic symptoms; otherwise, sleep generally is not refreshing.

It requires a level of fitness, in terms of fuel regulation, to successfully go 11-12 hours without eating. The liver, pancreas, adrenal glands, and muscle must all be in relatively good working order to get a good night's sleep resulting in proper fat burning. If at first this cannot be done, follow the information in this book to improve overall fitness of the body and work towards the ideal that is described in this chapter.

BLOOD-SUGAR LEVELS AND SLEEP

Hyperglycemic symptoms prior to bed generally feel like the body or mind is working too fast. These symptoms occur even though the person is tired or even exhausted. One can experience an uncomfortable racing feeling that prevents sleep. The heart can feel jittery, skipping a beat or pounding as the person lies down to go to sleep. It is not a normal feeling of energy; it is an uncomfortable feeling of energy. This feeling can come about simply as a lack of fitness in terms of not eating properly and not doing enough relaxing exercise. This racing feeling is easily magnified by stress.

Hyperglycemic-prone individuals often process the details of their life stressors before they go to bed. Their minds can be busy trying to figure everything out and have a plan ready for the next day. In essence, they generate a stress response, releasing adrenaline and cortisol before bed. This fuels the hyperglycemic reaction. Having an argument before bed is not good as it automatically puts a person in a hyperglycemic mode.

Hyperglycemic states before bed are driven by emotional stress, physical wear and tear, and/or leptin resistance. Because stress hormones are frequently involved, they interfere with falling to sleep, staying asleep, and sleeping deeply. They make an individual prone to have to go to the bathroom frequently during the night. Hyperglycemic issues cause a person to have problems with fuel regulation the next day thereby setting up a vicious circle.

Hyperglycemic individuals tend to burn fat inefficiently while they are sleeping. This causes an excess amount of ketones to form at night. This may cause nightmares. They may wake up with nausea, heartburn, or a queasy feeling in the middle of the night or in the morning.

When such individuals wake up nauseous or with heartburn, they typically find that if they eat a few crackers they can go back to sleep, as the rise in insulin from the carbohydrates turns off the hyperglycemic problem and stops the ketones from forming that cause digestive distress. While this works as a temporary solution, it does not help weight loss.

Some hyperglycemic individuals may become hypoglycemic during the night. This is because:

1) The liver's reserve of glycogen is not adequate; thus, they do not have a stable supply of blood sugar that is important for the proper burning of fatty acids, or

2) There is excessively high insulin from insulin resistance and leptin resistance that suppresses the proper release of glucagon; thus, the liver does not get in gear making energy before blood sugar drops.

3) The high cortisol level at bed blunts leptin function and disrupts sleep. By the time leptin gets going it blunts cortisol in the morning. The chaotic rhythms cause energy fluctuations that are abnormal, including hypoglycemia.

In any case, this may lead to waking up with extreme hunger, nightmares, excess sweating, and/or headaches during sleep or upon awakening.

Most individuals who go to sleep hyperglycemic wake up hypoglycemic. This causes them to feel heavy in the head, and their mood is irritable when blood sugar is low; in turn, we have the morning grouch.

When individuals wake up hyperglycemic, meaning blood-sugar numbers are high by test, then the pancreas fails to sense the rise in morning cortisol or leptin resistance has blunted the morning rise in cortisol. In either case, it is a more serious problem of hormone imbalance than waking up hypoglycemic.

Individuals who are hyperglycemic before bed generally find that if they have a small carbohydrate snack before bed, their uncomfortable racing feeling will calm down, and they will be able to go to sleep. This is better than not getting a good night's sleep, but it does not promote weight loss and does not solve the source of their problem.

Such individuals should avoid a high-protein/low-carbohydrate dinner, since the extra metabolic drive of such a dinner can push them into a hyperglycemic pattern as protein stimulates glucagon release. Individuals prone to hyperglycemia at bed tend to do best on a dinner that is higher in carbohydrate and somewhat lower in protein. Such individuals usually do better on higher protein earlier in the day.

A less common issue is the person who is hypoglycemic before bed. Such individuals feel dull in the head; they cannot remember things easily, and their brains feel foggy and disconnected. These symptoms occur because blood sugar is not adequate to keep the brain in a normal range of function. It is a different feeling than normal tiredness. It is more common that individuals wake up hypoglycemic in the middle of the night or in the morning than starting out that way before bed.

This type of individual ends up eating too much before bed in an effort to solve the hypoglycemic feeling. This also interferes with optimum fat burning. In many cases, this problem can be resolved by eating a high-protein dinner with moderate carbohydrates. This is the opposite dinner recommendation for the person who is prone to hyperglycemia at bed.

Taking any kind of medication to help sleep is undesirable over the long run, as they deaden nerves and pose problems to the liver. Correcting problems of leptin resistance, insulin resistance, hyperglycemia, and hypoglycemia solve most sleep problems. Many sleep medications are functionally addictive, meaning that once they are started, sleep problems are magnified when they are discontinued.

Hyperglycemic and hypoglycemic problems at bedtime, during sleep, or upon waking are key signs that overall fuel regulation is out of balance. Because nighttime is generally the longest time to go without food, it serves as an excellent metabolic test of the health of this system, especially overall liver fitness. It is essential to get it in good working order to properly lose weight. A good sign that this issue is improving is the ability to pop out of bed in the morning and get going with a good energy level without the need for caffeine or some other stimulant.

When a person is out of balance or if there has been an unusually stressful day or period of days, it is common that there is difficulty with fuel regulation and sleep quality. Steps need to be taken to get this issue on track as quickly as possible as well as improve the overall situation so that sleep is better. Disrupted sleep, whether due to fuel-regulation issues, stress, or no time for sleep, is a fast track to poor health. Over the years, there is no greater form of wear and tear than a lack of refreshing sleep.

MELATONIN, SLEEP, LEPTIN, AND THE FAT STOMACH

When there is good sleep, meaning that energy levels are stable through the night, other hormones have the potential to work properly because the body is in natural balance. When fuel balance does not work well, it shuts off the proper function of these hormones and causes a poor quality of sleep.

Melatonin is an important hormone that is released during sleep. It must peak at the proper time in order to ensure adequate deep sleep. Melatonin levels decline with age. Melatonin released correctly during the night is essential for proper leptin rhythm during the day.

Proper melatonin release helps establish proper leptin rhythm. When melatonin is released incorrectly, leptin is thrown out of rhythm.[285] Furthermore, supplementing melatonin can restore normal leptin rhythm.[286]

An animal study showed that melatonin prevents the accumulation of stomach fat and lowers leptin, independent of the diet.[287] Melatonin improves diabetes in animal studies by eliminating insulin resistance.[288]

It is interesting to note that scientists are demonstrating that low leptin levels in the brain, whether due to leptin resistance or the starvation metabolic pattern, are the actual cause of most hypothyroid problems. We will discuss this in detail in Chapter 36.

Too little leptin, the hallmark of the anorexic-like starvation metabolic pattern, causes a drop in serotonin function leading to depression and other more serious mental disorders.[289,290] We know that individuals with anorexia have low serotonin, making them more prone to depression. The low-leptin, hypothyroid, and low-serotonin picture prevents the proper formation of melatonin, which is normally made from serotonin.[291] Therefore, one of the fastest ways to become depressed and to disrupt sleep is to eat too little fat to have normal leptin in circulation.

In addition to the importance of melatonin in facilitating proper biological rhythms, melatonin also exerts a positive influence on the source of inflammation. It directly lowers TNFa by turning down excess NF kappaB. This improves the inflammation associated with irritable bowel[292] as well as helps lower high blood pressure.[293]

We frequently use .5 mg melatonin capsules, in dose ranges of 1-6 per night, to help individuals sleep better. On a proper dose, an individual notices better sleep. A proper dose of melatonin at night can improve leptin issues during the day, helping to normalize leptin rhythm and reduce food cravings. This is another tool to help reduce abdominal obesity.

SUMMARY

Too many Americans are sleep deprived. It is difficult to compensate for a lack of sleep. A lack of sleep accelerates wear and tear and pushes the body out of natural balance and rhythm.

In addition to not enough sleep, many individuals have trouble getting quality sleep. It is not possible to separate daytime energy regulation, blood sugar, eating patterns, eating habits, exercise, and stress from sleep issues. Central to sleep problems are fluctuating blood-sugar levels, both hyperglycemia and hypoglycemia. At the root of such blood-sugar related sleep problems is leptin resistance, insulin resistance, and adrenaline resistance.

For many individuals, a low dose of melatonin can promote more restful sleep and can help restore more normal leptin rhythms.

Quality of sleep is a key metabolic sign that fuel regulation is working well. It is prime fat-burning time. Shorting sleep or going to bed stressed not only handicaps repair, it interferes with the best time for losing those extra pounds.

31

Increasing Growth Hormone, Naturally

*G*rowth hormone (GH) is one of the most talked about hormones of modern times. Infomercials touting the benefits of taking human growth hormone saturate the media. It is promoted as the fountain of youth. In the hands of the uninformed, it may just as well be the fountain of death.

There is no question that GH levels decline with age. Likewise, over-weight individuals have seriously handicapped GH function. Lack of GH activity promotes weight gain around the midsection, the worst possible type of weight to gain.[294] As GH levels decline, the cardiovascular risk picture significantly worsens.[295]

GH can be measured in the blood to establish a lack of the hormone. GH can be given with the intent of replacing the lacking hormone and returning the GH blood test to a normal score. This is how Western medicine likes to operate; when the number on paper improves, it is thought that the body is back to normal.

Unfortunately, in the case of GH replacement, the short-term risk of this therapy is diabetes; the long-term risk is increased cancer risk. This serves as an example of the shortcomings of the Western medical approach to measure improvement and to monitor the function of the body.

It may seem hard to understand why a hormone that is essential to the body and declines with age can be involved as a primary factor in certain types of cancer.

A general way to understand the issue is to say that when a person takes GH and is already in an out-of-balance situation, GH may stimulate the growth of cancer even though the level of GH looks normal in the blood. Since most individuals who seem to need GH replacement are out of balance, taking GH is very risky. Taking GH does not fix the problem as to why GH is low and may in fact cause serious health problems.

The reason GH levels decline with age is because leptin and the inflammatory signals TNFa and IL-6 block the function of GH, causing GH resistance and depressed GH function. GH is depressed in response to these problems; it is not in control of them. The way to enhance GH function in the body is to solve leptin issues and reduce excess inflammation, not take GH drugs.

WHAT IS GROWTH HORMONE?

GH is produced in the pituitary gland of the brain. Its production is activated by growth hormone releasing hormone (GHRH), produced in the hypothalamus gland. GHRH is one of the oldest hormonal signals in human evolution. As the gene encoding GHRH evolved, its "children" became insulin, glucagon, and various other signals that affect reproduction.[296] Thus, the activity of GH is intimately involved with fuel utilization and reproduction, essential features that allow survival of the species.

When GH is released by the pituitary gland, it travels to the liver where it activates a family of hormonal signals that help carry out repair in the body. True to the family tree, these signals look almost identical to insulin. The primary signal made by the liver that reflects GH activity is called insulin-like growth factor 1 (IGF1). IGF1's main role in a healthy person is to facilitate growth, repair, and cell proliferation.[297] It is a driving force behind building up the body and maintaining it, in terms of physical structure.

The recent discovery of ghrelin, the hormone secreted by the stomach that initiates hunger, is a major breakthrough in understanding the function of GH. Ghrelin binds to cells containing GH, initiating the release of GH into the circulation. This finding is of extreme importance, one that is revolutionizing research in the GH field. We discuss it more in-depth later in this chapter.

GH and IGF1 are primarily anabolic hormone signals that help the body use protein to build and repair. This is essential for body growth. This is how growth hormone was named in the first place. In adults, GH is essential for body repair. Thus, it is a prime hormone that helps an individual recover from the wear and tear of living.

GH and IGF1 are closely associated with insulin, both in terms of structure and function. When insulin works properly in the body, it transports calories into storage, an anabolic activity. In a healthy person, this means insulin helps deposit calories in body tissue so that the tissue can use them as a fuel source or as a building material. Thus, there is synergistic harmony between GH, IGF1, and insulin when a person is in a state of natural balance.

By comparison, the stress hormone cortisol is a catabolic hormone. Cortisol promotes the breakdown of body fuel supplies, and potentially of body structural tissue, to use for fuel to meet the demands of stress.

There is a natural ebb and flow in the body between anabolic activity and catabolic activity. Anabolic activity repairs the body; catabolic activity provides energy for the body to meet demands. The ability to sustain natural balance between these two activities is essential for health.

GROWTH HORMONE AND CANCER

So far, the notion of replacing lacking GH sounds like a good idea. In reality, a person should seek to restore natural GH function by getting the body back into a state of natural balance and rhythm. This is not a quick fix, like taking a GH pill or injection.

There are two types of primary side effects from replacing GH in a medical context: diabetes and cancer. These issues are being discussed and warnings are being posted in major medical journals.

When a person develops insulin resistance then IGF1 levels become resistant to normal repair activity as well. This resistant condition causes higher levels of circulating insulin and IGF1. A deleterious side effect of this problem is that excess and nonfunctioning IGF1 will cause cancer to grow, especially breast cancer. This is why insulin resistance is reflective of breast cancer risk, issues we discuss in Chapter 44.

Higher than normal levels of IGF1 are associated with breast, prostate, colorectal, and lung cancer.[298] There are numerous scientists reporting these problems from a variety of research facilities worldwide.

Breast and prostate cancer cells use GH to fuel their own growth.[299] It is well documented that high IGF1 is associated with colorectal cancer and specifically acts to block cell death in colorectal cancer cells, helping them to survive and spread.[300]

GHRH is a primary growth stimulator of endometrial cancer.[301] Blocking GHRH activity suppresses the growth of cancer cells derived from reproductive tissue.[302] It is recognized that GH and IGF1 activity are major determinants of breast cancer.[303] Blocking GHRH activity reduces the spread of cancer cells and induces cell death in MDA231 breast cancer cells.[304]

GHRH activity is prevalent in human prostate cancer cell activity,[305] which explains why GHRH-blocking drugs reduce prostate cancer activity. Furthermore, GH and IGF1 are both associated with an increased activity of prostate cancer cells.[306]

A review published in 2002 of 1,848 patients treated with human pituitary growth hormone from 1959-1985 showed "significantly raised risks of cancer mortality overall... incidence of colorectal cancer was also greatly raised...and of Hodgkin's disease mortality."[307] In a smaller recent study treating 30 AIDS patients with recombinant human growth hormone (rhGH) in an effort to reduce their stomach fat, four of them developed diabetes and three of them developed cancer.[308]

GROWTH HORMONE AND DIABETES

Problems with GH and IGF1 lead to insulin resistance and diabetes.[309] Remember that GH and insulin come from the same family tree and look almost identical. Scientists found that the reason GH causes insulin resistance is that it binds to insulin receptors, clogging their function.[310]

Girls with Turner's syndrome, a condition of a lacking X chromosome that causes GH impairment resulting in short stature and sexual underdevelopment, are commonly treated with GH therapy. GH treatment helps correct the lack of GH, but the medical therapy has a major adverse side effect; it causes insulin resistance and greater risk for diabetes and heart disease.[311] When long-term GH therapy is discontinued, their insulin resistance goes away and their lipid values and cardiovascular risks improve.[312]

The *Journal of the American Medical Association* recently published the results of a 26-week long double-blind study to test the effects of GH therapy in healthy older adults. It was conducted with 57 women and 74 men, ages 65-88, to see if GH therapy could help improve strength. As expected, the researchers found a decrease in fat mass in both sexes. However, there was only a marginal strength increase in men and no significant improvement in strength or aerobic fitness in women.

The conclusion of the study is alarming "Because adverse effects were frequent, importantly, diabetes and glucose intolerance, GH interventions in the elderly should be confined to controlled studies."[313]

GH serves as an excellent teaching lesson for the Health Asset Manager.™ Here we have a hormone that is lacking as a person grows older. It is depressed more readily in overweight individuals, contributing to many of the health risks associated with obesity. Traditional straight-line thinking, the type on which drug dispensing is based, says that when a number is low on paper, prescribe a drug to bring the score back to normal.

When this line of reasoning is followed with GH, the short-term adverse effect is insulin resistance and diabetes; the long-term adverse effect is significantly increased cancer risk.

THE NATURAL BALANCE OF GROWTH HORMONE

In order to get GH to work properly, it is essential to be in a state of natural balance. Lacking GH is a consequence of the entire body being out of balance, with a loss of natural rhythm.

GH is a cornerstone of the drive of the body to fix and repair itself. When the hormone is given the opportunity to do its work, then it works in harmony with other hormones. When the body is out of balance and not communicating properly, then GH activity is depressed or malfunctioning.

We have explained how leptin is produced during the day in numerous rhythmic pulses, creating a "leptin tone" in the circulation. Overall leptin rises throughout the day and peaks at about midnight. Proper leptin function allows metabolism and energy to run at a proper level. When there is leptin resistance or not enough leptin, energetic drive is handicapped.

Similarly, GH is released in 10-20 pulses per day. The pulsing activity of GH secretion is reflective of its rhythmic tone. As blood levels of GH fall, the hypothalamus gland sends out GHRH to induce a surge of GH production by the pituitary gland. The largest amount of GH in a 24-hour period is released at night, several hours after the leptin peak.

When the GHRH surge is not there, the system loses its tone, GH cells in the liver lose their physical size, and GH production is seriously depressed.[314] GHRH is responsible for the quantity of the surge of GH production.[315]

GH and leptin have "opposing tone," when leptin levels are high, GH levels are correspondingly lower. Thus, leptin and GH have an ebb and flow relationship that is an essential part of natural balance. It is a synergy of coexistence. Leptin's main effect on GH is to restrict it.[316]

In terms of a general trend in the body, GH acts to lower leptin activity in fat cells,[317] leading to a reduction in fat mass, particularly abdominal fat.[318] However, GH does not seem to affect leptin genes in overall white adipose tissue,[319] meaning that GH effects on leptin seem to be concentrated in the abdominal fat area.

LEPTIN RESISTANCE AND GROWTH HORMONE

Once leptin resistance sets in and there is excess leptin in the circulation, then GH production is depressed. This is the true cause of the low GH problem.

For example, diabetic girls entering puberty have a significant problem with leptin resistance and blunted growth due to interference with GH.[320] This data shows that leptin has dominance over GH in terms of their relationship.

In overweight individuals, the daily pulsing of GH release is missing, signifying the leptin-resistant and GH-resistant state.[321] Once abdominal obesity and insulin resistance set in, there is disruption in the normal rhythms and relationship between leptin, insulin, and GH.[322] When rats are genetically bred to have low GH levels, they rapidly develop leptin resistance and obesity.[323]

TIMING AND STRESS AFFECT GROWTH HORMONE

Excess cortisol from stress stimulates the formation of excess fat in the abdominal area. Once GH is lacking, there is no metabolic force to help reduce abdominal fat, and it will keep accumulating as part of a leptin and insulin-resistant picture.[324]

Normal-weight young women with polycystic ovarian syndrome (facial hair growth, acne, disrupted menstruation) have lost their natural GH pulsing rhythm that enables proper ovarian function. Instead, they have higher and more consistent surges of GH, more typical of a male pattern of GH secretion.[325] This is a situation of too much GH at the wrong time.

The proper amount of GH in women must be present at the right time in the right amounts for normal function of the ovaries, sexual development, and sex drive.[326]

During fasting, GH levels rise, but this is not due to the brain stimulating GH production. Rather, in a fasting state, the stomach hunger hormone, ghrelin, promotes extra GH production.[327] This is a natural adaptation to stress. Patients who genetically, or due to a pituitary tumor, overproduce GH have depressed ghrelin levels and no normal ghrelin response to a meal, indicating a loss of natural rhythm due to excess GH.[328]

THE GHRELIN BREAKTHROUGH

Understanding ghrelin may be the key to the great paradox of GH. Ghrelin acts to stimulate the secretion of GH from cells that contain it, thus it is called a growth hormone secretagogue (GHS).

In aging individuals, it is not just a case that GH levels decline. It is a case that the stimulation of the production of GH in the brain declines (lack of GHRH) and the secretion of available GH does not occur (lack of GHS). GH itself is in a state of resistance, similar to leptin resistance. GH is in a state of stressed-out tension because it has lost its natural rhythm and ability to communicate.

GHS in drug form is being tested. It can help offset the lack of GH production in aging as it helps the body release its own GH. This is the forefront of GH research.[329] Since the long-term safety of drugs in this regard is unknown, it will be years before consumers are tempted with a new quick-fix pill or shot.

However, since drug companies and scientists have figured out that GH replacement is a risky proposition, the focus for drug development turns to GHS. In the meantime, even though the dangers of GH are known, the public continues to be bombarded by the promotion of GH until the next class of drug is ready. The marketing of an unsafe therapy continues until there is a new drug that can financially take the place of the older and less effective drug, regardless of potential adverse health consequences to those receiving the therapy.

The Health Asset Manager™ must back up and realize that the body already has a natural way to make GHS; it is called ghrelin. Why do we need a drug for something we already have? Let us get what we already have to work properly.

We pointed out in Chapter 22 that overweight individuals have less than normal ghrelin before eating.[330]

In normal-weight individuals, ghrelin levels drop when food is ingested. In overweight individuals, ghrelin levels stay elevated after food is eaten, leading to excess consumption of food.[331] Overweight individuals have a blunted response to ghrelin working as it should.

Once again, it is an issue of efficiency. Ghrelin loses its normal rhythmic function in overweight individuals. It does this because leptin is too high. As soon as high leptin levels come down, ghrelin goes back into natural balance and normal appetite patterns of ghrelin reappear.[332]

This information means that we can restore natural GH function by lowering leptin and getting it back into natural balance and rhythm.

THE INFLAMMATION CONNECTION

Individuals with serious physical trauma, sepsis, or burn develop GH resistance. Even though they have adequate GH, their bodies tend to go into a wasting pattern. The stress of such issues causes excess amounts of TNFa and IL-6. Researchers have shown that it is these inflammatory markers that bind to GH receptors and turn them off.[333] Inflammation signals have an opposite effect on the secretion of GH compared to ghrelin.

This information has been confirmed in other studies. TNFa is shown to be elevated in sepsis, causing GH resistance and body wasting.[334] Mice that genetically make too much IL-6 have normal or high levels of GH, yet have growth retardation, reflecting the problem of growth hormone resistance. The excess IL-6 production of these mice reduces the GH receptor function of the liver in half.[335]

Patients with fibromyalgia, a painful condition of muscle aching, have a nighttime surge of GH that is only about one-third that of normal.[336]

Patients with cancer and cachexia lose weight and muscle even when they eat, reflecting a condition of GH resistance. Researchers demonstrated that the level of IL-6 predicts the seriousness of the GH resistance and consequent body wasting.[337]

In these serious health conditions, the body is usually in a highly catabolic state with excess cortisol and low levels of leptin. The TNFa and IL-6 are inflammation signals coming from the disease process itself, causing GH resistance by blocking the activity of GHS. This science allows us to understand why obesity causes a depression of GH function.

As we explained in Chapters 6 and 27, extra pounds of fat contain immune cells that generate excessive amounts of TNFa and IL-6. Since excess amounts of these immune messengers cause the disruption of GH, turning them off is part of the key to getting back in balance.

Some of this can be accomplished in the short term. For example, taking fish oils reduces the output of TNFa and IL-6. Nutritional support can be used to help turn down acute inflammatory signals that disrupt GH and natural balance. This opens the door for weight loss, instead of being stuck in a metabolic trap.

Furthermore, as weight is lost, the actual number of fat cells making pro-inflammatory signals go away, resolving the issue of depressed GH.

THE UNIQUE CLA

CLA (conjugated linoleic acid) is a type of fat that naturally occurs in dairy products and meat when cows graze on grass. Grass contains linoleic acid. Enzymes in the digestive system of cows readily convert it to CLA. Most cows involved in our food supply do not graze on grass; therefore, there is not as much CLA in the diet as there used to be.

CLA is one of the most intensely researched nutrients in the world, and has been for the last 20 years ever since researchers at the University of Wisconsin discovered it while looking for carcinogens in cooked meat. Instead, they found a compound that seemed to stop cancer quite readily. They named this nutrient CLA. The potential role of CLA in nutrition is rather impressive with considerable science relating to its ability to reduce cancer, reduce hardening of the arteries, prevent diabetes, and reduce body fat.[338]

CLA is one of the most powerful nutrients known to stop leptin resistance and reduce the inflammatory signals coming out of fat cells. Thus, a person who is overweight has a greater need for CLA. The need is relative to the result of overcoming leptin resistance and shrinking the excess fat.

CLA changes the way the body processes fat and protein, shifting the body away from fat storage,[339] enhancing the formation of body protein,[340] and improving insulin resistance so that muscles more effectively take up calories.[341] CLA helps unclog stuck fat in the liver that blocks normal liver function,[342] a prime place for proper GH activation. These findings indicate that CLA helps GH work properly.

CLA reduces the amount of leptin that is produced by fat cells.[343] CLA can reduce leptin production by as much as 42 percent, and when it does this, it increases the burning of fats as fuel.[344] In essence, CLA and GH have similar effects on fat cells, causing them to shrink.

As CLA lowers leptin, it also lowers the inflammation generating TNFa.[345] In addition to lowering TNFa, CLA also reduces COX_2 and nitric oxide signals coming from the immune cells of the extra fat pounds.[346] As the fat amount shrinks, so does the amount of inflammatory messengers that mess up the body as a whole and depress GH.

CLA is of great assistance in terms of getting GH back on track, reducing leptin resistance, reducing food cravings at night, and speeding up the weight-loss process. Unlike GH therapy, CLA significantly reduces cancer risk and is widely being studied regarding its role in preventing diabetes. Because CLA is a polyunsaturated fatty acid, it is prudent to take CLA with vitamin E so that the CLA is not oxidized in the blood before it has a chance to work on fat cells.

THE IMPORTANCE OF SLEEP AND GH

Since nighttime is the most important time for the largest surge of GH, getting sleep back into natural balance is of primary importance to restore proper GH function.

If an individual has leptin resistance, their leptin and insulin levels will stay too high for too long, including during sleep time. For example, in individuals with insulin resistance, GH is depressed during the early part of sleep.[347] Since GH controls the rate of nighttime repair, this interferes with the general repair functions of the body. As repair does not happen at the rate it should, the fuel needed to carry out repair is not in demand. The normal rise of insulin and glucose in early sleep is blunted.

As morning approaches, the level of cortisol rises in the blood. The purpose of cortisol is to turn on all the light switches in every cell of the body to wake it up and get it ready for the day. In a normal-functioning person, as cortisol begins to rise, it signals the pancreas to stop making insulin, in turn lowering blood glucose and ending the sleep process.

In a person with insulin resistance, the pancreas ignores this signal, causing a person to wake up with higher than normal insulin and glucose levels.[348] If the liver is unable to store and release enough fuel to get through the night due to insulin resistance, the individual may wake up with low-blood sugar. In either case, it means a poor energy level in the morning and being tired and irritable. It is like getting up on the wrong side of the bed. Sleep is not refreshing.

When sleep is out of rhythm, insulin, glucose, leptin, and GH are out of rhythm as well. Insulin and glucose occur in the wrong amounts at the wrong time of the night. The individual wakes up with a poor blood-sugar condition that starts the day on the wrong foot. Therefore, waking up tired and in a bad mood are signs that GH is out of balance with the other hormones that influence energy and repair.

By following the *Five Rules*, leptin and insulin levels are in better balance when entering sleep, and they do not suppress the release of GH. This permits GH to be released at the right time with a normal surge, thus promoting a better condition of natural balance.

THE ALC SOLUTION

It was recently discovered that taking the nutrient ALC (Acetyl-L-Carnitine) before bed can help the hypothalamus gland stimulate the production of GH during sleep.[349] ALC enhances the release of GH as well as prevents hormonal depletion from stress.[350] ALC helps offset the effects of stress that induce sleep problems.

In a landmark study, ALC was found to help get rid of leptin resistance in the brain.[351] ALC can help the brain correctly sense the true amount of leptin, thus overcoming leptin resistance. This is a major discovery and signifies an unquestionable ability of nutrient support to prevent serious health issues by restoring natural balance.

Much of the early research on ALC was done regarding cognitive issues, wherein ALC consistently showed an ability to improve cognitive function, mood, and behavior in difficult situations, even Alzheimer's.[352,353,354,355,356,357] It has been proven effective in serious depression, actually restoring normal stress response and stress tolerance patterns. [358,359,360]

Amazingly, ALC can metabolize stuck cholesterol out of brain cells, thereby helping to return them to more normal and functional brain cells.[361,362,363] A new chain of discoveries shows that ALC can normalize glucose utilization in the brain,[364] thus helping to provide the energy for normal nerve transmission.[365,366]

ALC is a nutrient that acts in the nervous system to promote the return of normal communication between hormones, a key underlying issue at the center of "resistance," regardless of the hormone we are discussing. This includes enabling the brain to answer phone calls from leptin, meaning it helps leptin resistance go away. It also enhances the ability of the brain to make GH at night.

EXERCISE AND GH

We have mentioned in this chapter that GH is released during the day in a pulsing manner. It needs to maintain this "tone of fitness" in order to function properly.

Exercise by itself does not restore GH to youthful levels; however, it is one thing a person can do to help maintain proper daily tone and fitness in the GH system of the body.[367] While any exercise helps, consistent resistance training is the best for promoting healthy GH function.[368,369,370]

SUMMARY

There are no short cuts, quick fixes, surgeries, or drugs that will ever restore normal and natural balance in the GH system.

Current GH therapy, in an effort to replace the seemingly lacking hormone, significantly increases the risk of diabetes and cancer. It is a classic example of the shortcomings of Western medicine evaluation, wherein a lab test shows a bad number on paper and a drug is given to improve the number.

The only way to reverse the trend of declining and ineffective GH is to get the body back in natural balance. Many factors work against GH, including stress and inflammation. A primary factor that blocks GH is excess leptin due to leptin resistance.

By following our *Five Rules*, eating some carbohydrates to ensure ghrelin release, being consistent with strength-building exercise, and sleeping better, a person will improve leptin function and GH function at the same time. Nutrients such as fish oil, CLA, melatonin, and ALC can be used to help this process along, if needed.

Even serious and life-long problems with obesity can be improved by following a consistent path. We have helped countless people who think they have tried everything. Turning to diet drugs or gastric bypass surgery have serious and long-lasting effects on metabolism and overall health. There is a healthy way to solve these issues. It begins with understanding the body and how it is supposed to be working. It continues with the application of what is learned on a consistent basis. Only in this way can a Health Asset Manager™ solve the problems of leptin.

32

Male Hormone Fitness

Testosterone is the primary male hormone, the behavioral essence of a man's competitive drive. Estrogen is the primary female hormone. Men and women have both hormones, and it is the balance of these hormones working properly in harmony with other hormones that is essential for health.

Too much leptin puts the breaks on testosterone. A man suffering from leptin resistance has too much leptin in his circulation forcing down his testosterone. As he gains weight from the problem, especially weight on the lower half of the body, he converts testosterone into estrogen in the fat cells that are accumulating.

Leptin resistance and depressed testosterone are reflected by weight gain around the midsection. Higher estrogen draining testosterone is reflected by weight gain on the buttocks and thighs, the traditional female places for common weight gain. Many men have a combination of both problems.

TESTOSTERONE, LEPTIN, AND AGING

Andropause, the decline of testosterone as aging takes place, is now considered a multi-system disease state.[371] There is nothing "natural" about lacking testosterone. As testosterone declines, so does masculine motivational drive, sex drive, and sexual-performance ability. Furthermore, declining testosterone is related to increased risk for cardiovascular disease.[372,373,374,375,376,377,378]

The general trend of aging in men, even "healthy" men, is increased body fat and body weight and declining testosterone levels. In this context, the term "healthy" implies "free of abnormal disease," but it is far from optimum health. Men with significant andropause problems lose testosterone faster than the agreed upon rate of "normal." Such men have hypogonadism, excess weight in the midsection, and higher leptin levels than normal.[379]

As body fat accumulates, leptin levels increase and testosterone levels decrease.[380] When there is a lack of testosterone, leptin is inappropriately elevated.[381] There are leptin receptors in the testicles of men, meaning that there is intended communication between leptin and the male system. Higher leptin levels tell the male system not to synthesize male hormones.[382] High male hormones suppress leptin levels.[383] Replacing testosterone in lacking men lowers leptin levels.[384]

Leptin communicates to the male hormonal system. Scientists are trying to figure out exactly what it is doing. Some amount of leptin is essential for stimulating the production of male hormones. Too much leptin in the seminal fluid is present in men with infertility.[385]

Leptin controls other hormones. In many situations, the fundamental role of leptin is to permit other hormones to function. Just as the brain senses leptin to determine the allowable metabolic rate, many specific body areas require a certain amount of leptin to permit metabolic function.

It is not surprising that leptin is involved with reproduction in both men and women. Reproduction is one of the most energy intense activities possible. It makes sense that the primary hormone governing the use of energy has an active role in this endeavor.

The idea is not to get rid of leptin, as the proper leptin amount allows correct metabolic function including sex drive and fertility. The idea is to have the right amount of testosterone and leptin in relation to each other.

We have mentioned throughout this book the triad of problems called insulin resistance, leptin resistance, and adrenaline resistance. We have discussed how too much cortisol and not enough GH relates to abdominal weight gain. In the case of men, as aging takes place, the issue of low testosterone is consistent in this picture.[386]

There is low sexual function in any man with these leptin-driven set of problems. Judging by the sales of Viagra, this is quite a few men.

In fact, the problem of low testosterone and high leptin is passed on genetically by parents who have problems, specifically leptin resistance and diabetes. It is proven that first-degree relatives of individuals with diabetes are likely to have this problem of low testosterone and high leptin.

Male children with parents or relatives who are leptin resistant or diabetic are more likely to experience low testosterone and become diabetic due to this problem.[387] This type of hormone problem is not passed along this way to women, only to men. Furthermore, male hormone replacement prevents the problem from evolving, lowers leptin, prevents insulin resistance, and prevents diabetes.[388]

Andropause is not a pretty picture. Serious cases cause loss of sexual function, hypogonadism, heart disease, diabetes, and increased cancer risk. Milder cases see the male system deteriorate more slowly. The pivotal hormone in this picture is testosterone. It is governed by leptin function.

SOLUTIONS FOR LOW TESTOSTERONE

In addition to improving the efficient function of leptin to lose excess weight and enhance testosterone status, another approach is to give nutritional precursors to either help form or help transport testosterone.

Zinc is an important mineral in the formation and transport of testosterone.[389,390] Animal studies show that marginal zinc deficiency can reduce testosterone formation by 40 percent, whereas serious zinc deficiency can reduce it by 60 percent. Furthermore, when male animals go through puberty with zinc deficiency, testosterone expression is depressed and a significant increase in feminizing characteristics takes the place of the proper male traits.[391]

Tribulus Terristrus is an herb that has been used for centuries in India to treat male sexual problems. Animal and human studies show that it raises luteinizing hormone in the brain that in turn stimulates testosterone production in the testes. It increases sexual stamina, sex drive, helps get rid of impotence, and increases ejaculatory volume, sperm concentration, and sperm mobility.[392,393,394,395]

DHEA and androstenedione are testosterone building blocks. There are numerous studies pointing to the benefits of DHEA, including weight loss,[396] immune enhancement,[397] and increased energy and sex drive in men.[398] DHEA acts as a major anti-stress hormone, helping the body to adapt to change more efficiently to offset wear and tear. Additionally, it converts in part to androstenedione. Androstenedione raises testosterone.[399,400,401]

The neurotransmitter dopamine turns out to be a main stimulus to the male sex drive and function.[402] In Chapter 21, we explained that leptin is a key to the dopamine drive system and there needs to be a certain amount of fat in the diet to ensure there is a normal leptin level. Dopamine production is reinforced by the amino acid tyrosine. This shows that a certain amount of leptin in balance with testosterone is essential for male drive.

In addition to lowering leptin, a man can take nutritional support that helps build up testosterone. Combine this with strength training for a good fitness program to reduce leptin, build muscle, improve GH, and enhance the function of testosterone. This approach provides options to improve the amount of testosterone and help offset the declining trend of aging.

THE ANTI-TESTOSTERONES

It is one thing to build up testosterone; it is quite another to maintain test-osterone. There are various factors, both environmental and internal, that create an anti-testosterone situation. Remember that too much leptin is a primary anti-testosterone factor.

There is a natural enzyme in the body called aromatase; it is highly active in white adipose tissue on the lower half of the body. It has an effect on determining the fate of testosterone. In essence, it siphons off testosterone into other activities. Specifically, it converts testosterone into estrogen. This is normal, and a certain amount of this activity is needed for proper male function and drive.

Unfortunately, many men get an excess production of aromatase, a problem that becomes more prevalent as a man grows older and gains lower body weight. This tends to make men stay fat and de-energized, contributing to the loss of male function.[403]

It is normal for fat cells to change some testosterone to estrogen; this is a main reason why women have more fat than men.[404] However, progressive increase in body fat in a man tends to lock in an abnormal level of estrogen production, thus keeping testosterone depressed. This is caused by the activity of the aromatase enzyme inside fat cells. As a man gets heavier, there is more of the aromatase enzyme that is active. The extra pounds of fat are the cause of the problem.

Animal studies demonstrate that blocking the aromatase enzyme reduces the conversion of testosterone to estrogen, thereby leaving the testosterone level higher.[405] This helps correct the lack of male drive associated with too much estrogen coming from the aromatase enzyme.

It sounds like if we could just get rid of the aromatase enzyme and suppress it, men would have more than enough testosterone and all would be well. As is the case with virtually everything in the human body, there is an appropriate amount of aromatase that is needed for proper male sexual function.[406] The problem is the out-of-balance situation caused by extra fat on the buttocks and thighs that excessively convert testosterone to estrogen.

Male mice genetically programmed to make excess aromatase develop female breasts. This issue can be reversed by giving them aromatase inhibitors.[407]

When a man gains weight on his buttocks, there is an increase in aromatase conversion of testosterone to estrogen. This is because there is ten times the amount of aromatase activity in fat cells of the buttocks, compared to fat cells of the abdominal area. Thus, a man gains excess midsection weight due to high leptin, insulin resistance, adrenaline resistance, excess cortisol, lacking GH, and lacking testosterone. He gains weight on his buttocks and thighs due to excess testosterone conversion to estrogen by aromatase.[408] Green tea is a powerful inhibitor of the aromatase enzyme.[409]

Atrazine, the most commonly used herbicide in the U.S. and probably the world, decreased testosterone in male frogs ten fold at a dose exposure common to our current environmental levels. It induced demasculanzing effects in the frogs.[410] It does this by increasing the activity of aromatase. This is a serious issue and serves as the other main reason for increased aromatase activity in men besides extra pounds of fat. Too many chemicals in our environment make men lack testosterone.

CALCIUM FOR MEN

A recent study with old male rats showed that a lack of calcium caused an increase in testicular aromatase activity 2.4 times above normal, resulting in an elevation of estrogen four times normal in their blood.[411]

Additionally, calcium is a solution for men with erectile dysfunction. The main activator in the brain of male sex drive is the melanocortin 4 receptor.[412] When these receptors are activated, penis erectile activity is dramatic. Anything that gets in the way of this receptor in the brain will turn off sexual function.

As it turns out, a primary blocker of this receptor is the agouti gene. Since agouti is easily controlled by adequate calcium intake, getting enough calcium permits the proper nerve signal to flow from the brain and induce an erection. This is good news for men.

Remember that agouti is best friends with neuropeptide Y, the main signal in the brain that makes a person hungry. An excess of NPY directly blocks the function of testosterone.[413]

There are several different pathways in the brain that relate to appetite, especially involving excess consumption of carbohydrates, that block male sexual function. A long-term pattern of excess carbohydrate consumption, reflected by the extra pounds of fat that progressively accumulate and do not go away, takes its toll on male function, sooner or later. Any man who has lost his sex drive and function should lose his sweet tooth and eat fewer carbohydrates.

SUMMARY

Testosterone is an important hormone for proper male function, energetic drive, and cardiovascular health.

Too much leptin depresses testosterone. Not enough leptin causes metabolism to slow down, including male function. Thus, there is a proper amount of leptin that is needed by any man.

Problems occur when hormones are out of balance. Low testosterone is involved with weight gain around the midsection. Higher than normal estrogen causes excess weight on the buttocks and thighs. Many men have both problems.

In addition to balancing hormones and reducing leptin, a man can take steps to build up testosterone and reduce the conversion of testosterone to estrogen. Strength training is the best form of exercise for men to get GH and testosterone to work together to stabilize the male energy base.

When everything heads in the right direction, weight is progressively reduced and male energy is progressively enhanced.

33

Female Hormone Balance

*W*omen have three times the amount of leptin as men; this is normal. Even when body fat differences are adjusted, women still have more leptin than men. In fact, it appears that the amount of testosterone in women is the key factor that separates leptin levels in men and women, not body fat.[414]

The comparative lack of testosterone in women enables a permissive relationship between estrogen and leptin, allowing for a combination of higher circulating leptin, estrogen, and body fat. This not only defines a key difference between men and women, it is essential for reproduction and survival of the human race.

Leptin allows for the accumulation of body fat, enabling energy-demanding events to take place, including puberty, pregnancy, and lactation. Extra amounts of leptin are even produced by the placenta during pregnancy.[415] Leptin is essential for survival, not only for preventing starvation, but also for the reproductive function of women.

When a woman is in a state of natural balance and feeling good, then leptin, estrogen, testosterone, and body fat are in proper amounts and in harmonious function. Puberty occurs at the proper time, and there is no excess weight gain associated with it. Menstrual cycles run without symptoms and are in a regular pattern. Pregnancy is possible, and healthy pregnancy is typical. Transition is not accompanied by extra weight gain before, during, or after. Bone health, heart disease, and breast and female cancer are not issues.

Too much leptin or too little leptin causes serious problems for women. Leptin resistance means that the leptin message is not responded to by the brain or ovaries. This causes serious problems even if a woman is not overweight. Leptin efficiency, leptin timing, and the right amount of leptin are important for the female system to work properly.

LEPTIN AND FEMALE PROBLEMS CAN BEGIN EARLY

Girls who start their menstrual cycle early have leptin problems. They typically have higher body fat and are overweight, causing them to have twice the level of leptin as normal for their age.[416]

This may lead to excess androgen, male hormone production, and polycystic ovarian syndrome in their teens and early twenties.

This leads to at least a 40 percent increased risk of breast cancer, simply because of more estrogenic exposures due to more menstrual cycles in the course of a lifetime.

Girls who begin their menstrual cycles early make estrogen much earlier than they should. However, this problem may quickly shift to low estrogen production in their teens or early twenties.

LEPTIN HELPS REGULATE THE MENSTRUAL CYCLE

In the first half of the menstrual cycle, ovarian follicles are stimulated and an egg is ripened. This happens under the influence of a signal coming from the brain called FSH (follicle stimulating hormone). As the egg ripens, it gives off estrogen. The estrogen enters the general circulation.

When estrogen levels in the blood reach a certain level, the brain knows the egg is ripe. The brain now produces an androgenic signal called LH (luteinizing hormone). New information shows that the rise in estrogen parallels a rise in leptin, and it is the rising leptin that triggers the release of LH.[417] LH stimulates the release of the egg to go down the fallopian tube. The corpus luteum, that was previously holding the egg, now makes progesterone for the second half of the menstrual cycle to help proteins attach to the wall of the uterus in case there is a pregnancy.

If there is no pregnancy, then progesterone production stops and the wall of the uterus is sheathed off, resulting in menstruation. The process repeats itself, generally in a 28-day pattern.

Returning to the story of the leptin-void *ob/ob* mouse; it has great difficulty reproducing. This was the first clue that leptin played a significant role in the menstrual cycle.

We know that there is a normal circle of communication between the brain and the ovaries that involves leptin. Leptin acts as a primary regulator of proper menstrual rhythm. Problems with leptin resistance or the anorexic-like, low-leptin starvation metabolism disrupt the correct function of the menstrual cycle.

LEPTIN PROBLEMS DISRUPT MENSTRUATION

There are leptin receptors on the ovaries. Just as leptin resistance can occur in the brain, it can also occur in the ovaries. In the first half of the menstrual cycle, estrogen production occurs when there is a proper amount of leptin binding to the ovaries. When there is leptin resistance in the ovaries, estrogen is produced incorrectly. This causes higher levels of leptin in the follicular fluid surrounding the ovaries, compared to the levels of leptin in the blood.[418]

In this situation, the ovarian follicles are stimulated but may not fully mature, meaning that an egg does not properly ripen, or it requires much more effort than normal to ripen an egg. Minimally, this causes excess friction in the female system. In more extreme cases, no egg is ripened at all. These problems significantly affect 20 percent of menstruating women.

Once there is leptin resistance in the ovaries, the brain becomes out of balance and starts to produce excess luteinizing hormone.[419] This leads to excess production of male androgens. This causes acne related to menstruation.

If the problem becomes more significant, there is facial hair growth. This can lead to disrupted, irregular, skimpy, or missing menstrual cycles.

Remember that leptin resistance provokes insulin resistance. Insulin resistance aggravates the issue and further magnifies the problem of excess male androgen production.[420]

This is why leptin resistance that triggers early menstruation is such a problem. Excess fat prior to puberty accelerates female development and causes early onset of menstruation. It does this by inappropriately magnifying estrogen production via the aromatase enzyme inside of fat cells. This throws off female hormonal timing in relation to overall lifespan. Since leptin resistance drives this problem, once the menstrual cycle starts, there is a high risk for developing leptin resistance in the ovaries. This may happen right away or it may develop over a period of a few years.

Women who start menstruation later than normal generally have a low-leptin situation or non-obese leptin resistance due to erratic eating patterns or genetic leptin issues passed down from one or both parents. The result is a lack of leptin-driven stimulation to the ovaries, thus female development may be delayed. An extreme example of this is the female gymnast explained in Chapter 28.

POLYCYSTIC OVARIAN SYNDROME (PCOS)

When problems of excess male androgen production are ongoing and significant, there is serious clinical disruption of the menstrual cycle. This is a medical condition known as polycystic ovarian syndrome (PCOS).

Leptin problems cause PCOS. There are two types of PCOS, the obese and non-obese versions.

A fascinating study was conducted with young, normal-weight women with PCOS and those who did not have PCOS. Overnight blood sampling every 20 minutes was done to monitor the levels of leptin, luteinizing hormone, and androgen levels. Because this study was done using women who were not overweight, the general leptin issue was not yet developed to the point of obesity. However, the women had PCOS, reflected by their abnormally light or infrequent menstruation and other symptoms.

In all women, leptin levels were about the same. In healthy women, leptin release lagged behind the release of luteinizing hormone and androgen by about 20 minutes. In PCOS women, this timing relationship was absent.[421] This inability to have proper timing in hormonal rhythms is caused by resistance to the hormonal signals. It means that the ovaries and the brain do not sense leptin correctly, and leptin resistance takes place in the ovaries and possibly in the brain as well.

Insulin resistance and leptin resistance occur in women with PCOS. These issues coincide with abnormally low ghrelin levels.[422] Low ghrelin is reflective of abnormal GH activity in relation to the food that is eaten. Additional studies show that women with PCOS have abnormal GH responses to eating food.

Overweight women with PCOS have a blunted GH response to food. Normal-weight women with PCOS have an exaggerated GH response to eating food.[423] In women who do not have PCOS, GH is depressed in response to eating food. The reason it is elevated prior to food consumption is to help induce a normal hunger signal to eat. Once food is eaten, the proper response is to turn off the GH-related signal to eat food. This does not happen in women with PCOS.

Data on GH levels in overweight women with PCOS shows that their GH level is reduced by 60 percent and there is a 75 percent loss of pulsing rhythm in GH release.[424]

In normal-weight women with PCOS, the GH level is higher than normal in terms of consistent production, but they lack the pulsing rhythm that is seen in normal-weight women without PCOS. This abnormal GH release pattern causes excess LH and androstenedione, the precursor to testosterone, to be elevated in direct relation to the improperly timed release of GH.[425]

The overall level of GH is about half that of normal women.[426] Thus, we see the release of a hormone at the wrong time, in an out-of-balance way. Even though the total amount of hormone is only half that of normal women, the improper timing is enough to fuel excessive production of male androgens.

LEPTIN AND PMS

Estrogen and leptin are directly related to one another. Leptin enables a greater amount of body fat. Fat cells, in turn, can increase the metabolic activity of estrogen. When a woman attains natural balance between leptin and estrogen, there is an unmistakable feeling of smoothness and calm. There is also an ability to maintain normal body weight.

Unlike men, who must have a base level of testosterone drive in order to feel normal, women need a rhythmic balance between leptin and estrogen. When women have this working for them, there is a sense of being at emotional ease and in harmony.

Some women go their entire life and do not feel this way, just as some men never have much drive. Instead of being at ease and in harmony, there is an unsettling internal feeling that is magnified in different phases of the menstrual cycle. There may be a certain number of "good days" per month and then there are the bad days. Even the good days are generally defined as an absence of the uncomfortable feelings, rather than the existence of a sense of being at ease and in a state of harmony. Leptin levels are higher in women experiencing PMS, reflecting the issue of leptin resistance.[427]

Research shows that leptin levels can be raised in the second half of the menstrual cycle by estrogenic stimulation.[428] Overweight women have elevated leptin levels in the second half of their menstrual cycles whereas normal-weight women do not.[429] Thus, women who are overweight have more problems with leptin adversely affecting their menstrual cycles in terms of PMS symptoms. The combination of high leptin and low serotonin set up powerful sugar and carbohydrate cravings prior to menstruation.

LEPTIN, PREGNANCY, AND INFERTILITY

A woman entering childbearing years with leptin resistance may have difficulty getting pregnant. If she does get pregnant, she is at higher risk for miscarriage or complications of pregnancy.

Properly communicating leptin is involved with the correct development of the fetus, in part by its synergistic release of TNFa that may play a role in fetal growth or development. This is a "good" role of TNFa in the right amount at the right time, as opposed to excess TNFa causing inflammation and disease.

When there is too much leptin, there is a risk for high blood pressure. Remember the issue of adrenaline resistance discussed earlier. When adrenaline resistance happens during pregnancy, it causes fluid retention and results in a fairly common and potentially serious medical condition called preeclampsia. This condition is associated with excessively high leptin levels.[430] The excessive production of TNFa due to coexisting high leptin causes insulin resistance during pregnancy and increases the risk for gestational diabetes.[431]

The reason for high leptin levels in the female system is one of leptin resistance in the actual female organs. For example, fertility specialists have demonstrated that in-vitro fertilization is not likely to work in the presence of high leptin, indicating a clear leptin resistance preventing pregnancy from occurring.[432]

These findings are consistent with other research showing that leptin in fluids reflecting ovarian status were high, even though blood levels were normal in unexplained fertility. There is a female organ leptin resistance that is central to the problem of infertility.[433]

In fact, a certain amount of leptin must exist, along with estrogen, in order for pregnancy to begin. If there is a lack of leptin, then a woman may not get pregnant. If she does, there is a much higher likelihood of a miscarriage.[434]

LEPTIN AND ENDOMETRIOSIS

High leptin due to leptin resistance has a tendency to promote high estrogen compared to a relative lack of progesterone in the second half of the menstrual cycle. Warning signs of excess estrogen include heavy blood flow, frequent periods, breast swelling/tenderness, and PMS. This problem may lead to abnormal cell proliferation such as endometriosis. It can also set the stage for estrogenic stimulated cancer.

There are leptin receptors on the wall of the female endometrium,[435] meaning that leptin has a direct method of communicating to this tissue.

In a study comparing a group of women with various degrees of endometriosis to a control group, women with endometriosis had significantly higher leptin levels than women without it.

Furthermore, the high leptin levels correlated with inflammatory markers and were highest at the onset of the problem compared to end stage disease. Excessive inflammation caused by too much leptin is likely a causative factor in endometriosis.[436]

These findings have been confirmed by a more recent study showing that leptin is highly active in endometriosis and likely a major factor causing it to proliferate.[437] In Chapter 44, we discuss the breast-cancer risks associated with high leptin triggering excess TNFa and its companion, NF kappaB. At this point, it is worth noting that excess NF kappaB is the key elevated signal that causes endometriosis.[438]

THE POWER OF LEPTIN

The female hormonal system requires a tremendous amount of energy to run normally. The week prior to a menstrual cycle, during which time a significant amount of protein is placed on the wall of the uterus in case of pregnancy, is the equivalent of eight hours of construction work per day, on top of whatever else the woman does.

If there is a lack of energy for any reason, it shows up at this time of the month. The primary hormone in the human body that regulates energy use is leptin. Leptin allows the use of energy to go forward in the female hormonal system. Women with leptin resistance have impaired energy regulation.

Likewise, women with the anorexic-like starvation metabolism do not have enough leptin to allow normal energy expenditure to run their menstrual cycles.

In addition to allowing a proper energy level and metabolic rate, leptin is involved with governing the female hormonal system. Leptin resistance signifies a breakdown in communication between the brain, ovaries, and other female organs.

SUMMARY AND SOLUTIONS

Every health principle in this book, especially the *Five Rules*, consistent and refreshing exercise, and quality of sleep form the core health program for any woman. This lifestyle serves as a foundation for solving the cause of the numerous female problems discussed in this chapter and promotes natural rhythm and balance in all hormones in the body, including female hormones.

Any nutrient recommendation given in this book, such as higher essential fatty acids and calcium, is relevant to supporting female health as these recommendations support improved leptin communication and leptin function.

For example, acetyl-l-carnitine (ALC) enhances the correct rhythmic release of growth hormone as well as prevents hormonal depletion from stress.[439] Major female hormonal improvement was noted in women with missing menstrual cycles who took ALC.[440] ALC works by restoring proper communication of leptin, thus helping to resolve leptin resistance.[441]

Anything done to support more natural rhythms and function in any hormonal system, such as the ability to tolerate stress more efficiently, has a synergistic benefit on female hormones.

Trying to manipulate female hormones with drugs is a testament to the lack of skill of the general medical profession in solving common issues facing well over 50 percent of women.

For example, many physicians prescribe birth-control pills to stop menstrual symptoms. This approach provides a steady state of external hormones that override natural function. They may spare a woman the turmoil of experiencing how out of balance her menstrual cycle is, but they are far from anything resembling an actual solution.

Similarly, antidepressants are the "gold standard" for treating PMS.[442] It is easy to see that serotonin levels are low in women with PMS, reflecting a symptom of the problem of leptin issues. It is a sad commentary on the skill level of the medical profession when they think they are solving PMS by giving an SSRI medication.

While such symptom suppression may make a woman feel better for a while, SSRI medications frequently have weight gain as a side effect.[443] Another common side effect is sexual dysfunction, hardly a desirable result in correcting female hormone issues.[444] These medications are known to override body rhythms and can induce sleep disorders.[445,446]

If a medication causes weight gain, induces sexual dysfunction, and throws the body out of rhythm, it can hardly be considered a proper solution for the cause of PMS. The short-term symptom suppression does not address the cause of the problem, and may in fact make the cause of the problem worse.

Even naturally oriented health-care practitioners may make the mistake of focusing on hormone manipulation of the menstrual cycle. This can involve natural hormone support or various herbs that are known to help hormonal regulation. This strategy may have some value, but it is only symptom management if the underlying issue of leptin resistance or lacking leptin is not worked on and solved.

Regardless of whatever strategy a woman uses to help manage her hormonal symptoms, she should have her eye on changing the true cause of the problem. Invariably, hormonal symptoms have some aspect of leptin problems as a primary cause.

34

The Estrogen Confusion

*T*he recent development in the medical world of taking women off conjugated estrogens derived from horse urine leaves many women of transition age in a quandary about the subject of estrogen replacement. This type of estrogen drug, in combination with synthetic progesterone, was found to cause more disease than they were able to prevent.[447]

These problems have been obvious for many years. Western medicine was in denial of the dangers of the medications they were using. In fact, the only reason the problem came to light was because a drug company was funding a study to prove these drugs helped heart disease. It was quite a shock to them when the study data came back proving the opposite.

Many women are confused about the subject of estrogen and the appropriate use of it in the context of an overall health program, for women at any age.

THE THREE TYPES OF ESTROGEN
There are three primary types of estrogen:

1) **Estradiol (E2)** - Estrogen made in the ovaries and is the primary type produced during the menstrual cycle. It is the type of estrogen that was given in the above study as estrogen replacement therapy, the study that demonstrated an increase risk of life-threatening disease from its use.

2) **Estrone (E1)** - Estrogen made mostly in fat cells under the influence of aromatase enzyme. The body can convert estrone to estradiol.

3) **Estriol (E3)** - The protective estrogen. It is made in the ovaries and by conversion of adrenal hormone precursors. The placenta makes significant amounts during pregnancy to protect the developing baby. The

body does not convert estradiol or estrone into estriol. The body only slightly ever makes estriol into estrone or estradiol; it is not a primary or common metabolic path.

The general medical profession considerably misunderstands estriol calling it a "weak estrogen." It got this name because it has a very slight effect on stimulating the growth of the endometrium. In this regard, estradiol (E2) is 80 times more potent than estriol. Estrone (E1) is seven times more potent than estriol. This perceived potency or strength value is more reflective of potential risk, meaning that estradiol or estrone are more likely to cause inappropriate stimulation of estrogen receptive tissue (breast, cervix, uterus) leading to abnormal growths or cancer.

THE VALUE OF ESTRIOL

There have been several lone voices in the main medical journals pointing out the value of estriol over the years.[448] As far back as 1966, the *Journal of the American Medical Association* published research that showed women with breast cancer had much less estriol than women without breast cancer.[449] New interest in estriol research is fueled by the proven dangers of estradiol and estrone replacement therapy.

Recent discoveries shed light on the essential value of maintaining a proper level of estriol as an important aspect of healthy aging, a topic we discuss more in depth in our next chapter. This new science reshapes the way we think about hormones.

Estriol is the primary estrogen made during pregnancy. Its role during pregnancy is to act as a powerful antioxidant to protect the nervous system of the fetus.[450] A low level of estriol places a woman more at risk for postpartum depression.[451] Other female hormones, such as estradiol or progesterone, were not predictive of this problem; thus, estriol is a protective hormone in the female system. We pointed out that the condition of high blood pressure during pregnancy is caused by leptin resistance. In severe cases, there is a lack of protective estriol.[452]

Higher levels of estriol are protective against MS,[453] whereas higher estradiol may actually promote MS. Treating women who have MS with 8 mg of estriol per day, a dose similar to pregnancy levels, significantly reduces the problems of MS.[454]   Researchers find that brain imaging shows significantly fewer brain lesions while women are on estriol. When estriol was stopped, brain lesions increased. When estriol was resumed, brain lesions went away again. Thus, the lack of estriol is a major finding relating to autoimmune disease. As we mentioned in Chapter 28, leptin resistance is also a primary cause of autoimmune disease.

There is a synergistic relationship between the proper amount of leptin and estriol, both have a protective role in the brain and the female system. During leptin resistance, brain and/or ovarian levels of leptin drop. If estriol levels also drop, there are major problems. If leptin levels and estriol levels reinforce each other in a supportive role, then both the brain and female organs are offered major protection.

Women that have seizures prior to menstruation have lower levels of estriol, whereas women who have seizures at any time of the month have lower estriol and lower progesterone.[455]

The by-products of an AIDS infection can be neurotoxic. Not only does estriol protect brain cells from such toxicity, it is the most important form of estrogen in terms of protecting brain cells from calcium displacement (which causes natural balance in the brain cells to be disrupted).[456]

Another interesting study found that estriol was able to stop toxin-induced injury to brain cells, acting as an antioxidant in the brain, almost twice as effectively as estradiol.[457]   This study showed that estriol protects dopamine receptors, the same type of receptors that are protected by leptin.

This makes it clear that estriol is the estrogen of choice for protecting the brain, and in this regard, is much more powerful than estradiol. In this case, it is the estradiol that has a "weak effect." New science is turning the tables on our previous definition of weak estrogen.

ESTRIOL AND OVARIAN FUNCTION

In an interesting study, it was discovered that estriol maintains a constant level inside of ovarian follicles.[458] This is much different than estradiol, which rises and falls as eggs ripen in the follicles. It has been known since 1993 that estriol protects the ovaries from developing PCOS.[459]   As we mentioned in the previous chapter, PCOS, and varying degrees of it, is a major problem for many women. Estriol acts as a protective buffer so that the female system can run without the symptoms of PCOS.

Thus, a sign that estriol is lacking is any degree of PCOS, such as hormonal-related acne. Using estriol from days 3-14 and possibly longer in the menstrual cycle, in the dose of 2 mg per day, is helpful at stabilizing this problem.

Using natural micronized progesterone in the second half of the menstrual cycle can help improve symptoms of PMS or estrogen excess.[460,461,462] Medical researchers like to say that the results of using progesterone to improve PMS are statistically significant but not clinically important.[463] They say this so they can justify using SSRI medication, which has a higher degree of symptom suppression, but numerous adverse side effects that may make the problem worse.

To the contrary, our personal use of micronized progesterone with hundreds of women over a 15-year period shows it to be quite helpful much of the time. However, progesterone can easily be converted into stress-fighting hormones, a main reason why it is lacking in the first place. Thus, women get the most benefit from using progesterone in combination with an overall hormone-balancing program.

FERTILITY ISSUES AND PROBLEMS IN CHILDREN

Many women with leptin issues and some level of PCOS have trouble getting pregnant. In some cases they happen to become pregnant by chance, although it is harder than normal. In other cases they turn to fertility specialists to help them get pregnant.

A healthy pregnancy is based on properly communicating leptin and estriol. The placenta makes extra amounts of both of these hormones during pregnancy to protect the nervous system of the developing fetus. It is likely that proper function of these hormones during pregnancy provides stability and protection in a child's nervous system after delivery.

It has been our observation in working with children who have autism or Tourette's Syndrome that mothers frequently had issues with fertility, leptin resistance, and/or PCOS. This is not 100% of the time, as the placenta can make these hormones during pregnancy. However, if a pregnancy is not going smoothly it is common that there is a deficiency of these important protective hormones.

Children born under such circumstances have a higher risk for being neurologically adversely affected by chemicals in food, air pollution, toxins from any infection – especially low grade ongoing GI tract infections, and immunizations. A focus of helping such children is protecting their brain with adequate antioxidants, as well as minimizing the exposure to potential irritants.

A focus of helping a mother who is pregnant and has this risk pattern is ensuring there is proper estriol and leptin levels to sustain a healthy pregnancy, both to help the mother during pregnancy as well as to help protect against developing neurologic problems in the child.

This information also places emphasis on a mother having a lack of leptin resistance, PCOS symptoms, and a smooth running menstrual cycle before conceiving. Every effort should be undertaken to sort this out naturally before becoming pregnant. Caution and care should be taken if using medical fertility assistance, as it is essential to maintain proper hormone balance during pregnancy to offer the best chance of a healthy life to one's child.

SUMMARY

Natural balance in the female hormonal system requires an adequate amount of leptin that is efficiently communicating. Not enough leptin or leptin resistance pose major problems to female hormone function.

Estriol and micronized progesterone are useful hormonal support to help balance symptoms in the female system. These are body identical hormones derived from natural sources. They need to be used in conjunction with proper leptin management to ensure a true resolution of any problem.

Once leptin is properly balanced, especially in younger women, additional hormone support may no longer be needed. This is because the female hormonal system is back in natural balance.

As transition approaches, natural hormonal support can help ease the symptoms of transition. It is especially important to have an effective stress-management and leptin-management program in place; otherwise, no level of natural hormone support may stop out-of-balance transition symptoms.

35

Menopausal Weight Gain

*A*s a woman enters her forties, her estrogen levels rise. This is because the brain does not sense when an egg is ripe as well as it did when she was younger. These higher estrogen levels increase leptin production and make a woman more prone to gain weight in her forties, even if she did not have a weight problem before. In mild cases, it is only 5-10 pounds, but it does not respond to previous strategies she used to manage her weight.

A recent study comparing fat metabolism in healthy pregnant women, healthy pre-menopausal women, and healthy postmenopausal women showed that pre-menopause and pregnancy were significant high times for fat storage. There was a reduced ability to burn fat as fuel, directly related to the higher estrogen at these times. By comparison, postmenopausal women had an increased ability to burn fat but had higher insulin levels.[464]

This explains why women gain weight before menopause; higher estrogen leading to higher leptin.[465] But why do many women gain weight after menopause? The answer is leptin resistance.

LEPTIN RESISTANCE AND TRANSITION

The drop in estrogen in the female system creates a communication breakdown between leptin and estrogen. The natural rhythm and pattern of estrogen and leptin are disturbed.

Animal experiments show that the drop in estrogen causes leptin resistance in the brain, with an increase in neuropeptide Y.[466] Leptin resistance may develop as a result of a drop in estrogen, a contributing factor in the cause of weight gain in postmenopausal women. Since NPY also goes up, hunger is more common and more carbohydrates are eaten. During a hot flash, NPY is elevated by 34 percent.[467] A high level of calcium is not only helpful for bones, it also helps turn off hot flashes by lowering agouti that in turn lowers NPY.

In a study comparing pre-menopausal and postmenopausal women, it was found that postmenopausal women are more likely to gain weight in their abdominal area, as compared to the hips and buttocks, which are typical estrogen weight-gain areas.[468] The drop in estrogen causes a relative male androgen excess, even if blood levels of testosterone are low, thereby promoting weight gain around the stomach.

After transition, both leptin and estrogen levels drop.[469] Seemingly, this should help weight loss. However, leptin resistance increases due to a concurrent increase in insulin resistance. Even though there is less leptin, it does not work as well in the absence of its friend, estrogen. The degree of this abdominal weight gain in postmenopausal women is reflective of the level of leptin and insulin resistance.[470]

IL-6, the inflammatory messenger that disrupts hormone balance, is significantly higher in postmenopausal women.[471] Its partner in crime, TNFa, is also elevated in specific white blood cells. As estrogen drops, these immune cells start to hyper secrete TNFa, posing a specific risk of inflammatory driven bone loss.[472]

Once again we see the pattern of leptin resistance, insulin resistance, and inflammatory immune signals fueling the weight gain problem after transition.[473]

PREPARING FOR TRANSITION

How smoothly a woman handles transition depends on her overall level of physical fitness, her pre-existing body fat when entering her forties, her stress level, and her hormonal history.

In general, estrogen levels rise during her forties and leptin levels go up in response. If she is already leptin resistant and overweight, it is likely there will be a significant struggle with weight during this time. A woman who enters her forties with normal body weight will still struggle with these issues, typically showing up as a problem with 5-15 pounds of extra weight that had not been a problem before.

Both weight gain prior to menopause and after menopause are caused by leptin resistance. Prior to menopause there is an increase in estrogen that helps fuel the weight gain. As estrogen drops there is relatively more andro-gen, causing weight gain around the midsection. This basic pattern has many variables for any woman, based on her personal history with leptin, body weight, female hormones, and stress.

A woman who takes good care of herself for the 15 years prior to transi-tion will have much less trouble before, during, and after transition. The ability to stay fit, eat well, manage stress, and maintain a state of natural rhythm and balance are the cornerstones of health.

SOLUTIONS FOR MENOPAUSAL WEIGHT GAIN

In Chapter 27, we discussed the approach to solving weight gain around the midsection. We discussed the importance of essential fatty acids, pantethine, and calcium. In Chapter 31, we talked about CLA and Acetyl-L-Carnitine, two additional useful nutrients for weight loss. These nutrients are especially helpful in seeking to improve weight gain relating to transition, primarily an increase in abdominal weight.

As the issue of menopause is about changing levels of female hormones, especially a drop in estrogen with a correspondingly higher level of "male" hormones, it is important to know that estriol is a safe and effective way of naturally supporting hormone estrogen balance. This is much different than the dangerous form of estrogen, estradiol. These differences were explained in the previous chapter.

We have already pointed out in this chapter that leptin resistance is the key problem of postmenopause, with a relative higher level of "male" hor-mones due to the drop in estrogen. Keep in mind that this issue is not accurately reflected on blood or saliva tests for hormones. It is common that a post-menopausal woman will get such tests back and they will show low testosterone. However, testosterone is relatively higher than estrogen and there is resistance in the hormones working efficiently. If a woman takes testosterone to prop up her test scores, she will just get facial hair growth and more stomach fat, and may not experience any improvement at all in energy level, regardless of what lab tests say.

As we also pointed out in the previous chapter, a lack of estriol coexists with problems of leptin resistance. As we pointed out in this chapter, transition-related weight gain is primarily an issue of leptin resistance that happens as estrogen levels drop. It is logical to conclude that estriol is a supportive estrogen to help maintain proper body weight during and following transition, safely restoring a better harmony between estrogen and testosterone.

There is additional information to support this view. We know from the information presented in this book that there is greatly increased cardiovascular risk for any person who has leptin resistance. By comparison, estriol was recently proven to reduce atherosclerosis.[474] Furthermore, estriol levels are higher in healthy older women over age 85. Estriol specifically enhances circulation.[475] This indicates there is a lack of cardiovascular problems in women who have adequate estriol, meaning there is a lack of evidence for adrenaline resistance.

Estriol supplementation given to postmenopausal women causes a significant decrease in triglycerides, indicating improved function of insulin and fat transport throughout the body. Since insulin resistance is a key part of the postmenopausal weight gain, estriol helps this issue as well.

Estriol is proven to prevent a rise in total cholesterol.[476] On the other hand, conjugated estrogens containing estradiol, the type of estrogen that is dangerous to use for estrogen replacement, can lower cholesterol but they raise triglycerides, indicating that they make the overall metabolism of fat less efficient.

Only estriol has scientific data to support a favorable relationship in terms of helping to prevent leptin resistance, adrenaline resistance, and insulin resistance. Since the stress of menopause is a drop in estrogen with a relative increase of androgen, estriol is the estrogen of choice to help keep hormones in balance.

OTHER POSTMENOPAUSAL BENEFITS OF ESTRIOL

Additional benefits include that estriol can restore bone density in older women.[477] Estriol can also help relieve urinary incontinence and urinary tract infection.[478,479,480] It can return vaginal flora to normal in postmenopausal women, thus getting rid of itching and other problems of abnormal discharge.[481,482]

Because estriol binds tightly to vaginal estrogen receptors, it can have a significant impact on correcting vaginal dryness and thinning of the vaginal wall. One study showed a complete resolution of vaginal atrophy in 80 percent of women within four months of estriol use.[483] Another study demonstrated significant improvement in vaginal dryness and atrophy.[484]

In addition, estriol can significantly help improve the symptoms of transition, including hot flashes.[485]

ESTRIOL SAFETY, CANCER-RISK REDUCTION

A recent study with estriol and 241 postmenopausal women (125 taking estriol, 116 controls) found: "No clinically relevant difference between the endometrium status of postmenopausal women on long-term oral estriol therapy and untreated controls. This trial supports the endometrial safety of maintenance treatment with oral estriol."[486]

In a study comparing the now infamous estradiol with estriol, breast density was measured by mammography. The estradiol group had a 40 percent increase in breast tissue density, a result that alarmed the researchers. Estriol had only a 6 percent increase.[487]

In another study with 53 postmenopausal women taking 2 mg estriol daily for one year, there was a satisfaction rating of 83 percent to 95 percent that included reduction of symptoms. The results also showed "Histological evaluation of the endometrium in all women of Group I and ultrasound assessment of the breasts following 12 months of estriol treatment found normal results in all women. Therefore, estriol appeared to be safe and effective in relieving symptoms of menopausal women."[488]

Estradiol, the dangerous form of estrogen replacement, is shown to magnify the effect of a toxin to promote ovarian cancer, whereas estriol actually reduces the activity of the toxin and prevents cancer.[489] Several animal studies show the ability of estriol to inhibit breast cancer, even when breast tissue is exposed to known carcinogens.[490,491] Estriol binds to estrogen receptors in breast tissue, thus reducing excess amounts of stimulative estrone and estradiol from binding to the same receptors.[492]

In a groundbreaking study, estriol was found to work by down regulating NF kappaB.[493] Researchers were actually looking into why estriol helps multiple sclerosis. This unexpected discovery is of major importance, as excess NF kappaB is the prime cause of virtually all types of cancer, including female cancers, as we explain in Chapter 44. The bottom line is that adequate estriol may be a key component of any woman's cancer risk-reduction plan.

Estrone and estradiol produce estrogen sulfates that in excess cause cancer. This effect of estrogen sulfates can be blocked by progesterone, which is one reason why natural progesterone is also helpful to women.[494] Not only is this therapy effective, it is safe, as demonstrated in a large trial with over 900 women.[495]

SUMMARY

The evidence shows that estriol is the core estrogen of immense importance to maintaining health in any woman. Not only is estriol safe and effective for a variety of age-associated female complaints, it appears to be a key hormone that can help prevent leptin resistance and abdominal weight gain in post-menopausal years.

It may also be the case that women who do not have leptin resistance and do not have abdominal weight gain have been able to naturally maintain a higher level of estriol. For those who have not been as fortunate, estriol supplementation is a definite option.

Any support of female hormones works best with other hormones in a better state of natural balance. Thus, a woman who learns and applies the leptin managing skills of a Health Asset Manager™ will have an easier time keeping female hormones and health intact as she grows older.

36

Thyroid Problems Finally Resolved

*T*he liver is the metabolic factory of the human body; it is safe to consider it the brain of the physical body. Metabolic rate is largely determined by the rate of activity of the liver. Thyroid hormone, by comparison, is like a gas pedal on metabolism. The liver is the engine. Leptin is in charge of both of them because the brain tells the liver and thyroid what metabolic rate to employ based on the brain's perception of leptin (Figure 11).

Many individuals have the symptoms of hypothyroid function yet the thyroid lab tests come back normal. When it is understood that leptin is in control of the metabolic rate via the liver, it is logical to assume that thyroid hormones play a secondary role in overall body metabolic rate. We have already explained that if the body thinks it is starving, whether this perception is correct or not, then the metabolic rate slows down for the purpose of survival.

Research relating to thyroid function and leptin shows that thyroid hormones are not in control of leptin levels. It is true that leptin levels are higher in obese, hypothyroid individuals, but it was not the hypothyroid state that caused the levels to be higher.[496] These observations are confirmed by multiple studies,[497,498] and lead to the conclusion that any thyroid hormone impact on leptin levels is secondary or of minor importance.[499] This data means that thyroid problems do not cause leptin problems.

What is evident in these studies with thyroid hormone and leptin is that it is the percentage of body fat that determines the amount of leptin.[500] It is the combination of insulin resistance and high body fat that is the main factor associated with high leptin.[501] Leptin exists as a primary regulator of metabolic rate. When leptin resistance occurs, the body thinks it is starving

Normal Metabolic Rate & Thyroid Function

Figure 11

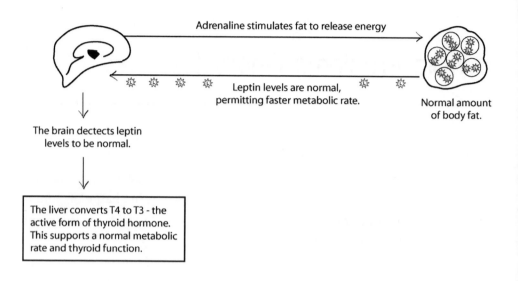

Adrenaline stimulates fat to release energy

Leptin levels are normal, permitting faster metabolic rate.

The brain dectects leptin levels to be normal.

Normal amount of body fat.

The liver converts T4 to T3 - the active form of thyroid hormone. This supports a normal metabolic rate and thyroid function.

Abnormal Metabolic Rate & Poor Thyroid Function Figure 12

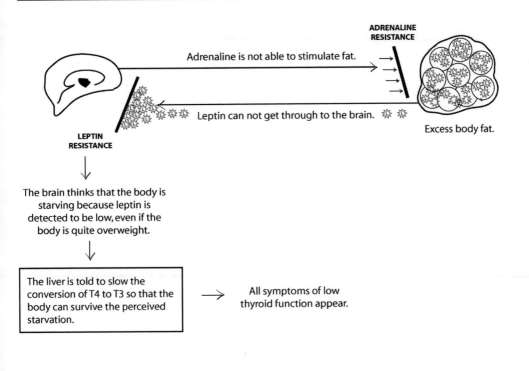

ADRENALINE RESISTANCE

Adrenaline is not able to stimulate fat.

LEPTIN RESISTANCE

Leptin can not get through to the brain.

Excess body fat.

The brain thinks that the body is starving because leptin is detected to be low, even if the body is quite overweight.

The liver is told to slow the conversion of T4 to T3 so that the body can survive the perceived starvation.

All symptoms of low thyroid function appear.

even though there is plenty of fat on hand. The liver stops converting thyroid hormone into active thyroid hormone because of the leptin-resistance issue, the true cause of the seeming thyroid problem (Figure 12).

LEPTIN CONTROLS THYROID HORMONE ACTIVATION

T3 is active thyroid hormone. Normally, most T3 is made in the liver, which converts T4, the hormone made by the thyroid gland, to T3, the metabolically active form of the hormone. When the liver is told a starvation situation exists, it slows down metabolism by reducing the production of T3. Researchers have shown an inverse relation between T3 and leptin.[502] This proves that the liver is in control of metabolic rate as a primary role.

It also means that the huge numbers of individuals suffering from hypothyroid symptoms suffer from leptin resistance and sluggish liver function, following the instructions of the subconscious brain that unfortunately perceives the situation incorrectly.

It is interesting to note that T4 to T3 conversion works differently in the brain. Whereas the liver handles the majority of T4 to T3 conversion for the body, the brain is under its own control. Every cell in the brain can convert T4 to T3.

If the individual is in a starvation situation, the liver metabolic rate slows down to save nutrition for the body. However, if the brain slows down too much, the person cannot function. Thus, the brain activates its own thyroid hormone independent of the liver so that the brain can keep a higher level of metabolic function during times of food deprivation.

This also explains a common, adverse, and now recognizably serious problem with thyroid medication. Blood levels of thyroid hormone are reflective of overall body metabolism and not brain metabolism. Even a person with clinically definable low thyroid is likely suffering from primary leptin issues.

If a person takes too much replacement thyroid hormone in an effort to get "blood scores into better range," adverse effects may occur in the brain long before blood scores begin to look normal. If a person takes more hormone than the brain needs, the head feels heavy and out of sync, literally creating a worse hypothyroid problem in the brain.

We bring this up because the common behavior of endocrinologists is to continue raising the dose of thyroid hormone until the numbers look good on paper. The fact is, they are not even looking at numbers that mean anything as far as how one's head feels or how one's actual liver-driven metabolism works. If leptin resistance can be corrected, thyroid problems will likely go away. Leptin is the boss, and thyroid answers to it.

STRESS AND THYROID PROBLEMS

There are two other main variables that get in the way of metabolic rate, stress and toxic waste.

Stress causes internal friction and inflammation, causing body tissue to become "hot." This is why ice is applied to an injury. However, in the case of stress wear and tear, the heat is all around in the body as multiple tissue areas have "micro injuries" that generate heat. This type of heat comes from inflammation, not as a by-product of normal metabolic energy production.

In the case of metabolic symptoms, it is like having a sprained metabolism. If metabolism tries to keep up a normal pace, then further overheating and damage occurs, just like running on a badly sprained ankle.

Instead of leptin resistance slowing down metabolism, this is a case of stress overload slowing down metabolism. The conversion of T4 to T3 by the liver is slowed down by high stress.[503,504,505,506] This is a natural defense mechanism against burning up.

Thyroid lab scores may or may not be low, but the typical symptoms of hypothyroid are present. If a person takes thyroid medication to force their body to go faster, the result can be harmful to health. This problem is even recognized in the medical literature. A recent study warns doctors not to give thyroid hormone to seriously ill patients, even if their thyroid lab scores are low, as significant problems can easily result.[507]

TOXINS AND THYROID PROBLEMS

Another major contributor to poor metabolism is the increase in environmental pollution. It is known that environmental pollution aggravates thyroid problems.[508,509,510,511,512]

Troublesome levels of pollution exist across the United States in groundwater.[513] Rodents eating contaminated fish from the Great Lakes region had significant adverse thyroid problems, even at lower doses of exposure than studied in most toxicology testing.[514]

Nitrates can interfere with thyroid function.[515] Thyroid function is deregulated by radiation exposure.[516] Infants can have impaired thyroid function from second-hand cigarette smoke from their parents.[517]

The most recent major study in this area, conducted in Canada, confirmed the serious thyroid problem from typical pollutants containing a variety of contaminants and heavy metals.[518] Not only do these pollutants disrupt thyroid function, they have a major impact on disrupting brain function.[519]

This constant burden of excess chemical pollution poses an ongoing metabolic challenge for any person. If the body cannot keep up with elimination of the toxins, then they are sure to overload metabolism and cause metabolism to slow down. It is like pouring sand into the gas tank of a car. It does not matter if the car is old or new, when the engine gets clogged, it will not run correctly. The liver must clear all such chemicals.

When the liver cannot keep up, there is a backlog of toxins in the blood. A person feels poisoned, fatigued, irritable, and has dark circles under their eyes. The lymph system gets backed up causing stiff upper shoulders, head pressures, excess mucous, and numb arms, especially when sleeping. These are plumbing problems indicating an overload of waste products. Such individuals eventually become sensitive to environmental chemicals and/or have been diagnosed with fibromyalgia.

It has been our consistent clinical experience that individuals with the most severe collection of hypothyroid symptoms also have the most toxic symptoms. This makes weight loss even more complex, as the body frequently tries to get extra toxins out of circulation by stuffing them into fat. Thus, a toxic person has great difficulty losing weight because the body does not want to give up the toxins stored in fat as doing so will re-expose the person to the chemicals. The liver, lymphatic, and bowel elimination systems must be improved so that toxins can be more efficiently eliminated, the constraint on metabolism can be removed, and weight loss can occur.

High levels of leptin, as are present in the leptin-resistant situation, induce liver damage.[520] Even more alarming, these high-leptin situations magnify the potential damage to the liver done by toxins.[521]

This is a significant reason why a combination of extra fat and environmental pollution is involved with the diseases associated with obesity. It is a major Catch-22 that must be solved. While an individual can certainly support detoxification and enhance thyroid function, the primary solution is to master leptin and overcome leptin resistance.

SUMMARY

The symptoms of hypothyroid are common in any person who is overweight and not feeling well. These issues are magnified by stress and chemical environmental pollution.

The primary cause of the problem is leptin resistance that forces the body into an inappropriate hibernation state. Fixing leptin resistance fixes the source of the problem.

If the problem is not fixed, then health deteriorates because the ability to tolerate emotional or physical stress is reduced, leading to accelerated wear and tear from common stress. Furthermore, the high levels of leptin magnify the damage caused by environmental pollution, that in and of itself is another primary burden to thyroid metabolism.

We have found that individuals with the most hypothyroid symptoms also have the most difficulty with chemical sensitivity and general "toxic symptoms," eventually resulting in fibromyalgia.

Since it is virtually impossible to escape environmental pollution, and stress may or may not be able to be reduced, the one ticket to health is resolving leptin resistance. Mastering leptin is the key to improving thyroid function, restoring metabolism, and being more able to withstand the stress factors in our lives and the environment.

Understanding that leptin resistance is the true cause of virtually all hypothyroid symptoms is a major advancement in our understanding of metabolism.

In Chapter 38, we give additional information on thyroid hormone function in the context of weight-loss plateaus and how to get out of a stuck starvation metabolic problem.

37

Solving Fibromyalgia; Is Your Metabolism Worn Out or Clogged?

*U*p to this point of this book, we have discussed the role of various hormones and placed them in the overall view of leptin management. The major reason for understanding any individual hormone is to help it work better. As each hormone works more efficiently, then all hormones as a group work in improved harmony. This enables an improved condition of natural balance.

There are many shades of gray between optimum health and a diseased state. We have explained how failing to manage leptin results in progressive problems with body weight, insulin resistance, inflammation, hormone issues, and so on. There are many levels of less efficient function heading from optimum fuel regulation towards type II diabetes.

A key indicator a person is heading for trouble is problems with leptin. This can be a problem of leptin resistance leading to obesity or a problem of a lack of leptin causing anorexic-like starvation metabolism. Since proper leptin function permits other hormones in the body to work properly, it is fundamental to health.

A person who is overweight is likely to have other hormonal problems, as being overweight is reflective of a lack of proper hormone balance thus setting the stage for progressive decline. However, normal-weight or underweight individuals can easily have trouble with hormones, including inefficient function of leptin.

Fibromyalgia is a problem in the hormonal balance system that is quite serious. In terms of natural balance, significant fibromyalgia is reflective of worn out metabolism. Any person who struggles with any hormone imbalance is more at risk for developing fibromyalgia.

The key defining symptom of fibromyalgia is body pain, particularly in the muscles. This leads to disrupted sleep and consequent fatigue.[522] The more intense the pain, the worse the sleep, and the more severe the case of fibromyalgia.

Every person knows how fibromyalgia feels. It is like having a nasty flu bug. The body feels as if it has been run over by a truck. Now imagine feeling that way without having the flu. There are varying degrees of fibromyalgia. There is always some level of abnormal pain, disrupted sleep, and increased fatigue.

Similarly, individuals with leptin resistance have some level of disrupted sleep and abnormal fatigue. Progression into fibromyalgia is simply adding pain to this equation. The best way to avoid getting stuck in the chronic pain of fibromyalgia is to master leptin. The tools of mastering leptin are also the way out of the fibromyalgia rut.

WESTERN MEDICINE IS OF LIMITED VALUE

The medical approach for fibromyalgia treatment is to modulate pain where possible and hope for improvement in other issues because pain is lessened. The use of tricyclic antidepressants such as amitriptyline and SSRI antidepressants are the common medical treatment specifically for pain.[523] This approach has a degree of workability since lowering pain improves sleep and helps fatigue.

This bandage approach of using pain-related medications to improve quality of life has a degree of value, but it does nothing to restore natural balance to the hormonal systems. A person in intense pain and unable to sleep has a benefit from medication that lowers pain and improves sleep.

However, the actual cause of the pain is not solved. This is reflected by the fact that many patients find the benefits of drugs like amitriptyline wear off after a month.[524] This is not unexpected, since the medications are not directed at the cause of the problem but rather at the suppression of the symptom called pain.

Fibromyalgia is not an easy problem to solve. State-of-the-art nursing care in Europe involves getting patients to understand that they will never get better, thus they are relieved of the stress of trying to find a solution.[525]

A primary reason why medical people have trouble figuring out the nature of fibromyalgia is hormone levels in the blood frequently look normal. Medical people have great difficulty understanding a problem if they cannot see problems in lab scores on paper. This typically leads them to conclude it must be in the mind of the patient.[526]

However, fibromyalgia is a classic condition of hormonal resistance and improper hormone timing, the hallmarks of an out-of-balance system. Frequently, lab scores on paper look normal enough, yet the proper function of those hormones is far from normal. This is because hormone levels in the blood or saliva do not reflect hormone resistance or improper hormone timing, which are the actual problems.

When lab scores come back normal and a person hurts all over, is fatigued, and does not sleep well, they get a diagnosis of fibromyalgia by default.

The reason modern medical treatment has no solutions for fibromyalgia is because it is not a disease with a traditional cause. It is a breakdown in homeostasis or natural balance. The solution is to fix natural balance. This is not so easy in the case of fibromyalgia, as fibromyalgia is a problem wherein the natural balance system has become worn out. It is similar to being anemic, only the problem is anemia of hormonal regulation.

Once a person is in this situation, they are handicapped in terms of dealing with various forms of stress. For example, if they get an infection, they have difficulty mounting a proper immune response to get rid of it. If they have an emotional problem in their life, they may have great difficulty solving it. If they break a bone, they may have trouble healing it.

Thus, while fibromyalgia is its own problem, any other problem is more difficult to solve. Under traditional medical care, this leads to a longer list of medications in an effort to manage the body's inability to bounce back on its own. Each time there is a new problem, a new medication is added.

Generally, the medications have adverse consequences to natural balance making the underlying problem worse. Thus, increased medication use places a person between a rock and a hard place. Such individuals feel bad on medication and feel bad off medication; they frequently have to figure out which "bad feeling" they would rather have.

We have helped thousands of people with fibromyalgia. Unraveling these problems takes work, but it can be done. It is easier to prevent fibromyalgia than it is to deal with the issue. Thus, we hope that many readers who struggle with leptin but have not yet progressed into fibromyalgia heed our warnings and learn to master leptin and keep hormones in a healthy condition of natural balance. Unlike the European nursing profession and general medical community, we offer hope of a true solution for the problem.

THE HORMONE IMBALANCE OF FIBROMYALGIA

Fibromyalgia is a loss of hormonal fitness; it is reflective of a hormonal system that does not bounce back and recover from stress properly.[527] There is a picture of hormonal tiredness and consequent inefficiency related to the hypothalamus gland in the brain.[528] The command and control center is too worn down to do its job.[529]

Fibromyalgia patients have generally lower levels of growth hormone, cortisol (the main stress hormone), and androgens (the main energetic drive hormone for both sexes) compared to normal.[530] However, if a person with fibromyalgia has acute stress, they get an exaggerated release of stress hormones, as if desperately trying to solve the stress but nothing in the body responds properly.

This is reflective of their path into fibromyalgia, wherein they have been overloaded by stress. Keep in mind that such stress triggers can be emotional or physical in nature. There is typically a major stress turning point, an event or period of time that acts like the straw that breaks the camel's back.

Thirty percent of patients with fibromyalgia have a definable level of GH deficiency.[531] Patients with fibromyalgia do not release GH in response to exercise, as do normal people. The scientists investigating this issue surmised that the GH regulatory system had lost its "tone"; in other words, it is tired and not working anymore.[532]

Corticotropin-releasing hormone (CRH) is the central hormone in the hypothalamus gland of the brain that initiates the stress response. When this hormone is injected into fibromyalgia patients and healthy individuals, there are different responses. In fibromyalgia patients, the hormone stays elevated in the blood and commands no appropriate reaction, reflective of general hormone resistance across the board in adapting to stress.[533]

As we have been pointing out all along in this book, leptin, adrenaline, NPY, agouti, and numerous other signals are processed in this brain center.

Fibromyalgia is a condition of hypothalamus gland fatigue. The hormone regulation system is worn out.

BACKED-UP PLUMBING

The consequence of this problem is physical pain and the accumulation of waste products due to clogged plumbing in the body. The longer the plumbing stays clogged, the greater the amount of localized tissue damage.[534]

Clogged plumbing in the body is like clogged plumbing in a house; the restrooms need to be used on a regular basis, but the waste products are backed up. This is certainly the case with fibromyalgia, as the backed-up waste products get in the way of hormones and cellular energy production, magnifying the obstacles that must be overcome to return natural balance. This is why it is such a difficult problem to solve; there is no drug that does housecleaning. There are no plumbers to call.

WEIGHT LOSS IS MORE DIFFICULT

Leptin-resistant and overweight individuals who have fibromyalgia have an even more difficult time. This is because the body seeks to get toxic waste out of circulation. Since normal plumbing routes are clogged, a secondary place to stuff toxic waste is fat cells. This at least gets them out of the circulation and away from key body organs. The formation of fat is enhanced by the condition of fibromyalgia as a natural defense system.

In order to lose weight, such a person must get the plumbing to work better. The toxins in the body, as well as the stored toxins that come out of fat cells as weight is lost, must have some place to go. The body is reluctant to break down toxic fat if there is no place for the toxins to go.

NERVE PAIN

There are three primary reasons for the pain of fibromyalgia; all need to be improved to solve this problem. The first one is nerve pain.

Nerve pain is a result of a worn-down nervous system. A normal response to stress involves the release of cortisol as well as sympathetic nerve stimulants such as adrenaline and dopamine. At the same time, the body releases beta-endorphins to improve pain tolerance and regulate the inflammation involved with stress.

When stress is ongoing, a person enters a phase of excess sympathetic nerve activity or surplus adrenaline. This leads to adrenaline resistance, insulin resistance, and leptin resistance with a corresponding lack of "relaxation reserves."

At the point where the natural-balance systems run out of energy, fibromyalgia sets in. In this worn-down condition, the nerves hypersecrete inflammatory signals at their ends, causing pain in muscles.[535] The phone poles and phone wires that make up the nervous system are now in a broken down condition. Any energy going through them, even too much positive emotion, can induce a flare-up of painful symptoms.

At the same time, the overall analgesic that helps a person normally tolerate pain, beta-endorphin, is exhausted and not available. This is easily seen in the lack of a refreshing response to exercise, wherein the normal rise of beta-endorphin does not occur and, in fact, too much exercise or physical activity in the day overloads the already exhausted system and induces pain that may last for days.

Conversely, the ability to get a refreshing response to exercise, to perform more physical activities during the day, and to tolerate positive energy going through the nerves without rebound negative setbacks of pain are key signs that a person is solving fibromyalgia.

The antidepressant medications the medical profession uses target these nerve-related pain signals and blunt the pain-related communication system. This is potentially helpful to the degree that pain is out of control. However, the actual cause of the problem is worn-down nerves.

SOLUTIONS FOR NERVE PAIN

The approach to solve this problem is to restore nutritional energy to the nervous system while at the same time being consistent with an amount of exercise the person can perform.

B vitamins are the most fundamental nutrients for nervous-system function. We use a specially formulated multiple vitamin that contains high amounts of the coenzyme forms of B vitamins. These are a tremendous advantage for anyone with fibromyalgia, as they require no energy to make them active in the body as do regular B vitamins. This formulation is also high in malic acid, an important cofactor for energy production in cells and the clearance of lactic acid. It contains no citric acid, which may induce immediate fatigue and headache in fibromyalgia patients.

In addition to the basic multiple vitamin, we use a unique form of calcium called calcium AEP. Calcium is important for nerve function; however, calcium AEP is special. This form of calcium builds up the myelin sheathing of nerves, enabling the nerves to carry more energy, a key problem of fibromyalgia.

There are other nutrients that can be used to help nerves, such as Acetyl-L-Carnitine, Phosphatidylserine, DHA, Carnosine, and many others. These nutrients may be quite helpful. However, a person with fibromyalgia cannot tolerate a great deal of stimulation, including nutrient stimulation.

Whatever program is embarked upon, it is essential to find an amount of support that helps nerves have some energy without crossing a line into too much stimulation too fast. The best way to gauge this is to combine nutrition with a consistent amount of exercise that can be done without inducing pain.

Some people start out with five minutes of walking. As they begin to improve, exercise gradually increases and higher amounts of nutritional support help to strengthen the nerves at a quicker rate.

As nerve-related pain declines, sleep automatically improves. As part of a fibromyalgia program, melatonin can be used to help the sleep process. The dose can range anywhere from .5 mg a day up to 5 mg a day, taken before bed.[536]

CLOGGED PLUMBING PAIN

The primary internal plumbing system of the human body revolves around the functioning of the lymphatic system. The lymphatic system is the fluid between all cells of the body leading through various channels and glands to its two major thoracic ducts that drain on both sides of the shoulders back into the veins. Waste then flows to the liver and hopefully into the GI tract on its way out of the body.

The lymph system is a one-way pressure system. Thus, when it is clogged, there are unmistakable symptoms. A person may not have every one of these symptoms, but there is a collection of them to a greater or lesser degree. The shoulder area builds up pressure that does not easily go away. This is like having constipation, but instead of the bowels, it is the lymph system that is stuck.

Such pressure tends to go backwards when the thoracic ducts are clogged. A person may feel pressure going up the back of their head; it may feel like the top of the head is going to blow off, and/or there may be recurring sinus or ear pressures not necessarily related to a sinus or ear infection.

Once the lymph is clogged, the body looks for alternative ways to get rid of waste. This usually involves making extra mucous and trying to excrete it through the sinuses. Thus, clearing the throat, especially after eating, are signs of lymphatic congestion. This can also cause ear popping, ear ringing, and ear noises, as the fluids in the ear cannot drain properly and there is a backup. In some people, this can be severe, causing pressure on the inner ear and dizziness.

Because the lymph system is most active while asleep, many individuals wake up with excess congestion, mucous, and body aches. As the lymph swells during sleep, it pushes on nerves that go to the hands or arms; thus, it is common for individuals with lymph congestion to wake up with an arm or hand asleep. This can also happen during the day as the wear and tear of the day overloads the lymph system.

Because the lymph system is a pressure system, it responds to environmental pressure changes. Prime examples are flying in an airplane or a change in weather fronts. A secondary example is the full moon or no moon. These environmental influences of pressure change are felt as symptoms of congestion, aches, and backed-up plumbing by a person with a sluggish lymph system.

Once the lymph system is backed up, then lactic acid tends to accumulate more easily in the muscles, aggravating the pain of fibromyalgia. This is especially true when the person tries to exercise. In serious fibromyalgia, it feels like a marathon has been run when all one did was go for a walk. Fibromyalgia individuals "hit the lactic acid wall" with normal everyday activities.

Medical professionals generally do not understand this problem, do not know how to help it, and frequently make it worse with medications.

SOLVING CLOGGED PLUMBING PAIN

Stagnation is the enemy of the lymph system. Overdoing it is also a problem. In significant fibromyalgia, there is sometimes very little difference between stagnation and overdoing it, an issue that must be resolved in order for a person to get better.

Thus, we seek to get a person to do a baseline of exercise that is possible. It is important to be consistent, not intense. As a person improves, they will be able to consistently do more.

The most effective compound we have found for helping the lymph system move along is arabinogalactan. This unique nutrient wakes up the macrophages in the lymphatic system and puts them back on cleaning duty, as well as facilitates other aspects of immune function to work better.[537] Doses may range from one-half teaspoon to one heaping tablespoon, one to four times a day. Once again, finding a dose that helps lower clogged plumbing symptoms is the key. More is not necessarily better.

We also use magnesium malate to help clear lactic acid from muscles. It is also important to help the liver process the waste that goes to it. We use a "liver multiple nutrient" for this job, one that has a good base of sylimarin and other toxin-clearing nutrients. Of course, if a person is constipated, the bowels must move or waste products back up in the body.

When an individual improves the lymph system and related plumbing, the pain of fibromyalgia can be greatly reduced. Just like plumbing in a house, this plumbing is always in use. It is not that a person goes through a detoxification and is then free of fibromyalgia. Efficient function of one's plumbing on a daily basis is essential; otherwise, a backlog has serious repercussions to hormonal balance.

TISSUE DAMAGE PAIN

Individuals with fibromyalgia have much higher levels of advanced glycation end-product (AGE) modified proteins. The proteins of muscle fibers are cemented together in abnormal structures and no longer work properly. This is a form of tissue damage that causes pain. Unfortunately, this tissue damage flares up excess production of NF kappaB that contributes to the pain and perpetuates the damage.[538]

This AGE-induced tissue damage occurs once the antioxidant reserves of the muscle are used up. When nerve pain is initially directed at the muscles, the muscles activate their cellular defense mechanisms in an effort to withstand the problem. As the problem continues, the antioxidant defense system is used up. At this point, excess NF kappaB is activated in an inflammatory manner. This in turn causes a progression of the local tissue damage and resulting pain.

The longer a person stays in the fibromyalgia pain condition, the more likely it is that damage is being done to the muscles.

SOLVING TISSUE DAMAGE PAIN

The solution for this type of pain is to stop fibromyalgia hormone imbalance in the first place. However, this may take some time, even on a good program. In the meantime, we cannot simply stand by as tissue is damaged.

There are various nutritional strategies that can be employed. Lipoic acid, a potent antioxidant, has proven to stop AGE-associated damage by turning off the excess production of NF kappaB.[539] There are numerous studies demonstrating the ability of lipoic acid to turn off the production of excess NF kappaB.to□ [540,541,542] Lipoic acid is an excellent antioxidant for the nervous system; thus, it is helpful for the nerve pain and nerve inflammation of fibromyalgia.[543,544] Lipoic acid is a primary nutrient to help stop the progression of tissue damage. The most effective form of lipoic acid for supplementation is called R alpha lipoic acid.

There is also hope for repairing tissue damage that has already been done. We use the enzymes bromelain and papain to help dissolve abnormal tissue protein damage.[545,546] We combine them with quercetin and curcumin to further reduce inflammation and help turn off excess NF kappaB.[547,548,549]

We may add a nutrient such as hyaluronic acid. Hyaluronic acid signals genes to help synthesize new cells as well as act as a connective tissue raw material itself.[550] Our goal is not only to reduce pain but also to improve the response to exercise, especially to find a level of support that helps a person do strength-training exercise.

When we can get a person with fibromyalgia onto a strength-training program and get a good response to that program, we can fix their problem. This works in part by enhancing the release of growth hormone, helping to put the hormone balance issue back into natural function.[551]

However, in order to get a good response to even mild strength training, a person must be able to repair tissue damage induced by the exercise. Unfortunately, fibromyalgia patients may already be in a condition of tissue damage that they are not able to repair. If they try to do strength training, they may make their overall problem worse, which is not hard to tell judging by the amount of pain they are in after they work out.

For example, a normal person who does an exercise they are not conditioned to perform may experience muscle tissue breakdown and stiff muscles for 2-3 days. This stiffness goes away or is shortened once the person is conditioned. A person with fibromyalgia may induce the same sort of pain response, but the pain may last 1-2 weeks! Furthermore, doing the exercise again may result in the same problem, not in improved conditioning.

Thus, anti-inflammatory and structural nutritional support is important for a person with fibromyalgia to improve their muscle fitness and ability to recover from tissue damage. This enables them to begin to get a good response to improved muscle fitness. At the same time, it signifies they have enough nutritional support to prevent excess muscle tissue damage and enhance the repair of muscle.

SUMMARY

Fibromyalgia is the problem of a worn-down hormonal system. It is especially reflective of the commander in chief of the subconscious brain, the hypothalamus gland, being too tired to carry out its work properly. Since its work is primarily the job of ensuring that natural balance takes place, this is a major problem.

Leptin resistance and related issues set the stage for this problem. When these problems exist, the body struggles to maintain natural balance. Fibromyalgia is a progression of these problems into a state of hormonal regulation exhaustion. There are still hormones in the blood; however, hormones do not work the way they once did. Quality, timing, and overall efficiency of the hormonal system is lacking.

Refreshing response to aerobic exercise and a healthy muscle response to strength-training exercise are important steps on the path to recovery from fibromyalgia. Doing whatever it takes to solve these issues helps solve fibromyalgia. Re-energizing the nervous system, improving the plumbing operation, and restoring physical fitness are imperative to solving fibromyalgia.

By taking it a step further and learning to be a Health Asset Manager™, a person can prevent sliding back into a problem of fibromyalgia or from ever having the problem in the first place.

38

Rapid Weight Gain and Yo-Yo Diets

*I*ndividuals can rapidly gain weight from eating too much food. Some individuals gain weight from eating a normal amount of food. This is especially true when a person finishes dieting and starts eating more food. This typically results in gaining back the weight that was lost and frequently 5-10 additional pounds.

These issues are caused by leptin. In the person who is overeating, leptin resistance fuels the excessive weight gain.

In the person who gains weight back after dieting, the natural response of leptin following a diet is to replenish the supply of fat. It is this survival instinct of leptin that causes dieters to have so much trouble.

The more history a person has with weight gain and weight loss, the greater the degree of leptin resistance and leptin problems the person is likely to have. The body does not trust them anymore; it is all too eager to put extra fat back in place just to be on the safe side. The body considers the scarcity of food to be an extreme threat to survival. The subconscious brain does not know that when the diet is over there is food available on every corner.

When individuals lose weight by following the *Five Rules* and a consistent exercise program, that weight loss tends to be permanent. Any time a person tries to lose weight by eating reduced calories, they are prone to gain it back once they start eating more. That is the nature of leptin.

EATING MORE SAFELY

Many individuals keep themselves in anorexic-like starvation metabolism because they want to look thin, and they are afraid that if they eat too much they will gain unwanted weight.

If a person follows the *Five Rules* and exercises, they will not gain inappropriate weight as they begin to eat more. Rather, they gain energy, strength, proper immune function, and improved sex hormone balance.

However, individuals with a yo-yo diet history have trained their nervous system and leptin response into a bad habit or routine. Thus, some individuals have an ingrained negative training due either to their own experience or as a "gift" from their parents.

While such individuals know they should follow the *Five Rules* and exercise consistently, and in fact may even do so once they realize they should, they are more easily thrown into leptin problems resulting in weight gain. For example, they do fine until they get under stress. All of a sudden they start to eat more. They cannot get out of the pattern; they are sucked back into leptin-resistant weight gain.

Such individuals have a real problem with leptin running their life, as opposed to them managing leptin.

CLA TO THE RESCUE

CLA is an effective compound for keeping leptin under control. CLA is an effective weight-loss nutrient for many people as part of an overall program of natural balance; however, it excels at helping to keep leptin under control.

One common use of CLA is to tame the out-of-control eating urges at night. We introduced CLA in Chapter 31 and explained its role in this capacity.

Another important use of CLA is to prevent extra weight gain when a person starts to eat more food. This helps to train the body into the correct utilization of food, keeping leptin under control so that it does not tell the food that is being eaten to store as fat.

As a person becomes consistent over a number of months eating more food, maintaining the *Five Rules*, exercising consistently, and getting adequate sleep, the body will build a new set of healthy rhythms. At this point, CLA is no longer needed to maintain the state of natural balance. Rather, it was used as a tool to help train leptin to behave correctly.

CLA can also be used to help keep a person in balance while under the influence of stress. Thus, if a person is under more stress and prone to poor eating patterns and eating too much food, CLA can be used to stop the leptin urges that subconsciously drive the eating behavior.

CLA reduces the amount of leptin that is produced by fat cells.[552] CLA can reduce leptin production by as much as 42 percent, and when it does this, it increases the burning of fats as fuel.[553] As CLA lowers leptin, it also lowers the inflammation generating TNFa.[554]

In clinical practice, we use doses ranging from 3–6 grams a day. Our basic dose is three grams a day for the prevention of gaining back too much weight after a period of dieting. Remember, this needs to be done in conjunction with the *Five Rules*, exercise, adequate sleep, and stress management.

SUMMARY

Yo-yo dieting is very unhealthy. Not eating enough food so as not to gain weight, essentially staying malnourished, is also unhealthy.

The base for solving these problems is implementing the *Five Rules*, consistent exercise, adequate sleep, and hormone management skills.

Some individuals need additional physical assistance to keep leptin levels under control so they do not gain back weight after a period of weight loss. CLA is an effective nutrient for this purpose.

39

Solving Stubborn Weight-Loss Problems

*W*e have extensively discussed the anorexic-like starvation metabolism. This problem may exist as the dominant metabolic pattern in an individual. Such a person can eat like a bird and still not lose weight.

Anorexic-like starvation metabolism may also be encountered in the dieting process. It causes a person to hit a plateau or be unable to get rid of the last few pounds. When this happens, a person gets stuck at a weight and does not progress.

Remember, the subconscious brain does not look in a mirror and has no clue how overweight a person may be. The subconscious brain determines where calories head based entirely on one thing, the perception of leptin.

If the subconscious brain does not receive a perception of leptin that permits active metabolism to occur, it enforces starvation metabolism on the person, regardless of how much fat is already in storage. This is the reason a person cannot get past a certain weight.

VARYING DEGREES OF DIFFICULTY

This perceived state of starvation comes in different levels of severity. Many individuals who follow our *Five Rules*, exercise consistently, and get adequate sleep will be able to solve this problem easily. Remember, these steps are essential for anyone to follow even if they have a more severe problem.

A person may do these basic leptin management skills correctly in terms of eating and exercise, but their weight still will not budge or they hit a plateau and have trouble getting past it. This is a more serious problem.

It does not mean that our approach is not correct; it simply means that the underlying hormonal system is too out of balance to respond to the fundamentals. If a person goes against the basic lifestyle approach, they will simply get worse. However, they need more help to get their metabolism in gear and out of the perceived state of starvation.

THE GREAT WEIGHT-LOSS MYSTERY

Understanding the problem of perceived starvation is the key to overcoming stubborn weight-loss issues.

Thyroid hormone is blocked during perceived starvation. In perceived starvation, there are elevated levels of reverse T3, the form of T3 that puts the brakes on metabolism. Overweight people who are not in starvation metabolism do not have elevated reverse T3, only people who are overweight and in perceived starvation.[555]

This is true even if the basic thyroid lab tests say there is no problem, as most thyroid tests do not look for reverse T3, and it can continue to be the case even if a person takes thyroid hormone. A person is either in a perceived state of starvation or they are not, regardless of what the thyroid lab tests says, or in some cases, the thyroid medication that is being consumed. Thyroid medication is definitely not the answer to this problem.

It should be pointed out that anorexic individuals also have this same problem of elevated reverse T3. In the case of a true malnutrition, starvation, or anorexia situation, we can understand the increase in reverse T3 as the body tries to slow down metabolism so that it does not waste away. However, why would a person who is 50 pounds overweight get stuck in a perceived state of starvation?

We have already stated in Chapter 36 that the cause of most thyroid problems is leptin resistance. It difficult metabolic situations, some aspect of the leptin resistance will not budge; otherwise, following the *Five Rules*, exercise, and adequate sleep would have solved the problem.

THE CAUSE OF THE REVERSE T3 PROBLEM

It has been known since 1990 that TNFa causes an increase in reverse T3.[556] It has been known since 1996 that IL-6 causes an increase in reverse T3.[557] We are not saying TNFa and IL-6 simply coexist with the problem of elevated reverse T3, we are saying that science clearly proves TNFa and IL-6 actually cause elevated reverse T3.

In the case of true anorexia, the elevated reverse T3 comes from the inflammatory wasting process.

The great discovery of leptin and consequent scientific exploration into the structure of fat cells shows that fat cells produce IL-6 and TNFa. The more pounds of fat on hand, the greater the likelihood of excess production of these two pro-inflammatory immune signals.

Now we understand why an overweight person can get stuck in a perceived state of starvation. It is due to excess production of TNFa and IL-6 coming from the extra pounds of fat on hand, a nasty Catch-22. If they do not lose the extra pounds of fat, the elevated reverse T3 problem does not go away. On the other hand, the elevated reverse T3 prevents them from losing the extra pounds of fat by locking in the leptin resistance and causing perceived starvation.

Before explaining how to solve this problem, it is worthwhile to understand the significance of reverse T3 to overall health.

REVERSE T3, MORE THAN A WEIGHT-LOSS ISSUE

It is more expensive to determine reverse T3 on a blood test than the basic type of thyroid scores normally evaluated. Testing for reverse T3 is not needed to determine primary hypothyroidism. The fact that it involves increased cost and is not needed in order to determine if a doctor should give a patient thyroid medication, it is not done as a matter of routine.

As it turns out, testing for reverse T3 may be one of the most useful tests a doctor can order as part of a routine health check. This fact has been pointed out to doctors in their literature for over 20 years.[558] It is certainly helpful in our understanding of the overweight person who is stuck in perceived starvation.

This lab test demonstrates to what degree a person is stuck at a weight-loss plateau due to perceived starvation. It is a valuable tool for guidance in weight-loss issues, especially to those who have struggled with weight loss. However, it is much more than that.

We know that reverse T3 can be induced by stressful trauma. Being wheeled into an operating room for surgery can even start elevated reverse T3, in addition to the surgery itself.[559] Major stress trauma that involves elevated cortisol, including life stress, sets the stage for reverse T3. These are the "health turning points" in one's history.

Reverse T3 status is related to whether or not a person survives a heart attack.[560] The more elevated the reverse T3, the more likely it is that the person does not survive. The level of reverse T3 following a heart attack is related to the amount of cardiac damage.[561]

Another study was conducted with bone marrow transplant patients. Unlike heart attack patients, this enables a test wherein reverse T3 can be tested before the surgery as well as after. This information sheds light on the importance of the pre-existing nutritional status before stress, as well as the effects of the major stress itself. Researchers found that either poor nutritional status prior to the operation, as determined by elevated reverse T3, and the failure of reverse T3 to return to a lower level following the operation, was the determining factor of who lived and who died.[562]

This information is of immense importance to society. It tells us that by managing the problem of elevated reverse T3, we can significantly improve any person's chances of survival. A person who does not have elevated reverse T3 prior to a trauma has a much better chance of surviving it, because the energy regulation systems in the body work more efficiently and have an appropriate energetic response to the emergency.

It is not surprising to find elevated reverse T3 occurring in various inflammatory conditions and issues of poor health during the aging process.[563] It is interesting to note that the anorexia of aging, that is, the deterioration of the body as one grows older, is associated with elevated reverse T3 and lower levels of active T3.

Elderly people on the low-fat, low-energy diets are likely to be in self-induced perceived starvation metabolism with low levels of active T3, increased reverse T3, and in poor health.[564]

This is one more scientific fact that tells us that not eating enough calories for energy, including an appropriate amount of saturated fat, is cardiovascular counter-productive. Instead of being a cardiovascular protective measure, it can create a low-energy, low-leptin environment that makes a person less likely to survive a heart attack.

Thus, we have two primary risk groups for cardiovascular disease. One is the over-nourished individual, stuck with leptin resistance, adrenaline resistance, and insulin resistance, otherwise known as metabolic syndrome X.[565] The other is the low-leptin malnourished individual, whose LDL cholesterol may be too low due to malnutrition, and who is in an inflammatory or progressive wasting pattern. This problem also occurs in the dieting person who gets stuck at a plateau and is in the anorexic-like starvation metabolism. A key cardiovascular risk measurement is elevated reverse T3.

SOLVING PERCEIVED STARVATION

Solving perceived starvation requires a high degree of skill on the part of the Health Asset Manager.™ There are no shortcuts and there are many variables.

It is important to remember that there are degrees of this problem. The better the overall health and fitness of the person, the easier perceived starvation is to solve. Gradually improving fitness over time is essential.

In addition to the principles of the *Five Rules*, consistent exercise, and adequate sleep, following are the five most important additional issues to work on to improve and solve perceived starvation.

1) Reduce TNFa and IL-6 levels, prime causes of the problem. Since there is no getting away from the extra pounds of fat that generate these signals, these problems can be greatly assisted by nutrients that help turn them off.

   We have already mentioned the importance of essential fatty acids and CLA in this regard. Virtually any nutrient that acts as an antioxidant or anti-inflammatory aids this situation.

2) Provide nutrition to help the stressed out thyroid gland and to enhance the conversion of T4 to active T3. This includes nutrients such as selenium, manganese, tyrosine, iodine, and calcium.

3) Learn to more effectively manage stress and ensure there is enough nutritional support to feel on top of stress. Stress is a trigger that sends a person down the reverse T3 path. It is the elevated TNFa and IL-6 that lock in this problem over time.

However, if a person is under constant stress, they keep tilting their metabolism in the direction of elevated reverse T3, especially if there is a major stress event or an extended time period of stress.

If a person is losing weight and the weight loss stops, look for changes in stress. This can be emotional stress or physical stress such as an infection. Also look for changes in medications. These are common changes that interfere with the progression of weight loss.

Nutrient support for stress requires extra antioxidants, B-vitamins, calcium, magnesium, zinc, coenzyme Q10, Acetyl-L-Carnitine, and other possible choices including immune-boosting nutrition. A person needs enough nutritional support to feel on top of stress.

If there has been a medication change that coincides with weight gain or the inhibition of weight loss, find out to what extent it may be involved in the problem by working with one's doctor to find alternatives to the medication.

4) Move stagnant calories out of the circulation. Under the influence of reverse T3, especially in overweight individuals, it is common that cholesterol and/or triglycerides accumulate in the blood. It is like having trucks parked on a highway. These show up on a lab test.

Rather than trying to suppress the production of cholesterol with a drug that has unpredictable effects on natural balance, we like to take the approach of hauling the stagnant fat into metabolic action.

The best nutrients for this are pantethine, Acetyl-L-Carnitine, chromium, vanadium, and tocotrienols. Pantethine acts as an energetic carrier to move fat into action. Acetyl-L-Carnitine improves the ability of cells to burn fat for fuel and helps the brain sense leptin more accurately. Chromium and vanadium help calories enter cells to help lower insulin resistance. Gamma tocotrienol helps slow down the excess production of cholesterol, training the liver into a better metabolic pattern and out of the bad habit of making too much cholesterol. Alpha tocotrienol protects the arteries from damage.

The net effect of these nutrients helps natural metabolism clear the surplus of stagnant energy from the blood. Once this happens, it is a lot easier to get reverse T3 problems solved, as there is not so much "sludge" in the circulation.

5) Effectively manage all symptoms of fibromyalgia. Desired weight loss is not possible if the plumbing system gets backed up and the body is stuck in inflammatory pain. Toxins do not come out of fat if there is no place for them to go. Individuals who have fibromyalgia issues must address this issue as a priority.

Others encounter fibromyalgia-like issues as they try to lose fat that contains toxins. This is reflected in a distinct "poisoned," irritable, and possibly queasy feeling. Dark circles under the eyes appear. Headaches may also occur as part of this process.

Managing toxic symptoms is an important factor involved with weight-loss plateaus and the last 5-10 pounds, as this "core fat" is frequently the most toxic fat the body has difficulty losing.

We have provided extensive recommendations for this issue in Chapter 37 on fibromyalgia.

A person in perceived starvation metabolism may have problems in any one or all five of these areas. Improving any one of them tends to improve the others. As overall fitness improves, all of the five areas tend to improve at the same time. Thus, the best that some may be able to hope for is gradual improvement over time that corresponds to gradually improving fitness.

Addressing these areas can speed up weight loss and make weight loss possible for those prone to perceived starvation. How much any person must do is based on the result. Do enough to get into metabolic gear. Once in metabolic fat-burning mode, be thankful, resist the temptation to get off a plan that is finally working.

SUMMARY

The hallmark of frustration with weight loss is hitting the perceived state of starvation. Some individuals are in this condition before they begin to lose weight. Others encounter it during a weight-loss plateau or when they get down to the last few stubborn pounds that do not want to leave the body.

If a person gets frustrated and throws away their good eating patterns and exercise habits, they will simply gain back excess weight and be miserable. Thus, we need solutions for perceived starvation.

The mystery of the nature of this problem has now been identified. It is an issue of elevated reverse T3 fueled by chronically elevated TNFa and IL-6. Stress, toxins, fibromyalgia, and a buildup of stagnant fat in the blood, work against the situation and keep aggravating it.

The *Five Rules*, consistent exercise, and adequate sleep are the cornerstone solutions relating to leptin. In this chapter, we provided five additional areas of nutritional support that may be needed, including our basic recommendations that are capable of breaking a person out of perceived starvation and onto a path of better health.

Solving perceived starvation is a true test of the skills of a Health Asset Manager.™

Leptin, NF kappaB, and the Cause of Cancer

*E*xcess leptin sets the stage for too much inflammation and is a primary cause of this issue. This disrupts natural balance or homeostasis in the body. It can have a domino effect that may lead to virtually any disease; therefore, it is a general health principle of extreme importance. Extra pounds of fat are a pivotal causative issue in the quality of health.

New information uncovers the true significance of these discoveries. Leptin resistance leads to a situation that promotes major risk for cancer and numerous other diseases.

TNFa CAN BE FRIENDLY AND HELPFUL

So far we have painted TNFa as an enemy that generates inflammation. We also pointed out that TNFa is involved as a needed signal in the response to stress. Additionally, we should point out that TNFa, also known as tumor necrosis factor alpha, is a main signal in the body that kills cancer cells. This is how it originally got its name. The word necrosis means death to a cell; thus, tumor necrosis means death to tumor cells. TNFa is a known factor that kills tumor cells. How can that be a bad thing?

The answer to this question goes back to the underlying themes of this book. It is an issue of efficiency. When TNFa works properly, it helps regulate the immune response, the inflammatory response, the healing response, supports healthy pregnancy, and acts to knock out cancer. Timing is everything.

When TNFa is released at the right time for the right set of circumstances, implying that the body is in good natural balance as a baseline and then releases TNFa to deal with stress or to help reproduction, it is part of the body's perfect system of natural balance. When TNFa is released continuously due to excess fat pounds, the outcome of what it does is unpredictable. Instead of helping to kill cancer, it is unfortunately the case that excess TNFa causes cancer.

HOW TNFa LEADS TO CANCER

What determines if TNFa acts in a good way or in a cancer-causing way? Scientists have been studying this issue rather closely. In conducting experiments on cells that behaved differently in response to TNFa, it became clear that in cells leading to cancer progression, the TNFa activated a substance called granulocyte macrophage colony stimulating factor, GM-CSF.

GM-CSF is a growth factor that facilitates cellular growth, possibly to the point of being resistant to normal death mechanisms. If a cancer can hijack this mechanism in the human body, then it is extremely difficult, if not impossible, to kill. In cells that TNFa was killing, these cells do not generate any GM-CSF.[566]

Why does a cell generate excess amounts of GM-CSF that can perpetuate cancer and make it resistant to medical treatment? Answer - Excess production of NF kappaB.

HOW NF kappaB DOES ITS JOB

NF kappaB is the 911 switchboard of a cell's defense against stress. When a cell clicks along in a normal mode of healthy operation, then NF kappaB is dormant, much like a 911 operator at the police department who is not getting any calls. NF kappaB exists in every cell of the human body in this dormant state when things run as expected.

Under the influence of a stressful irritant, NF kappaB is activated. We are not talking about a simplistic biological mechanism. We are talking about a 911 activation system that has millions of years of genetic evolution to deal with a great variety of different types of stress. It can be chemical/pollution stress, infection stress, injury stress, or emotional stress. Literally, there can be a multitude of various stressors confronting a cell.

NF kappaB goes to the DNA of the cell and tells the DNA what proteins to make to fight the stress so that the cell can survive. This is a complex activity, one we are only beginning to understand. For example, if it is a chemical stress, the cell has to figure out how to deactivate or detoxify the chemical before its gets stuck to the DNA and induces mutation. If it is a viral stress, the cell has to figure out how to kill the virus before it kills the cell.

Exactly what the cell should do to defend itself is commanded by NF kappaB. NF kappaB contains the genetic intelligence to deal with stress as well as to adapt to new stress. The survival of any cell, and consequently the survival of the human body, is based on the efficient operation of NF kappaB.

NF kappaB also makes the tough decisions about who lives and who dies. Many of the activities of NF kappaB include survival mechanisms so that a cell can withstand stress. In other words, there may be an emergency need to make cellular components or tissue in order to withstand the type of stress the cell experiences. Thus, GM-CSP can be made to help sustain body structure under duress. Once the duress is over, the need for extra GM-CSP goes down and NF kappaB stops its production.

On the other hand, the cell may be overwhelmed by the type of stress it is experiencing. If a horribly malfunctioning cell mutates, it is likely to be in a cancerous form. Therefore, NF kappaB has to decide at what point sustaining the cell life is no longer a good idea. NF kappaB then initiates death signals that cause the cell to die, a situation known as apoptosis.

Thank goodness there are not a lot of politics involved with these decisions. They are tough life and death decisions. They are based on the potential ability of the individual cell to survive but not at the cost of inducing damage to other cells. It is an incredibly complex and sophisticated defense system.

When the body is in a state of natural balance, it works perfectly!

NF KAPPAB AS THE CAUSE OF CANCER

In March 2002, researchers from the Department of Pharmacology, University of California, published a paper called, *NF kappaB at the Crossroads of Life and Death.*[567] In July 2001, researchers at the Harold Simmons Cancer Center, University of Texas Southwestern Medical Center, published a paper called, *Role of the NF kappaB Pathway in the Pathogenesis of Human Disease States.*[568] These studies show that scientists are aware that excess NF kappaB is central to serious disease.

Cancer's goal is to survive while it destroys the human body. Cancer that is resistant to treatment has successfully hijacked NF kappaB and is using the cell's own perfect defense system to perpetuate its own survival and to kill other cells. This is a major breakthrough in our understanding of the nature of cancer.

The issues going on at genetic levels are complex. An easy way to understand this is as follows:

1) There is a normal activation of NF kappaB to deal with stress.
2) There is an abnormal constant elevation of NF kappaB that exists in cancer situations, wherein the cancer has hijacked NF kappaB and uses it to foster its own survival while the cancer destroys the body.

A key mechanism that causes NF kappaB to elevate is the excess production of TNFa. Excess TNFa keeps generating other excess gene signals (Bcl-2, Bcl-x(L)), which then feed the excess production of NF kappaB for no good reason, other than the survival of cancer.[569]

TNFa, the substance that is supposed to help the body kill cancer cells, has turned traitor. It becomes the key and pivotal signal that causes NF kappaB to be elevated as well as causes itself to continue excess production.[570,571]

NF kappaB, in turn, uses the body's own antioxidant defense system to protect cancer cells from destruction by TNFa.[572] Furthermore the excess NF kappaB keeps producing GM-CSP that makes the cancer resistant to the normal destruction by TNFa. This is completely upside down and backwards from what should be happening.

Excess NF kappaB is like a forest fire raging out of control. Once the forest fire is put out, meaning that the excess levels of NF kappaB can be lowered so that they are back to normal, then TNFa starts working again to kill cancer instead of helping perpetuate cancer.[573,574,575]

Pancreatic cancer, a very resistant type of cancer, is an example of this excess NF kappaB driven issue.[576] It was recently discovered that suppressing NF kappaB stops the progression of oral cancer.[577] Furthermore, suppressing NF kappaB makes cancer cells more susceptible to be killed by chemotherapy. This has recently been demonstrated with lung cancer.[578]

SUMMARY

The important point to understand is that the body's own defense system is being used against itself so as to perpetuate cancer. The exact mechanisms of how this works in all cancers are yet to be defined, but the overall picture is established.

A person's extra body fat generates excess amounts of TNFa. It is essential, as far as cancer is concerned, to have excess amounts of TNFa in order to generate excess amounts of NF kappaB. Extra pounds of fat are a primary risk factor for developing cancer. This does not mean that all overweight people develop cancer; it simply means that they have a much higher risk.

A person with normal body weight can get cancer quite easily. For example, a smoker can be at any body weight and have an increased risk for cancer. The constant poisoning of the body with toxins causes excess inflammation and excess NF kappaB production, leading to cell mutation and risk for any type of cancer. Lung cancer may develop that is resistant to treatment. Any type of excessive inflammatory condition, regardless of the individual's body weight, can increase the risk for cancer by constantly elevating NF kappaB.

We talk more about the leptin, NF kappa B, and cancer issue in Chapter 43 and Chapter 44. This principle is a dominant theme in cancer, especially those resistant to treatment. Solutions to this problem are key for improving the chances for a positive treatment outcome.

41

Leptin, NF kappaB, and the Cause of Disease

The purpose of this chapter is to give an overview of how leptin, TNFa, and NF kappaB, when in a condition of excess, contribute to virtually all types of disease associated with the aging process. This is a general and far reaching principle of health.

LIVER HEALTH

The liver is the metabolic factory of the body. Keeping it in excellent working order is of primary importance. Excess body weight leads to fatty liver issues, wherein the liver is infiltrated by excess amounts of fat that should not be there. These extra amounts of fat increase the production of TNFa.

Too much TNFa induces excess production of NF kappaB, setting the stage for significant liver injury and liver damage.[579] Furthermore, this issue is magnified when the body is exposed to pollution. Common pollution, such as air pollution, induces specific excess production of NF kappaB in the liver.[580]

The combined issues of extra body fat and exposure to common pollution cause a synergistic negative stress on the liver wherein the rate of liver damage accelerates and the risk for liver cancer increases. As every person in America is exposed to excess pollution and has no choice about the issue, the primary way to reduce this risk is to reduce body fat.

When a person consumes too much alcohol at any one time, liver cells are infiltrated with alcohol, causing NF kappaB levels to rise.[581] How much alcohol the liver can tolerate before this happens varies from person to person.

MORE ON CARDIOVASCULAR HEALTH

The general principles of the usefulness of NF kappaB to help regulate stress and the problems of excess NF kappaB in causing disease are definite factors in issues of heart health. Both TNFa and NF kappaB act to protect the heart from stress, just as they act to protect single cells from stress.[582,583] Therefore, if the body is in natural balance and is exposed to something that is a cardio-vascular stress, TNFa and NF kappaB behave in a healthy way and protect the heart from damage.

The endothelial lining is the Achilles' heel of the circulatory system. It is a "skin" or membrane of cells that acts as the buffer between what circulates in the blood and the structural walls of arteries, veins, and capillaries. The endothelial cells have a regulatory effect on blood pressure and many other aspects of circulatory function; they are not a passive structure. Damage to the endothelial cell lining leads to plaque accumulation in the lining of arteries and eventually leads to cardiovascular disease.

It has been known since 1999 that elevated leptin, as in the case of the leptin-resistant individual, induces excess production of free radicals that damage the endothelial lining of the circulatory system, thereby triggering plaque accumulation and setting the stage for cardiovascular disease. Part of the damaging free-radical process involved the excess production of NF kappaB.[584]

Around the same time, other researchers proved that inflammation leading to plaque formation involved excess production of TNFa and NF kappaB.[585] Both studies show that these issues can be reversed with antioxidants.

There is no question that excess inflammation is a prime cause of plaque accumulation. There is also no question that leptin resistance tilts the entire body into a more pro-inflammatory condition. Excess NF kappaB is at the core of this issue in terms of how much plaque forms. It is the prime causative mechanism behind the excess clotting that leads to a heart attack or stroke.[586]

Even in medical settings, the value of this new information may soon be put to advantageous use. For example, when an individual has balloon angioplasty, the entire endothelial lining is stripped and damaged. This is an unfortunate side effect of calling in a plumber to clean out a clogged artery.

In this emergency medical situation, it is essential to open up the clogged artery so that blood can flow.

The fact that the artery wall is damaged in the process is undesirable but viewed to be not as important as the clogged artery. After the operation, in a relatively short period of time, it is common for the artery to clog again, an issue called restenosis. This happens in a large part due to the injury caused by the medical procedure. Animal experiments show that suppressing the production of NF kappaB can prevent the artery from clogging after surgery.[587]

We are back to our bottom line issue. NF kappaB is essential for survival and defending the body against stress. Too much NF kappaB causes excess inflammation and progression of cardiovascular disease. Extra pounds of fat cause excess TNFa that in turn stimulates the excess NF kappaB leading to the problem. Extra body weight is therefore a major cause of cardiovascular disease.

ALZHEIMER'S AND MENTAL DECLINE

NF kappaB is essential to the healthy function of the human brain. It is involved with the survival of brain cells, especially when brain cells are exposed to some type of stress.[588]

It should come as no surprise that excess production of NF kappaB is a prime cause of Alzheimer's and mental decline.[589]

An out of control inflammatory situation in the brain is at the root of Alzheimer's and cognitive decline. This is confirmed by the evidence that excess amounts of TNFa and other inflammatory markers are all elevated along with the excess amount of NF kappaB.[590,591,592,593]

These studies show that this is not a trivial side issue that happens as a result of Alzheimer's. Rather, these are causative issues related to the severity of the problem and risk of death from Alzheimer's. In centurions, those that have the most cognitive decline have the highest amount of circulating TNFa.[594]

Furthermore, extra fat in the diet raises the deposition of Apo E in the brain, under the influence of leptin resistance, in direct correlation to weight gain.[595] High levels of Apo E are a primary risk factor for developing Alzheimer's disease.

While being overweight does not necessarily cause Alzheimer's, it certainly tilts body chemistry in a direction that increases one's risk for the disease, especially if a person has genetic predisposition to the problem.

A recent study with dogs demonstrated that air pollution activates all of the above inflammatory factors and leads to changes in the brain consistent with Alzheimer's disease.[596] Similarly, exposure to aluminum produces the same elevation of NF kappaB and TNFa leading to damaged brain cells.[597] Exposure to lead, methyl mercury, and aluminum are known to cause developmental issues in children and brain disease in the elderly.[598]

Alzheimer's is predicted to be a major health epidemic as the baby-boomer population ages. The cost to society will be staggering. There will be no easy cure for Alzheimer's. Worldwide pollution must be curtailed as a priority; otherwise, any person who is overweight and/or genetically at risk is likely to get Alzheimer's.

ARTHRITIS

Excess amounts of leptin increase the amount of immune cells that attack joints, otherwise referred to as rheumatoid arthritis.[599] Excess amounts of TNFa and NF kappaB are present in rheumatoid arthritis and multiple sclerosis, as causative factors of the problems.[600,601]

Feverfew is an herb that has been used traditionally to help arthritis and migraine headaches. The active component of this herb, parthenolide, is proven to work by lowering NF kappaB to reduce inflammation.[602,603,604] The herb is highly effective at getting straight to the gene signal causing the problem.

These findings are spurring other research into parthenolide, including cancer prevention and treatment. Parthenolide can change the way human leukemia cells progress so that the cells are changed into normal monocytes instead of cancer. This is done by altering the NF kappaB gene signal.[605]

Parthenolide also helps reduce the activity of breast cancer cells and makes them more susceptible to be killed by cancer drugs. Once again, this is due to being able to lower NF kappaB.[606]

Interestingly, parthenolide seems to have an ability to differentiate between appropriate cell death, as in helping to kill cancer cells, and inappropriate cell death. It has been shown to turn off inappropriate signaling of NF kappa B that causes T cells to be killed when they should not be.[607]

VIRAL INFECTIONS

Being sick with the flu is bad enough. Now we have to start looking at the effect of low-grade and chronic viral infections on our health. Everyone in America is exposed to a variety of viral infections, most are cousins and best friends of each other.

Many individuals suffer from low-grade viral activity on a regular basis. Some have more recognizable viral syndromes. Others are simply prone to catching bugs easily and get sore throats often, including waking up in the morning with them.

Numerous studies in the last two years are making a viral-cancer connection. From a cell's point of view, a viral invasion is a form of stress. This activates NF kappaB as would any initial stress. Chronic viral infections learn to coexist inside of cells, literally hijacking cells and altering their genetic function.[608] Unfortunately, the virus specifically stimulates the excess production of NF kappaB.[609]

Considerable evidence is mounting:

1) Hepatitis B and C both excessively raise NF kappaB, leading to increased risk for liver cancer. Several labs around the world recently confirmed the Hepatitis C and cancer connection[610] involving elevated NF kappaB.[611,612] Likewise, several other labs confirmed the Hepatitis B and cancer connection.[613,614]

2) The Epstein Barr Virus (EBV) activates NF kappaB in lymph cells, causing lymphoma.[615]

3) Human T-cell leukemia virus type I is the cause of adult T-cell leukemia/lymphoma. It is activated by excess NF kappaB production.[616,617]

4) Human papillomavirus (HPV), a commonly sexually transmitted viral infection that can lead to cervical cancer, actively promotes excess NF kappaB.[618]

5) The Kaposi's sarcoma herpes virus induces problems by excessively activating NF kappaB.[619]

Mounting a more efficient immune response against viruses and not getting so run down that viral issues flare up are key factors in cancer-risk reduction. It is evident that if a person is overweight and has extra leptin, TNFa, and NF kappaB already circulating, then a viral infection has an easier time hijacking a defense system that is already handicapped.

SOLUTIONS

Having the body in a less inflammatory condition is the fundamental way to prevent problems with excess NF kappaB. Following the *Five Rules*, regular exercise, stress management, and maintaining optimum body weight are keys to reducing risk for disease. Adopting a lifestyle conducive to healthy rhythms and feeling in sync is essential.

As a person gets into higher levels of ongoing inflammation and wear and tear, there is a concurrent excess production of TNFa and NF kappaB. If a person is overweight, the fat cells make this problem worse by generating increased amounts of these signals into the body, on top of other stress factors.

Excess TNFa and NF kappaB problems are reflective of a general condition of a lack of antioxidants, as NF kappaB sits underneath the antioxidant system. Improved antioxidant status is likely to cool down the tendency towards excess NF kappaB production. This is why a variety of antioxidants, such as vitamin E, shows improvement for issues such as Alzheimer's.[620] Having enough antioxidants prevents toxins from inducing liver damage by helping to prevent excess NF kappaB.[621] Even getting enough vitamin C can help reduce TNFa and NF kappaB.[622]

While antioxidants alone may not fully solve a NF kappaB problem, they are the first line of defense. The more "antioxidant reserves" an individual has, the higher their ability to tolerate issues that would otherwise lead to excessive production of NF kappaB. A comprehensive array of basic antioxidant nutrients is helpful for everyone, specifically for the prevention of disease. Even the *Journal of the American Medical Association* agrees with this fundamental recommendation for disease prevention.[623]

In Chapter 43 and Chapter 44, on breast and prostate cancer, we list additional nutrients that have powerful NF kappaB regulating effects. These not only apply to cancer issues, they apply to offsetting the wear and tear of life. The greater degree of stressful wear and tear a person experiences, the greater the need for protection. This is not hard to figure out. Use enough support to stay in balance, in sync, and keep up with the demands of life.

SUMMARY

Excess leptin causes many problems relating to body weight and the ability to attain and maintain a proper body weight.

Additionally, excess leptin is a major risk factor that sets the stage for disease. This is because it raises and reinforces the excess production of TNFa and NF kappaB. Carrying extra pounds of body fat that cranks out these inflammatory signals is a major risk factor for any disease. Whether a person gets cancer, heart disease, Alzheimer's, or some other issue depends on genetic risk as well as other stress factors that contribute to their health picture.

Antioxidants form the first line of defense against stress-related generation of excess NF kappaB. Those who have been advocating antioxidants for years based on its ability to deactivate free radicals, now have far more powerful scientific information to back up their use. They are the primary bank account of natural compounds that act as a buffer for the tolerance of stress. When the buffer is lacking or is used up by too much stress, then excess activation of the panic stricken NF kappaB can wreak havoc with health.

The jigsaw puzzle of who gets what and why, as well as how to exactly solve the issues, will be the great scientific discoveries of this century. Meanwhile, it is apparent that reducing body fat to a healthy level and keeping the body in a state of natural balance are the keys to disease-free aging.

42

A Major Breakthrough for Bones

*P*roperly functioning leptin is essential for the formation and health of bones. It is a primary hormone that must work properly for bone health.

Drug companies want to have a drug for everything. They see bone-loss issues as a big drug market, using drugs for prevention. Current drugs to help prevent bone loss have adverse side effects and are not even directed at the real issue – making new bone. They only address a secondary factor in bone loss. A recent scientific article seeking to promote new areas for bone-loss drug design said the following about current bone-loss drugs:

> These drugs have been identified by serendipity rather than rational drug design and are not ideal because of limited bioavailability, mode of administration, or other unwanted effects. There is still a place for even more suitable and effective resorption inhibitors than those currently available. The more compelling need in this field is an acceptable drug that is anabolic for bone, that safely and acceptably increases bone mass, and improves the disturbances in bone microarchitecture that characterize established and advanced osteoporosis.[624]

As it turns out, leptin fits the description of this ideal drug. A primary factor in bone health is to maintain leptin in good working order, not having too little leptin and not having leptin resistance.

STARVATION METABOLISM AND BONE LOSS

Underweight women are prone to osteopenia and osteoporosis.[625] It is documented that underweight women lose significant bone.[626] Bone loss can occur during dieting as leptin levels drop.[627] Furthermore, this problem is a more significant issue for older women.[628] This is one reason why proper leptin management and following the *Five Rules* is so important.

Bone loss occurs when the anorexic-like starvation metabolism is present. It accelerates in the presence of excess inflammation of any type.

LEPTIN HELPS BONE WORK PROPERLY

Healthy bones are a more complex issue than simply the amount of bone mass. Leptin is involved with the healthy workings of bone metabolism. Leptin is involved with the formation of blood cells, both red cells and white cells. This activity takes place inside of bones.[629] Leptin acts as a powerful hormone inside of bone that stimulates the formation of new bone.[630]

In fact, not only does leptin act inside of bones to help make bone, recent information shows that when leptin binds to the hypothalamus gland in the brain, it facilitates the hypothalamus gland to initiate new bone formation.[631,632] Furthermore, omega 3 fatty acids are essential for this leptin-regulated bone building to take place.[633]

HOW BONE BUILDING WORKS

There are two main types of cells in bone that act to repair and build bone, osteoblasts and osteoclasts. Osteoclasts work by taking down old bone or stressed bone. Essentially, this is demolition work. Osteoblasts work by building up new bone. They take raw materials, such as protein and calcium, and construct bone.

Proper bone health involves a synergistic balance between osteoclasts and osteoblasts. As older or stressed bone is removed, new bone is built in its place. This process goes on throughout life.

Problems occur when factors speed up the rate of bone loss or when there is difficulty making new bone.

The current bone-loss drugs are targeted at osteoclasts, hoping to slow down the rate at which bone is removed. This may slow down inappropriate bone loss, but it does not solve the problem of building new bone or the problem of why bone loss accelerates. Such medications are second-rate, temporary solutions.

As mentioned above, leptin is the key hormonal signal that works on bone as well as coordinates a signal from the brain to build bone. Leptin is the key anabolic hormone for bone building, helping osteoblasts to form new bone.

This is why starvation metabolism causes bone loss. Bone is not made fast enough because there is not enough leptin to help stimulate the formation of new bone.

INFLAMMATION AND BONES

The other side of the coin relates to factors that cause the loss of bone to accelerate in the first place. These are factors that speed up the rate at which osteoclasts take down bone.

Such factors fall under the general umbrella of stress and inflammation, issues we have discussed throughout this book.

A large body of scientific evidence shows that excess IL-6, TNFa, and NF kappaB speed up the activity of osteoclasts, causing bone to be lost at an excessive rate.[634,635,636,637,638]

Vitamin D helps bones by protecting the bone-building cells, osteoblasts, from inappropriate cell death.[639] However, excess TNFa and NF kappaB block the ability of vitamin D to protect osteoblasts, leading to excess osteoblast cell death.[640] These inflammatory signals interfere with bone building while at the same time accelerate bone loss.

SOLUTIONS FOR HEALTHY BONES

Tocotrienols, a special form of vitamin E, help improve bone mineral density.[641] Unlike regular vitamin E, tocotrienols work by lowering excess TNFa and NF kappaB, the true source of the accelerated bone loss.

Another important nutrient is magnesium. A lack of magnesium causes depressed osteoblast bone building and accelerated osteoclast bone loss. In the presence of lacking magnesium, growth plate of bone decreased 33 percent indicating a lack of bone building. At the same time, TNFa activity inside of osteoclasts increased up to 500 percent of normal. The lack of magnesium permits excessive inflammation in the bone, a problem that prevents calcium from building bone.[642]

The results of a four-year study with adults ranging in age from 69-97 years of age confirmed the value of magnesium, potassium, fruits, and vegetables in the diet in terms of significantly helping preserve bone mass in these older individuals.

This study also laid to rest one of the oldest arguments amongst nutritionists, that is, is dietary protein good or bad for bone? Researchers thought that too much protein would be bad for bone because it would cause an acid pH that would work against the alkalizing minerals, fruits, and vegetables. Much to their surprise, they found that higher protein consumption facilitated better bone density.[643]

This result is not at all surprising to us. For years, we have told our clients the value of protein to help build bone.

Strength-bearing exercise helps bones because it applies stress to bones, in essence promoting them to break down so they can be built up. It is based on the age-old principle, "if you don't use it, you lose it." This strategy only works well if a person has the energetic and nutritional capacity to repair bone and form new bone, including adequate dietary protein.

SUMMARY

Building healthy bone requires the proper activity of bone-building hormones, cells, and nutrients. These are the anabolic bone-building factors. They include proper function of the hormone leptin and various nutrients such as calcium, vitamin D, omega 3 fatty acids, and protein.

Maintaining bone requires an absence of inflammation that interferes with bone building and accelerates bone loss. Nutrients proven to specifically help this issue are magnesium, tocotrienols, and alkalizing fruits and vegetables.

There are many nutrient suggestions throughout this book that help reduce excess inflammation. There are also numerous lifestyle and dietary tips to reduce stress and inflammation. A person needs to do enough to get out of the wear and tear trend. The inflammatory wear and tear trend is the actual cause of accelerated bone loss.

43

Leptin, NF kappaB, and Prostate Cancer

*A*t this point, researchers find that insulin resistance is more predictive than leptin levels of significantly increased risk for prostate cancer.[644] This is consistent with how insulin resistance coexists with problems of excess IGF1, and the IGF1 helps fuels the production of prostate cancer. We explained this mechanism in Chapter 31 on growth hormone.

However, a close analysis of prostate cancer cells shows that they have active leptin receptors in them. Furthermore, it may not require too much extra leptin, only moderate levels, in order to stimulate prostate cancer.[645] The more advanced and aggressive the prostate cancer is, the higher the level of leptin fueling its growth.[646]

We know that leptin resistance and insulin resistance work together to generate excess amounts of TNFa and NF kappaB. We have explained that cancer that is resistant to medical therapy has excess production of NF kappaB. This is certainly true of prostate cancer.[647,648,649,650,651]

Studies show that excess NF kappaB activity is the prime cause of prostate cancer, and it is the mechanism that makes prostate cancer resistant to treatment. Furthermore, it is not a passive factor that happens to be occurring at the same time as prostate cancer. It is the prime cause.

NF KAPPAB CAUSES TESTOSTERONE PROBLEMS

On a cellular basis, NF kappaB means survival. On a male body basis, the hormone testosterone means survival. In prostate cancer, even in cancer that does not require testosterone for growth, testosterone is used to make the cancer resistant to death.[652] The mechanism that enables this hijacking of testosterone to work against a man is the improperly elevated level of NF kappaB.

The severity and invasiveness of prostate cancer is related to how much excess NF kappaB there is; the greater the amount of NF kappaB, the more severe the cancer.[653] Additionally, if NF kappaB is blocked, then the prostate cancer stops growing and spreading.[654]

It is recognized that excess NF kappaB causes excess TNFa and IL-6, the two classic excess immune signals coming from fat cells that are in higher circulation due to leptin resistance. Once the NF kappaB is knocked down, the TNFa and IL-6 go down. This makes a previously untreatable disease susceptible to treatment.[655]

The bottom line of any prostate cancer, and especially prostate cancer that cannot be stopped, is a hijacking of testosterone by NF kappaB and excessive NF kappaB used by the cancer to aid its own survival. The two most important survival systems in the male body have been turned against the body.

This opens the door to new solutions never before possible, focusing on reducing NF kappaB so that cancer can be killed. For example, researchers have demonstrated the deficiency of zinc enables excess production of NF kappaB and prostate cancer. When zinc is replenished, the excess NF kappaB decreases. The cancer cells that were resistant to medical drugs are now susceptible to being killed by medical drugs.[656]

RISK FACTORS FOR PROSTATE CANCER

There are a variety of irritants that can induce excess NF kappaB in the prostate. They include estrogenic chemicals in the food supply, pollution, fungal infections, excess alcohol consumption, and more. There may be a combination of irritants that set the stage for wear and tear and create a situation wherein NF kappaB increases to an excess level.

As mentioned above, there is evidence linking leptin resistance to the severity of prostate cancer. While it is certainly possible to get prostate cancer due to factors other than leptin, leptin resistance creates a situation that seriously weakens the male body and sets the stage for prostate cancer as a prime risk factor for a great majority of American men.

Leptin resistance causes excess fat to form around internal body organs, including the prostate gland. This excess fat generates pro-inflammatory immune signals, TNFa and IL-6. The excess fat also reduces normal circulation to the prostate, tilting the pH of the prostate to a more acidic condition wherein infections can thrive and healthy enzymes do not work correctly.

These inflammatory immune signals also ramp up NF kappaB, causing it to be overactive on a continuous basis, a chemistry issue essential for cancer to prosper. The excess leptin also depresses testosterone, causing a weakness in the male system. Throw in some environmental toxin irritants, and we have a recipe for problems.

NATURAL OPTIONS

A key theme to prevent prostate cancer and maintain optimum male function is to keep the body in overall natural balance. The most fundamental issues in this regard are to eat properly and exercise. This is the foundation of a healthy program for anyone and the cornerstone of a treatment plan for those with a health problem.

We previously raised the issue of what is a minimum daily need for various nutrients. We proposed that needs are based on functional results. Thus, there may be a need for supplemental nutrients that enable the body to maintain optimum weight loss or even to initiate the possibility of weight loss.

While such nutrients may not be needed to prevent a nutritional deficiency disease, such as the lack of vitamin C causing scurvy, specific nutrients may be essential to help a person overcome leptin resistance. This need varies from person to person.

What about the nutritional needs of someone who is at high risk for prostate cancer or who has prostate cancer?

In the preventive sense, there are two ways to look at this. One way is to use nutrition to help correct leptin resistance and insulin resistance, in turn, lowering the risk factor for the problem. The other way is to use nutrition to lower NF kappaB.

The reason traditional cancer therapy does not work on resistant cancer cells is due to excess NF kappaB. Nutritional support is one of the most effective and side-effect free ways to lower NF kappaB.

Nature has already provided answers. The scientific evidence is clear that nutritional supplements can lower NF kappaB and thereby make cancer cells more susceptible to killing. We have already mentioned the importance of zinc. In the context of this chapter, we talk specifically about prostate cancer; however, this information applies to any type of cancer.

In a scientific review of over 80 case-controlled studies, it was demonstrated that the greater the amount of cruciferous vegetables in the diet, the less the risk for cancer. The proposed mechanism of action is the I3C (Indole-3-carbinol) content of the cruciferous vegetables and their effects on detoxification and estrogen metabolism.[657]

Eating three ½-cup servings of cruciferous vegetables per week cut the risk of prostate cancer by 41 percent.[658] Even a small amount helps, and it is clear that more is better. New research shows that I3C helps to induce cell death in cancer cells.[659] Part of the mechanism is a reduction in NF kappaB. This led the researchers to conclude that "I3C may be an effective chemo preventive or therapeutic agent against prostate cancer."[660]

Another promising nutrient is curcumin, a natural spice. Curcumin can directly turn off NF kappaB in hormone sensitive and hormone independent types of prostate cancer, leading to the death of prostate cancer cells.[661] A recent study showed curcumin to make prostate cancer cells more susceptible to be killed, enabling chemotherapy to kill them when before it could not. This led researchers to conclude that "the incorporation of curcumin into cytotoxic therapies may be a promising strategy for the treatment of androgen-independent prostate cancer."[662]

Other nutrient strategies are also backed by solid science. Silymarin, an herb we mentioned for liver support, has the ability to lower NF kappaB and cause prostate cancer cells to become susceptible to medical treatment. Researchers once again conclude, "These results indicate that silibinin, the active component of sylimarin, can be used to enhance the effectiveness of TNFalpha-based chemotherapy in advanced prostate cancer."[663]

Another nutrient, NAC (N-Acetyl-Cysteine) is known to suppress NF kappaB. Scientists recently reported that it can be an effective compound for helping chemotherapy work more effectively during prostate cancer treatment.[664]

There is no longer any reason for nutritional and drug therapies to be at odds with each other when it comes to prostate cancer, or any cancer for that matter. Nutritional supplements not only excel at reducing risk for those individuals living with extra pounds of fat, they can make a medical treatment work that has little or no chance of working without them.

SUMMARY

Leptin resistance and extra body fat are important risk factors that cause wear and tear to the male system, weakening it and setting the stage for prostate cancer risk.

Taking effective steps to clear leptin resistance and lose unneeded body weight are at the forefront of quality of life for any man.

44

Leptin, NF kappaB, and Breast Cancer

/ t was reported in 1999 that leptin activity is present in breast cancer cells. [665] There was another report in 2000 showing that patients with breast cancer were found to have higher circulating leptin and TNFa. [666] Another 2000 study also confirmed higher circulating leptin correlating to higher breast cancer in pre-menopausal women. [667]

Studies in 2002 distinctly characterized leptin as a growth promoter of breast cancer. One study, using human breast cancer MCF-7 cells, showed that leptin fueled the growth of this type of breast cancer cell. [668] In another study, with cells from 20 breast-cancer biopsies, all 20 were found to have active leptin activity.

Additionally, this study shows that leptin significantly fueled the growth of another breast-cancer cell line, T47-D. [669] The most recent study shows that high leptin and high blood sugar, due to insulin resistance, fueled breast-cancer cell growth. [670] It is clear that leptin activity is associated with breast cancer, and that leptin activity fuels the growth of breast cancer.

This information does not prove that leptin causes breast cancer; it simply means that leptin is involved in the process. Since leptin is essential for reproduction and is associated with fat, leptin will always be present in breast tissue. A key question becomes, at what point does leptin turn against its helpful role and start becoming a life-threatening problem?

NF KAPPAB AND BREAST CANCER

Excess and ongoing NF kappaB activation must be present for breast cancer to occur. [671] For example, normal and healthy breast cells can induce cell death in a breast cell that starts to become cancerous. If a mutant breast cell escapes self-imposed death, then it can go on to cause cancer.

What enables breast cancer to happen is excessive and ongoing production of NF kappaB. This is what makes breast cancer resistant to normal body checks and balances as well as makes breast cancer resistant to drug treatment.[672]

It is unlikely that we will ever discover a single irritant that causes breast cancer. There are many estrogenic chemicals in the environment that can easily bind to breast cells and induce extra NF kappaB activation. Too much emotional distress activates excess NF kappaB. So can physical wear and tear. Insulin resistance leads to excess IGF1, in turn stimulating the growth of breast cancer cells. Combine this with higher estrogens and higher leptin associated with higher body fat and/or a certain time in a woman's life and we have an overall situation that can tilt the body into chronic NF kappaB activation. It is not one issue; it is a combination of factors that disrupt natural balance.

Some women have better genetic tolerance for these issues and never have a problem. Other women have poor genetic tolerance and are more susceptible to have a problem even from lower amounts of "stressors." Therefore, family history is a predictive factor of genetic ability of NF kappaB to not get overloaded.

Regardless of genetic predisposition, keeping leptin in natural balance is a key way to reduce risk factors associated with breast cancer.

A COMMENT ON TAMOXIFEN

Tamoxifen is a favorite drug used to suppress estrogen activity following breast cancer. The hope is that it will stop breast cancer from coming back by reducing estrogenic activity in breast tissue. On the surface, this argument sounds reasonable. A closer look, based on new information, raises doubts regarding the safety of the drug.

It was found that Tamoxifen raises the production of leptin from fat cells, with a steady increase during the first six months of use. Twenty-one out of the 30 women in the study also experienced an increase in body fat as a result of the treatment.[673]

In a study comparing 58 women who had breast cancer to 58 women who did not, it was found that the cancer patients had higher leptin levels. Furthermore, in the cancer patient group, those taking Tamoxifen had higher levels of leptin than those not taking Tamoxifen. This was true even after correcting for body fat. The researchers concluded, "high-serum leptin levels seen in breast-cancer patients are not related to the stage of the disease or to cancer itself but may be associated with the use of Tamoxifen."[674]

This information is alarming because a drug that elevates leptin levels promotes leptin resistance. In turn, this can increase inflammation and NF kappaB anywhere in the body. This has the net effect of increasing general cancer risk.

We have already explained that leptin resistance promotes insulin resistance. Women with insulin resistance are much more likely to get a recurrence of breast cancer than women who do not have insulin resistance.[675]

Tamoxifen increases fatty congestion in the liver, a primary problem of leptin resistance. We have discussed the nature of fatty liver problems, including the magnification of liver damage from toxic exposure. The problem goes away when the drug is stopped.[676]

Tamoxifen causes abnormal estrogenic cell metabolism on the endometrial lining of the uterus.[677] The initial results of a major Tamoxifen study have been released. Notable side effects of the therapy include endometrial cancer, vaginal bleeding and discharge, cerebrovascular events, venous thromboembolic events, and hot flashes.[678]

This is a typical situation where the medical profession feels the benefits outweigh the risks. More pointedly, the drug has a lot of adverse side effects, but it is going to be recommended until there is a more effective drug to sell, which is likely to be years.[679]

Unlike the drug trial that halted the widespread use of estrogen replacement, it is unlikely that the use of Tamoxifen will be halted until there is a better drug. Tamoxifen has a degree of workability, and thus a degree of justification for its use. However, it only moderately helps one potential reason for a recurrence of breast cancer. It also has many side effects, some very serious. In terms of the numbers game played by medical statisticians, rationalization for continued use can be justified. What this means to the health of an individual taking the drug is not so clear.

THE MOMENTUM FOR A NEW APPROACH

There is adequate science already available to put a variety of nutritional supplements to rigorous medical testing. Most of these nutrients have very few, if any, adverse side effects. The nutrients can be used in combination with Tamoxifen and other breast-cancer treatments. In some cases, they may work better, which needs more clarification.

Following is a significant array of compelling information that is sure to open new doors for breast-cancer risk reduction. It also lends a hand in helping medical doctors more effectively treat breast cancer, as well as help prevent a recurrence of the problem.

An individual reading this book should understand that reducing excess inflammation is a good idea. However, think twice before reaching for a bottle of acetaminophen. Acetaminophen increases the growth of breast-cancer cells by 40 percent, specifically due to increased production of NF kappaB.[680]

Tocotrienols, a special form of vitamin E, have powerful anti-proliferative and cancer-cell killing capability, an ability that regular vitamin E (d alpha tocopherol) does not have.[681] There are numerous cell studies that show the ability of tocotrienols to reduce the spreading or knock out breast- cancer cells.[682,683,684,685]

Unlike Tamoxifen, tocotrienols can block both estrogen-receptor positive and estrogen-receptor negative breast cancer cells. When tocotrienols are combined with Tamoxifen, there is synergistic benefit.[686,687] Tocotrienols have a far superior advantage to regular vitamin E because they are much better at lowering TNFa and NF kappaB.[688]

CLA, the nutrient we use to help control leptin, made its claim to fame by reducing the risk for breast cancer.[689] Numerous studies confirm its ability to stop breast cancer cells.[690,691,692,693,694] Women with higher CLA in their blood have an inverse likelihood of breast cancer.[695] CLA works by knocking out excessive activation of NF kappaB in breast-cancer cells.[696]

Green tea is a natural option to reduce both TNFa and NF kappaB.[697] Green tea modulates, in a positive manner, genetic signals that otherwise lead to an excess production of NF kappaB in breast-cancer cells.[698] Therefore, green tea has the ability to help the body kill cancerous breast cells, while leaving healthy breast cells undamaged.[699]

Trans-resveratrol, a powerful antioxidant found in some red wines and available as a nutritional supplement, binds to estrogen receptors in breast tissue and interferes with cancer.[700] Scientists have proven that resveratrol works by reducing NF kappaB, thereby stopping the breast-cancer activity.[701] There is plenty of science to show that resveratrol is a potent anti-breast cancer and highly protective nutrient.[702,703,704,705]

The bioflavonoid quercetin, found in fresh vine-ripened fruit and available as a nutritional supplement, induces death in breast-cancer cells.[706] Quercetin demonstrated the ability to prevent environmental chemicals from promoting estrogen driven breast cancer.[707]

Interestingly, quercetin is shown to be more effective than Tamoxifen at binding to type II EBS receptors. The same study also shows it to be very effective at stopping the progression of a human breast-cancer cell line.[708] There is data to support the use of quercetin and Tamoxifen together, helping to synergistically make cancer more susceptible to medical treatment.[709]

Indole-3-caribinol (I3C) is the active component of cruciferous vegetables, mentioned in the chapter on prostate cancer. Several studies conducted in the early 1990s demonstrated that 400 mg of I3C per day in women can normalize the way estrogen is metabolized so that it will not go down a pathway that could stimulate cancer.[710,711,712]

When researchers injected I3C directly into breast-cancer cells, I3C halted the cancer-cell division by blocking cancer-cell DNA duplication.[713] This lead to another study to see if the I3C was as effective as Tamoxifen. Researchers injected one group of human breast-cancer cells with I3C, another group with Tamoxifen, and a third with I3C and Tamoxifen. The cells injected with Tamoxifen alone experienced a 60 percent inhibition in DNA synthesis, the cells injected with I3C had a 90 percent inhibition, and the combination had a 95 percent reduction.[714]

If there were drugs that could knock out NF kappaB, while leaving healthy cells alone, they would be the "gold standard" of cancer treatment and heralded on the front page of every paper and magazine as the greatest breakthroughs ever made for the treatment of cancer. The fact that nature already provides a wide array of such substances should be of more than passing interest, even to the worst skeptic.

Medical authorities will need to wait for extensive testing of these helpful nutrients until broad public recommendations can be made. This will take years, especially since there is no financial incentive for any drug company to pursue the issue.

Adequate science now exists for any women to incorporate special nutritional support as part of a breast-cancer risk-reduction program or to assist in a positive outcome of medical treatment. This is quite a bit more than nutritional use in the context of basic nutritional needs. This is nutritional use based on the most recent genetic discoveries relating to how natural function turns against the individual.

This data shows that reducing NF kappaB slows down cancer and makes cancer that is resistant to medical treatment much more responsive to medical treatment. This is done by restoring a normal gene signal back into a state of balance. Due to the lack of adverse side effects of these nutrients, there is good reason for consumers and medical professionals to gain a better working understanding of these nutrients in actual practice.

SUMMARY

Leptin is essential for female health, reproduction, and proper estrogen balance. Problems with leptin cause problems in the female system, including increased risk for breast cancer.

Leptin resistance leads to an inflammatory condition of excess TNFa and NF kappaB, increasing cancer risk and the potential for cancer that is not responsive to medical treatment.

Mastering leptin is the answer to this problem.

The Anti-Aging Skills of the Health Asset Manager

*I*t takes a considerable amount of skill and personal knowledge about the human body to have the potential to be a competent Health Asset Manager.™ It takes an additional level of personal strength and integrity to make daily choices to keep oneself on track and in a healthy pattern.

Our *Five Rules* are the key points about how to eat in order to have a good energy level and avoid developing problems with leptin resistance.

Our emphasis is on establishing an entire lifestyle pattern that facilitates a state or condition of natural balance. When a person has a good underlying base of healthy habits, they have much more potential to tolerate stress, perform at a higher level of efficiency, and have an overall higher quality of health.

Leptin is a hormone signal relating to long-term survival. A program for mastering leptin must, by definition, be a program for the long haul. This means a way of approaching life, wherein true success is measured not only in the ability to overcome acute challenges but also by the true quality of health as years go by.

A person needs a basic way to approach life that facilitates this result. Our *Five Rules* are not a diet plan to follow for a few weeks to drop a few pounds only to return to previous poor habits. Those who implement our *Five Rules* as a lifestyle will have a tremendous advantage in maintaining their health.

Incorporating relaxing exercise, adequate sleep, and good stress management skills are other key factors that are essential to the basic leptin-management plan. Such variables easily transcend dietary principles, meaning that many factors in life come to rely on the ability to successfully manage leptin.

In essence, mastering leptin is an issue of managing energy. If the body gets out of balance, the subconscious brain may enforce survival instincts that are misguided for the actual situation. This leads to weight gain and other health issues.

The far-reaching impact of leptin on all hormones is a significant health breakthrough. Leptin is the most important single hormone in the body. Although leptin was not discovered until 1994, what first seemed like a key hormone that regulated the response to starvation, soon became the superstar of hormones. Leptin is in control; all other hormones answer up to leptin. Leptin is the energy broker for the body, literally providing the financial energy to make metabolism work.

It takes considerable skill to manage leptin effectively. If done well, health will benefit dramatically. Serious problems with leptin resistance, including obesity, sex hormone issues, weight gain around the middle, fatty liver disease, addiction problems, memory and brain problems, cardiovascular issues, and cancer risk can all be improved with an effective leptin-management plan.

In addition to good diet and exercise, there are nutrient solutions that help resolve leptin resistance, increase the metabolism of fat, and reduce excess levels of leptin.

If leptin issues are left unresolved, there is eventually an increased risk for cancer. This is because the genetic signal NF kappaB gets overworked and stays in a chronic state of activation. This is a serious consequence from a failure to master leptin. The risk for any disease of aging is significantly increased.

Failing to master leptin as the years go by increases internal friction, therefore increasing the rate of aging. Initially this is an out-of-rhythm feeling that goes along with increased wear and tear. It can develop into an exhaustion of the metabolic system, such as fibromyalgia, or it can end up in the body's own natural and essential survival systems being turned against oneself. The excess production of TNFa, NF kappaB, cancer causation, and accelerated aging all share the same common features.[715]

Generally, this does not happen over a period of a few weeks or months. It happens as a result of a lifestyle pattern based on leptin mismanagement over a number of years. This results in a loss of the natural balancing systems of health, otherwise known as homeostasis. This causes aging to happen faster than it should. In many cases the aging process can be slowed down. In some cases, damage can be repaired and reflect "reverse aging."

BECOMING A *HEALTH ASSET MANAGER*™

Who taught us to put our health in the sole hands of our doctors? Why were we never educated to take charge of our own health? Why was any health education we received as children and teens so simplistic it failed to arm us with vital information about our health?

The top priority of the pharmaceutical-based medical world is the sale of drugs. The top priority of public-health officials appears to be the dispensing and enforcement of immunization programs. Could more knowledge and education keep us off the drug path and on a health path whereby drugs are not needed in the first place? The person with the biggest vested interest in your health is you. Quality of health is at stake, your single most important asset.

Knowledge is power. As a reader of this book, one is empowered with knowledge that is not only of immense personal value, it is also practical to implement as a lifestyle. The fact that doing so can have such a profound effect on overall health, both in terms of fixing existing issues as well as preventing serious health conditions, opens the door to many benefits for individuals and reduced health-care costs for society. This is truly information that can be used as a life tool, and it enables one to educate their family as well. This is where the change begins.

The ability to skillfully return the body to a state of natural balance is the key to a healthy future. Mastering leptin is the single most important skill of the Health Asset Manager.™ Our information opens the doors to healthy solutions that have never before been possible.

INDEX

REFERENCES

[1] Surgeon General's Report on Nutrition and Health. US Department of Health and Human Services. Available on the WEB @ www.mcsspotlight.org/media/reports/surgen_rep.html

[2] Mokdad AH, Serdula MK, Dietz WH, Bowman BA, Marks JS, Koplan JP. The spread of the obesity epidemic in the United States, 1991-1998. *JAMA* 1999 Oct 27;282(16):1519-22.

[3] Mokdad AH, Bowman BA, Ford ES, Vinico F, Marks JS, Koplan JP. The continuing epidemics of obesity and diabetes in the United States. *JAMA* 2001 Sep12;286(10):1195-200

[4] Bridges EJ, Woods SL. Cardiovascular chronobiology: do you know what time it is? *Prog Cardiovasc Nurs* 2001 Spring;16(2):65-79.

[5] Smith DH. Pharmacology of cardiovascular chronotherapeutic agents. *Am J Hypertens* 2001 Sep;14(9Pt 2):296S-301S.

[6] Levi F. Giacchetti S, Zidani R, Brezault-Bonnet C, Tigaud JM, Goldwasser F, Misset JL. Chronotherapy of colorectal cancer metastases. *Hepatogastroenterology* 2001 Mar-Apr;48(38):320-2.

[7] Vandel P, Boiteux J, Sechter D. Bilogicial rhythms and psychiatric syndromes. *Rev Prat* 1997 Nove 1;47(17):1878-83.

[8] Nagayama H. Influences of biological rhythms on the effects of psychotropic drugs. *Pyschosom Med* 1999 Set-Oct;61(5):618-29.

[9] Okawa M, Uchiyama M, Ozaki S, Shibui K, Ichikawa H. Circadian rhythm sleep disorders in adolescents: clinical trial of combined treatments based on chronobiology/ *Psychiatry Clin Neurosci* 1998 Oct;52(5):483-90.

[10] Kagami M, Tomioka H, Nakazawa T, Yoshida S. Chronotherapy of bronchial asthma: circadian rhythms in asthmatic symptoms. Report I: Survey on chronobiology acrophase of asthmatic symptoms. *Arerugi* 2001 Jun;50(6):528-34.

[11] Kraft M. Corticosteroids and leukotrienes: chronobiology and chronotherapy. *Chronobiol Int* 1999 Sep;16(5):683-93.

[12] Turkoski BB. Medication timing for the elderly: the impact of biorhythms on effectiveness. *Geriatr Nurs* 1998 May-June;19(3):146-51.

[13] Stefanov R, Dimitrov BD. Cytomegalovirus infection in infants: an example of a chronopharmacological approach. *Folia Med (Plovdiv)* 1999;41(1):20-4.

[14] Fyfe AI. Transplant atherosclerosis: the clinical syndrome, pathogenesis and possible model of spontaneous atherosclerosis. *Can J Cardiol* 1992 Jun;8(5):509-19

[15] Stockfleth E, Ulrich C, Meyer T, Christophers E. Epithelial malignancies in organ transplant patients: clinical presentation and new methods of treatment. *Recent Results Cancer Res* 2002;160:251-8

[16] Zackheim HS, Koo J, LeBoit PE, McCalmont TH, Bowman PH, Kashani-Sabet M, Jones C, Zehnder J. Psoriasiform mycosis fungoides with fatal outcome after treatment with cyclosporine. *J Am Acad Dermatol* 2002 Jul;47(1):155-7

[17] Pielop JA, Jones D, Duvic M. Transient CD30+ nodal transformation of cutaneous T-cell lymphoma associated with cyclosporine treatment. Int J Dermatol 2001 Aug;40(8):505-11

[18] Zhang Y, Proenca R, Maffei M, Barone M, Leopold L & Friedman JM. (1994) Positional cloning of the mouse *obese* gene and its human homologue. *Nature* 372, 425-432.

[19] Trayhurn P, Beattie JH. Physiological role of adipose tissue: white adipose tissue as an endocrine and secretory organ *Nutrition Society* (2001) 60, 329-339.

[20] Wilding JP. Leptin and the control of obesity. *Curr Opin Pharmacol* 2001 Dec;1(6):656-61.

[21] Scarpace PJ, Tumer N. Peripheral and hypothalamic leptin resistance with age-related obesity. *Physiol Behav* 2001 Nov-Dec;74(4-5):721-7.

[22] Schwartz MW. Brain pathways controlling food intake and body weight. *Exp Biol Med Vol.* 226(11):978-981, 2001.

[23] Trayhurn P, Beattie JH. Physiological role of adipose tissue: white adipose tissue as an endocrine and secretory organ *Nutrition Society* (2001) 60, 329-339.

[24] Cannon WB Bodily changes in pain, hunger, fear, and rage. New York and London:D.Appleton and Co. 1929.

[25] Trayhurn P, Duncan JS, & Rayner DV (1995*a*) Acute cold-induced suppression of *ob*(obese) expression and circulating heptin levels in lean mice by the beta 3-adrenoceptor agonists BRL 35135A and ZD2079. *Biochemical and Biophysical Research Communications* 228, 605-610.

[26] Satoh N, Ogawa Y, Katsuura G, Numata Y, Tsuji T, Hayase M, Ebihara K, Masuzaki H, Hosoda K, Yoshimasa Y & Nakao K. (1999) Sympathetic activation of leptin via the ventromedial hypothalamus – Leptin-induced increase in catecholamine secretion. *Diabetes* 48, 1787-1793.

[27] Sinha MK, Ohannesian JP, Heiman ML< Kriauciunas A, Stephens TW, Magosin S, Marco C & Caro JF. (1996) Nocturnal rise of leptin in lean, obese, and non-insulin-dependent diabetes mellitus subjects. *Journal of Clinical Investigation* 97, 1344-1347.

[28] Licinio J, Mantzoros C, Negrao AB, Cizza G, Wong ML, Bongiorno PB, Chrousos GP, Karp B, Allen C, Flier JS & Gold PW. (1997) Human leptin levels are pulsatile and inversely related to pituitary-adrenal function. *Nature Medicine* 3, 575-579.

[29] Herrmann TS, Bean ML, Black TM, Wang P, Coleman RA. High glycemic index carbohydrate diet alters the diurnal rhythm of leptin but not insulin concentrations. *Exp Biol Med* (Maywood) 2001 Dec;226(11):1037-44

[30] Kalsbeek A, Fliers E, Romijn JA, La Fleur SE, Wortel J, Bakker O, Endert E, Buijs RM. The suprachiasmatic nucleus generates the diurnal changes in plasma leptin levels. *Endocrinology* 2001 Jun;142(6):2677-85

[31] Himms-Hagen J. (1999) Physiological roles of the leptin endocrine system: Differences between ice and humans. *Critical Reviews in Clinical and Laboratory Science* 36, 575-655.

[32] Trayhurn P, Hoggard N, Mercer JG & Rayner DV. (1999) Leptin: fundamental aspects. *International Journal of Obesity* 23, 22-28.

[33] Kieffer TJ, Heller RS, Leech CA, Holz GG, Habener JF. Leptin suppression of insulin secretion by te activation of the ATP-sensitive K channels in pancreatic B-cells. *Diabetes* 46: 1087-1093, 1997.

[34] Van Gaal Lf, Wauters MA, Mertens IL, Considine RV, DE Leeuw IH: Clinical endocrinology of human leptin. *Int J Obes Relat Metab Disord* 23 (Suppl 1): 29-36, 1999.

[35] Tatti P, Masselli L, Buonanno A, Di Mauro P, Strollo F. Leptin levels in diabetic and nondiabetic subjects. *Endocrine* 2001 Aug;15(3):305-8.

[36] Naimi TS, Brewer RD, Mokdad A, Denny C, Serdula MK, Marks JS. Binge Drinking Among US Adults. *JAMA* 2003 Jan 1;289(1):70-5

[37] Mokdad AH, Ford ES, Bowman BA, Dietz WH, Vinicor F, Bales VS, Marks JS. Prevalence of obesity, diabetes, and obesity-related health risk factors, 2001. *JAMA* 2003 Jan 1;289(1):76-9

[38] Kiefer F, Jahn H, Wolf K, Kampf P, Knaudt K, Wiedemann K. Free-choice alcohol consumption in mice after application of the appetite regulating peptide leptin. *Alcohol Clin Exp Res* 2001 May;25(5):787-9

[39] Kiefer F, Jahn H, Jaschinski M, Holzbach R, Wolf K, Naber D, Wiedemann K. Leptin: a modulator of alcohol craving? *Biol Psychiatry* 2001 May 1;49(9):782-7

[40] Nicolas JM, Fernandez-Sola J, Fatjo F, Casamitjana R, Bataller R, Sacanella E, Tobias E, Badia E, Estruch R. Increased circulating leptin levels in chronic alcoholism. Alcohol Clin Exp Res 2001 Jan;25(1):83-8

[41] Rojdmark S, Calissendorff J, Brismar K. Alcohol ingestion decreases both diurnal and nocturnal secretion of leptin in healthy individuals. Clin Endocrinol (Oxf) 2001 Nov;55(5):639-47

[42] Campillo B, Sherman E, Richardet JP, Bories PN. Serum leptin levels in alcoholic liver cirrhosis: relationship with gender, nutritional status, liver function and energy metabolism. Eur J Clin Nutr 2001 Nov;55(11):980-8

[43] Lin HZ, Yang SQ, Zeldin G, Diehl AM. Chronic ethanol consumption induces the production of tumor necrosis factor-alpha and related cytokines in liver and adipose tissue. Alcohol Clin Exp Res 1998 Aug;22(5 Suppl):231S-237S

[44] Kiefer F, Jahn H, Schick M, Wiedemann K ALCOHOL INTAKE, TUMOUR NECROSIS FACTOR-alpha, LEPTIN AND CRAVING: FACTORS OF A POSSIBLY VICIOUS CIRCLE? Alcohol 2002 Jul-Aug;37(4):401-4

[45] Hill DB, Barve S, Joshi-Barve S, McClain C. Increased monocyte nuclear factor-kappaB activation and tumor necrosis factor production in alcoholic hepatitis. J Lab Clin Med 2000 May;135(5):387-95

[46] Jokelainen K, Reinke LA, Nanji AA. NF kappaB activation is associated with free radical generation and endotoxemia and precedes pathological liver injury in experimental alcoholic liver disease. Cytokine 2001 Oct 7;16(1):36-9

[47] Nanji AA, Jokelainen K, Fotouhinia M, Rahemtulla A, Thomas P, Tipoe GL, Su GL, Dannenberg AJ. Increased severity of alcoholic liver injury in female rats: role of oxidative stress, endotoxin, and chemokines. Am J Physiol Gastrointest Liver Physiol 2001 Dec;281(6):G1348-56

[48] Saller R, Meier R, Brignoli R. The use of silymarin in the treatment of liver diseases. Drugs 2001;61(14):2035-63

[49] Capasso A. Involvement of nuclear factor-kB in the expression of opiate withdrawal. Prog Neuropsychopharmacol Biol Psychiatry 2001 Aug;25(6):1259-68

[50] Shalev U, Yap J, Shaham Y. Leptin attenuates acute food deprivation-induced relapse to heroin seeking. J Neurosci 2001 Feb 15;21(4):RC129

[51] Lee YW, Hennig B, Yao J, Toborek M. Methamphetamine induces AP-1 and NF kappaB binding and transactivation in human brain endothelial cells. J Neurosci Res 2001 Nov 15;66(4):583-91

[52] Larsen PJ, Vrang N, Tang-Christensen M, Jensen PB, Hay-Schmidt A, Romer J, Bjerre-Knudsen L, Kristensen P. Ups and downs for neuropeptides in body weight homeostasis: pharmacological potential of cocaine amphetamine regulated transcript and pre-proglucagon-derived peptides. Eur J Pharmacol 2002 Apr 12;440(2-3):159-72

[53] Kristensen P, Judge ME, Thim L, Ribel U, Christjansen KN, Wulff BS, Clausen JT, Jensen PB, Madsen OD, Vrang N, Larsen PJ, Hastrup S. Hypothalamic CART is a new anorectic peptide regulated by leptin. Nature 1998 May 7;393(6680):72-6

[54] Ludvigsen S, Thim L, Blom AM, Wulff BS. Solution structure of the satiety factor, CART, reveals new functionality of a well-known fold. Biochemistry 2001 Aug 7;40(31):9082-8

[55] Tsuruta Y, Yoshimatsu H, Hidaka S, Kondou S, Okamoto K, Sakata T. Hyperleptinemia in A(y)/a mice upregulates arcuate cocaine- and amphetamine-regulated transcript expression. Am J Physiol Endocrinol Metab 2002 Apr;282(4):E967-73

[56] Kask A, Schioth HB, Mutulis F, Wikberg JE, Rago L. Anorexigenic cocaine- and amphetamine-regulated transcript peptide intensifies fear reactions in rats. Brain Res 2000 Feb 28;857(1-2):283-5

[57] Kastin AJ, Akerstrom V. Entry of CART into brain is rapid but not inhibited by excess CART or leptin. Am J Physiol 1999 Nov;277(5 Pt 1):E901-4

[58] Whitfield JF. Leptin: brains and bones. *Expert Opin Investig Drugs* 2001 Sep;10(9):1617-22

[59] Figenschau Y, Knutsen G, Shahazeydi S, Johansen O, Sveinbjornsson B. Human articular chondrocytes express functional leptin receptors. *Biochem Biophys Res Commun* 2001 Sep 14;287(1):190-7

[60] Hardwick JC, Van Den Brink GR, Offerhaus GJ, Van Deventer SJ, Peppelenbosch MP. Leptin is a growth factor for colonic epithelial cells. *Gastroenterology* 2001 Jul;121(1):79-90

[61] Chen HC, Smith SJ, Tow B, Elias PM, Farese RV Jr. Leptin modulates the effects of acyl CoA:diacylglycerol acyltransferase deficiency on murine fur and sebaceous glands. *J Clin Invest* 2002 Jan;109(2):175-81

[62] Christou H, Serdy S, Mantzoros CS. Leptin in relation to growth and developmental processes in the fetus. *Semin Reprod Med* 2002;20(2):123-30

[63] Shanley LJ, Irving AJ, Harvey J. Leptin enhances NMDA receptor function and modulates hippocampal synaptic plasticity. *J Neurosci* 2001 Dec 15;21(24):RC186

[64] Dicou E, Attoub S, Gressens P. Neuroprotective effects of leptin in vivo and in vitro. *Neuroreport* 2001 Dec 21;12(18):3947-51

[65] Sriram K, Benkovic SA, Miller DB, O'Callaghan JP. Obesity exacerbates chemically induced neurodegeneration. *Neuroscience* 2002;115(4):1335-46

[66] Dunbar JC, Lu H. Chronic intracerebroventricular insulin attenuates the leptin-mediated but not alpha melanocyte stimulating hormone increase in sympathetic and cardiovascular responses. *Brain Res Bull* 2000 May 15;52(2):123-6

[67] Masuo K. Obesity-related hypertension: role of the sympathetic nervous system, insulin,and leptin. *Curr Hypertens Rep* 2002 Apr;4(2):112-8

[68] Esler M, Rumantir M, Wiesner G, Kaye D, Hastings J, Lambert G. Sympathetic nervous system and insulin resistance: from obesity to diabetes. *Am J Hypertens* 2001 Nov;14(11 Pt 2):304S-309S

[69] Bratanova-Tochkova TK, Cheng H, Daniel S, Gunawardana S, Liu YJ, Mulvaney-Musa J, Schermerhorn T, Straub SG, Yajima H, Sharp GW. Triggering and augmentation mechanisms, granule pools, and biphasic insulin secretion. Diabetes 2002 Feb;51 Suppl 1:S83-90

[70] Radziuk J, Pye S. Hepatic glucose uptake, gluconeogenesis and the regulation of glycogen synthesis. *Diabetes Metab Res Rev* 2001 Jul-Aug;17(4):250-72

[71] Powers, MA Handbook of Diabetes Medical Nutrition Therapy *Aspen Publishers* 1996:8-9

[72] Buczkowska EO, Jarosz-Chobot P. Insulin effect on metabolism in skeletal muscles and the role of muscles in regulation of glucose homeostasis *Przegl Lek* 2001;58(7-8):782-7

[73] Powers, MA Handbook of Diabetes Medical Nutrition Therapy *Aspen Publishers* 1996:8

[74] Powers, MA Handbook of Diabetes Medical Nutrition Therapy *Aspen Publishers* 1996:8

[75] Powers, MA Handbook of Diabetes Medical Nutrition Therapy *Aspen Publishers* 1996:8

[76] Powers, MA Handbook of Diabetes Medical Nutrition Therapy *Aspen Publishers* 1996:9

[77] Powers, MA Handbook of Diabetes Medical Nutrition Therapy *Aspen Publishers* 1996:9

[78] Zammit VA, Waterman IJ, Topping D, McKay G. Insulin stimulation of hepatic triacylglycerol secrection and the etiology of insulin resistance. J Nutr 2001 Aug;131(8);2074-7

[79] Diraison F, Dusserre E, Vidal H, Sothier M, Beylot M. Increased hepatic lipogenesis but decreased expression of lipogenic gene in adipose tissue in human obesity. *Am J Physiol Endocrinol Metab* 2002 Jan;282(1):E46-51

[80] Zhao AZ, Shinohara MM, Huang D, Shimizu M, Eldar-Finkelman H, Krebs EG, Beavo JA, Bornfeldt KE. Leptin induces insulin-like signaling that antagonizes

cAMP elevation by glucagon in hepatocytes. *J Biol Chem* 2000 Apr 14;275(15):11348-54

[81] Seppala-Lindroos A, Vehkavaara S, Hakkinen AM, Goto T, Westerbacka J, Sovijarvi A, Halavaara J, Yki-Jarvinen H. Fat accumulation in the liver is associated with defects in insulin suppression of glucose production and serum free Fatty acids independent of obesity in normal men. *J Clin Endocrinol Metab* 2002 Jul;87(7):3023-8

[82] Nemecz M, Preininger K, Englisch R, Furnsinn C, Schneider B, Waldhausl W, Roden M. Acute effect of leptin on hepatic glycogenolysis and gluconeogenesis in perfused rat liver.*Hepatology* 1999 Jan;29(1):166-72

[83] Harris RB. Acute and chronic effects of leptin on glucose utilization in lean mice. *Biochem Biophys Res Commun* 1998 Apr 17;245(2):502-9

[84] Hanefeld M, Kohler C. The metabolic syndrome and its epidemiologic dimensions in historical perspective *Z Arztl Fortbild Qualitatssich* 2002 Mar;96(3):183-8

[85] Gomez-Ambrosi J, Salvador J, Paramo JA, Orbe J, de Irala J, Diez-Caballero A, Gil MJ, Cienfuegos JA, Fruhbeck G. Involvement of leptin in the association between percentage of body fat and cardiovascular risk factors. Clin Biochem 2002 Jun;35(4):315-20

[86] Unger RH. Lipotoxic diseases. *Annu Rev Med* 2002;53:319-36

[87] Hosker JP, Burnett MA, Mathews DR, Turner RC. Suppression of insulin secretion by falling plasma glucose levels is impaired in type 2 diabetes. *Diabetic Med* 1988;5:856

[88] Gerich JE. Is reduced first-phase insulin release the earliest detectable abnormality in individuals destined to develop type 2 diabetes? *Diabetes* 2002 Feb;51 Suppl 1:S117-21

[89] Trayhurn P, Hoggard N, Mercer JG & Rayner DV. (1999) Leptin: fundamental aspects. *International Journal of Obesity* 23, 22-28.

[90] Kieffer TJ, Heller RS, Leech CA, Holz GG, Habener JF. Leptin suppression of insulin secretion by te activation of the ATP-sensitive K channels in pancreatic B-cells. *Diabetes* 46: 1087-1093, 1997.

[91] Van Gaal Lf, Wauters MA, Mertens IL, Considine RV, DE Leeuw IH: Clinical endocrinology of human leptin. *Int J Obes Relat Metab Disord* 23 (Suppl 1): 29-36, 1999.

[92] Masuo K, Mikami H, Ogihara T, Tuck ML. Familial obesity, sympathetic activation and blood pressure level. *Blood Press* 2001;10(4):199-204.

[93] Law C. Adult obesity and growth in childhood. *BMJ* 2001 Dec 8;323(7325):1320-1.

[94] Breier BH, Vickers MH, Ikenasio BA, Chan KY, Wong WP. Fetal programming of appetite and obesity. *Mol Cell Endocrinol* 2001 Dec 20;185(1-2):73-9.

[95] Wang J, Obici S, Morgan K, Barzilai N, Feng Z, Rossetti L. Overfeeding rapidly induced leptin and insulin resistance. *Diabetes* 2001 Dec;50(12):2786-91.

[96] Guyton A. Specific dynamic action of protein. *Textbook of Medical Physiology* WB Saunders Company 1991:793-4.

[97] Receputo G, Rapisarda R, Motta L. Centenarians: health status and life conditions *Ann Ital Med Int* 1995 Jan-Mar;10(1):41-5

[98] Bray GA. Reciprocal relation of food intake and sympathetic activity: experimental observations and clinical implications. *Int J Obes Relat Metab Disord* 2000 Jun;24 Suppl 2:S8-17

[99] Astrup A. Thermogenic drugs as a strategy for treatment of obesity. *Endocrine* 2000 Oct;13(2):207-12

[100] Boozer CN, Daly PA, Homel P, Solomon JL, Blanchard D, Nasser JA, Strauss R, Meredith T. Herbal ephedra/caffeine for weight loss: a 6-month randomized safety and efficacy trial. *Int J Obes Relat Metab Disord* 2002 May;26(5):593-604

[101] Sachan DS, Hongu N. Increases in VO(2)max and metabolic markers of fat oxidation by caffeine, carnitine, and choline supplementation in rats. *0955-2863* 2000 Oct;11(10):521-526

[102] Ryu S, Choi SK, Joung SS, Suh H, Cha YS, Lee S, Lim K. Caffeine as a lipolytic food component increases endurance performance in rats and athletes. *J Nutr Sci Vitaminol* (Tokyo) 2001 Apr;47(2):139-46

[103] McCarty MF. Modulation of adipocyte lipoprotein lipase expression as a strategy for preventing or treating visceral obesity. *Med Hypotheses* 2001 Aug;57(2):192-200

[104] Sakamoto W, Nishihira J, Fujie K, Mizuno S, Ozaki M, Yukawa S. Coffee and fitness-coffee suppresses lipopolysaccharide-induced liver injury in rats. *J Nutr Sci Vitaminol* (Tokyo) 2000 Dec;46(6):316-20

[105] Lindaman BA, Hinkhouse MM, Conklin JL, Cullen JJ. The effect of phosphodiesterase inhibition on gallbladder motility in vitro. *J Surg Res* 2002 Jun 15;105(2):102-8

[106] Boekema PJ, Samsom M, van Berge Henegouwen GP, Smout AJ. Coffee and gastrointestinal function: facts and fiction. A review. *Scand J Gastroenterol Suppl* 1999;230:35-9

[107] Cammisotto PG, Bukowiecki LJ. Mechanisms of leptin secretion from white adipocytes. *Am J Physiol Cell Physiol* 2002 Jul;283(1):C244-50

[108] Ramsey JJ, Colman RJ, Swick AG, Kemnitz JW. Energy expenditure, body composition, and glucose metabolism in lean and obese rhesus monkeys treated with ephedrine and caffeine. *Am J Clin Nutr* 1998 Jul;68(1):42-51

[109] van Dam RM, Feskens EJ. Coffee consumption and risk of type 2 diabetes mellitus. *Lancet* 2002 Nov 9;360(9344):1477-8

[110] Lieberman HR, Tharion WJ, Shukitt-Hale B, Speckman KL, Tulley R. Effects of caffeine, sleep loss, and stress on cognitive performance and mood during U.S. Navy SEAL training. *Psychopharmacology* (Berl) 2002 Nov;164(3):250-61

[111] Yeomans MR, Ripley T, Davies LH, Rusted JM, Rogers PJ. Effects of caffeine on performance and mood depend on the level of caffeine abstinence. *Psychopharmacology* (Berl) 2002 Nov;164(3):241-9

[112] McClellan Stine M, O'Connor RJ, Yatko BR, Grunberg NE, Cousino Klein L. Evidence for a relationship between daily caffeine consumption and accuracy of time estimation. *Hum Psychopharmacol* 2002 Oct;17(7):361-7

[113] Kruger S, Braunig P. Abuse of body weight reducing agents in bulimia nervosa *Nervenarzt* 1995 Jan;66(1):66-9

[114] Sours JA. Case reports of anorexia nervosa and caffeinism. *Am J Psychiatry* 1983 Feb;140(2):235-6

[115] Shaul PW, Farrell MK, Maloney MJ. Caffeine toxicity as a cause of acute psychosis in anorexia nervosa. *J Pediatr* 1984 Sep;105(3):493-5 Shaul PW, Farrell MK, Maloney MJ. Caffeine toxicity as a cause of acute psychosis in anorexia nervosa. *J Pediatr* 1984 Sep;105(3):493-5

[116] Forman J, Aizer A, Young CR. Myocardial infarction resulting from caffeine overdose in an anorectic woman. *Ann Emerg Med* 1997 Jan;29(1):178-80

[117] Keijzers GB, De Galan BE, Tack CJ, Smits P. Caffeine can decrease insulin sensitivity in humans. Diabetes Care 2002 Feb;25(2):364-9

[118] Lane JD, Pieper CF, Phillips-Bute BG, Bryant JE, Kuhn CM. Caffeine affects cardiovascular and neuroendocrine activation at work and home. *Psychosom Med* 2002 Jul-Aug;64(4):595-603

[119] Halford JC, Blundell JE. Separate systems for serotonin and leptin in appetite control. *Ann Med* 2000 Apr;32(3):222-32

[120] Christensen L, Pettijohn L. Mood and carbohydrate cravings. *Appetite* 2001 Apr;36(2):137-45

[121] Christenese L, Somers S. Comparison of nutrient intake among depressed and nondepressed individuals. *Int J Eat Disord* 1996 July;20(1):105-9

[122] Sayegh R, Schiff I, Wurtman J, Spiers P, McDermott J, Wurtman R. The effect of carbohydrate rich beverage on mood, appetite, and cognitive function in women with premenstrual syndrome. *Obstet Gynecol* 1995 Oct;86(4 Pt 1):520-8

[123] Yoshimatsu H, Chiba S, Tajima D, Akehi Y, Sakata T. Histidine suppresses food intake through its conversion into neuronal histamine. *Exp Biol Med* (Maywood) 2002 Jan;227(1):63-8

[124] Mollet A, Lutz TA, Meier S, Riediger T, Rushing PA, Scharrer E. Histamine H1 receptors mediate the anorectic action of the pancreatic hormone amylin. *Am J Physiol Regul Integr Comp Physiol* 2001 Nov;281(5):R1442-8

[125] Morimoto T, Yamamoto Y, Yamatodani A. Brain histamine and feeding behavior. *Behav Brain Res* 2001 Oct 15;124(2):145-50

[126] Watanabe T, Yanai K. Studies on functional roles of the histaminergic neuron system by using pharmacological agents, knockout mice and positron emission tomography. *Tohoku J Exp Med* 2001 Dec;195(4):197-217

[127] Kang JH, Kim KS, Choi SY, Kwon HY, Won MH, Kang TC. Carnosine and related dipeptides protect human ceruloplasm against peroxyl radical mediated modification. *Mol Cells* 2002 Jun 30:13(3):498-502

[128] Tabakman R, Lazarovici P, Kohen R. Neuroprotective effects of carnosine and homocarnosine on pheochromocytoma PC12 cells exposed to ischemia. *J Neurosci Res* 2002 May 15;68(4):463-9

[129] Boldyrev AA, Yuneva MO, Sorokina EV, Kramarenko GG, Fedorova TN, Konovalova GG, Lankin VZ. Antioxidant systems in tissues of senescence accelerated mice. *Biochemestry (Mosc)* 2001 Oct;66(10):1157-63

[130] Dukic-Stefanovic S, Schinzel R, Riederer P, Munch G. AGES in brain aging: AGE-inhibitors as neuroprotective and anti-dementia drugs? *Biogerontology* 2001;2(1):19-334

[131] Horning MS, Blakemore LJ, Trombley PQ. Endogenous mechanisms of neuroprotection; role of zinc, copper, and carnosine. *Brain Res* 2000 Jan 3;852 (1) :56-61

[132] Niijima A, Okui T, Matsumura Y, Yamano T, Tsuruoka N, Kiso Y, Nagai K. Effects of L carnosine on renal sympathetic nerve activity in DOCA-salt hypertensive rats. *Auton Neurosci* 2002 May 31;97(2):99-102

[133] Wilding JP. Neuropeptides and appetite control. *Diabet Med* 2002 Aug;19(8):619-27

[134] Fekete C, Sarkar S, Rand WM, Harney JW, Emerson CH, Bianco AC, Lechan RM. Agouti-related protein (AGRP) has a central inhibitory action on the hypothalamic-pituitary-thyroid (HPT) axis; comparisons between the effect of AGRP and neuropeptide Y on energy homeostasis and the HPT axis. *Endocrinology* 2002 Oct;143(10):3846-53

[135] Claycombe KJ, Xue BZ, Mynatt RL, Zemel MB, Moustaid-Moussa N. Regulation of leptin by agouti. *Physiol Genomics* 2000 Apr 27;2(3):101-5.

[136] Zemel MB. Agouti/melanocortin interaction with leptin pathways in obesity. *Nutr Rev* 1998 Sep;56(9):271-4.

[137] Zemel MB, Shi H, Greer B, Dirienzo D, Zemel PC. Regualtion of adiposity by dietary calcium. *FASEB J* 2000 Jun;14(9):1132-8.

[138] Makimura H, Mizuno TM, Mastaitis JW, Agami R, Mobbs CV. Reducing hypothalamic AGRP by RNA interference increases metabolic rate and decreases body weight without influencing food intake. *BMC Neurosci* 2002 Nov 7;3(1):18

[139] Zemel MB. Caluium modulation of hypertension and obesity mechanisms and implications. *J Am Coll Nutr* 2001 Oct;20(5 Suppl):428S-435;discussion 440S-442S.

[140] Shi H, Dirienzo D, Zemel MB. Effects of dietary calcium on adipocyte lipid metabolism and body weight regulation in energy-restricted aP2-agouti transgenic mice. *FASEB J* 2001 Feb;15(2):291-3.

[141] Menendez C, Lage M, Peino R, Baldelli R, Concheiro P, Dieguez C, Casanueva FF. Retinoic acid and vitamin D(3) powerfully inhibit in vitro leptin secretion by human adipose tissue. *J Endocrinol* 2001 Aug;170(2):425-31.

[142] Holst JJ, Orskov C. Incretin hormones—an update. Scand J Clin Lab Invest Suppl 2001;(234):75-85

[143] Miyawaki K, Yamada Y, Ban N, Ihara Y, Tsukiyama K, Zhou H, Fujimoto S, Oku A, Tsuda K, Toyokuni S, Hiai H, Mizunoya W, Fushiki T, Holst JJ, Makino M, Tashita A, Kobara Y, Tsubamoto Y, Jinnouchi T, Jomori T, Seino Y. Inhibition of gastric inhibitory polypeptide signaling prevents obesity. Nat Med 2002 Jul;8(7):738-42

[144] Ninomiya Y, Shigemura N, Yasumatsu K, Ohta R, Sugimoto K, Nakashima K, Lindemann B. Leptin and sweet taste. *Vitam Horm* 2002;64:221-48

[145] Cone RD, Cowley MA, Butler AA, Fan W, Marks DL, Low MJ. The arcuate nucleus as a conduit for diverse signals relevant to energy homeostasis. *Int J Obes Relat Metab Disord* 2001 Dec;25 Suppl 5:S63-7

[146] Tschop M, Flora DB, Mayer JP, Heiman ML. Hypophysectomy prevents ghrelin-induced adiposity and increases gastric ghrelin secretion in rats. *Obes Res* 2002 Oct;10(10):991-9

[147] Beck B, Musse N, Stricker-Krongrad A. Ghrelin, macronutrient intake and dietary preferences in long-evans rats. *Biochem Biophys Res Commun* 2002 Apr 12;292(4):1031-5

[148] Caixas A, Bashore C, Nash W, Pi-Sunyer F, Laferrere B. Insulin, unlike food intake, does not suppress ghrelin in human subjects. *J Clin Endocrinol Metab* 2002 Apr;87(4):1902

[149] Volante M, Allia E, Gugliotta P, Funaro A, Broglio F, Deghenghi R, Muccioli G, Ghigo E, Papotti M. Expression of ghrelin and of the GH secretagogue receptor by pancreatic islet cells and related endocrine tumors. *J Clin Endocrinol Metab* 2002 Mar;87(3):1300-8

[150] Trudel L, Tomasetto C, Rio MC, Bouin M, Plourde V, Eberling P, Poitras P. Ghrelin/motilin-related peptide is a potent prokinetic to reverse gastric postoperative ileus in rat. *Am J Physiol Gastrointest Liver Physiol* 2002 Jun;282(6):G948-52

[151] Papotti M, Cassoni P, Volante M, Deghenghi R, Muccioli G, Ghigo E. Ghrelin-producing endocrine tumors of the stomach and intestine. *J Clin Endocrinol Metab* 2001 Oct;86(10):5052-9

[152] Volante M, Allia E, Gugliotta P, Funaro A, Broglio F, Deghenghi R, Muccioli G, Ghigo E, Papotti M. Expression of ghrelin and of the GH secretagogue receptor by pancreatic islet cells and related endocrine tumors. *J Clin Endocrinol Metab* 2002 Mar;87(3):1300-8

[153] Kanamoto N, Akamizu T, Hosoda H, Hataya Y, Ariyasu H, Takaya K, Hosoda K, Saijo M, Moriyama K, Shimatsu A, Kojima M, Kangawa K, Nakao K. Substantial production of ghrelin by a human medullary thyroid carcinoma cell line. *J Clin Endocrinol Metab* 2001 Oct;86(10):4984-90

[154] Cummings DE, Purnell JQ, Frayo RS, Schmidova K, Wisse BE, Weigle DS. A preprandial rise in plasma ghrelin levels suggests a role in meal initiation in humans. *Diabetes* 2001 Aug;50(8):1714-9

[155] Traebert M, Riediger T, Whitebread S, Scharrer E, Schmid HA. Ghrelin acts on leptin-responsive neurones in the rat arcuate nucleus. *J Neuroendocrinol* 2002 Jul;14(7):580-6

[156] Tschop M, Weyer C, Tataranni PA, Devanarayan V, Ravussin E, Heiman ML. Circulating ghrelin levels are decreased in human obesity. *Diabetes* 2001 Apr;50(4):707-9

[157] English PJ, Ghatei MA, Malik IA, Bloom SR, Wilding JP. Food fails to suppress ghrelin levels in obese humans. *J Clin Endocrinol Metab* 2002 Jun;87(6):2984

[158] Bagnasco M, Kalra PS, Kalra SP. Ghrelin and leptin pulse discharge in fed and fasted rats. *Endocrinology* 2002 Feb;143(2):726-9

[159] Mustonen AM, Nieminen P, Hyvarinen H. Preliminary evidence that pharmacologic melatonin treatment decreases rat ghrelin levels. *Endocrine* 2001 Oct;16(1):43-6

[160] Patten SB. Major depressive episodes and diet pills. *Expert Opin Pharmacother* 2002 Oct;3(10):1405-9

[161] Patten SB. "Diet pills" and major depression in the Canadian population. *Can J Psychiatry* 2001 Jun;46(5):438-40

[162] Orlistat: a second look. At best, a minor adjunct to dietary measures. *Prescrire Int* 2002 Feb;11(57):10-2

[163] Binkley K, Knowles SR. Sibutramine and panic attacks. Am J Psychiatry 2002 Oct;159(10):1793-4

[164] Nisoli E, Carruba MO. An assessment of the safety and efficacy of sibutramine, an anti-obesity drug with a novel mechanism of action. *Obes Rev* 2000 Oct;1(2):127-39

[165] Birkenfeld AL, Schroeder C, Boschmann M, Tank J, Franke G, Luft FC, Biaggioni I, Sharma AM, Jordan J. Paradoxical effect of sibutramine on autonomic cardiovascular regulation. *Circulation* 2002 Nov 5;106(19):2459-65

[166] Wen W, Shu XO, Potter JD, Severson RK, Buckley JD, Reaman GH, Robison LL. Parental medication use and risk of childhood acute lymphoblastic leukemia. *Cancer* 2002 Oct 15;95(8):1786-94

[167] Samenuk D, Link MS, Homoud MK, Contreras R, Theohardes TC, Wang PJ, Estes NA Adverse cardiovascular events temporally associated with ma huang, an herbal source of ephedrine. *Mayo Clin Proc* 2002 Jan;77(1):12-6

[168] Fobi M, Lee H, Igwe D, Felahy B, James E, Stanczyk M, Fobi N. Prophylactic cholecystectomy with gastric bypass operation: incidence of gallbladder disease. *Obes Surg* 2002 Jun;12(3):350-3

[169] Melinek J, Livingston E, Cortina G, Fishbein MC. Autopsy findings following gastric bypass surgery for morbid obesity. *Arch Pathol Lab Med* 2002 Sep;126(9):1091-5

[170] Blachar A, Federle MP, Pealer KM, Ikramuddin S, Schauer PR. Gastrointestinal complications of laparoscopic Roux-en-Y gastric bypass surgery: clinical and imaging findings. *Radiology* 2002 Jun;223(3):625-32

[171] Goldner WS, O'Dorisio TM, Dillon JS, Mason EE. Severe metabolic bone disease as a long-term complication of obesity surgery. *Obes Surg* 2002 Oct;12(5):685-92

[172] Cummings DE, Weigle DS, Frayo RS, Breen PA, Ma MK, Dellinger EP, Purnell JQ. Plasma ghrelin levels after diet-induced weight loss or gastric bypass surgery. *N Engl J Med* 2002 May 23;346(21):1623-30

[173] Pombo M, Pombo CM, Garcia A, Caminos E, Gualillo O, Alvarez CV, Casanueva FF, Dieguez C. Hormonal control of growth hormone secretion. *Horm Res* 2001;55 Suppl 1:11-6

[174] Cui GL, Syversen U, Zhao CM, Chen D, Waldum HL. Long-term omeprazole treatment suppresses body weight gain and bone mineralization in young male rats. *Scand J Gastroenterol* 2001 Oct;36(10):1011-5

[175] Bayes B, Pastor MC, Bonal J, Junca J, Hernandez JM, Riutort N, Foraster A, Romero R. Homocysteine, C-reactive protein, lipid peroxidation and mortality in haemodialysis patients. *Nephrol Dial Transplant* 2003 Jan;18(1):106-12

[176] Hasegawa T, Negishi T, Deguchi M. WBC Count, Atherosclerosis and Coronary Risk Factors. *J Atheroscler Thromb* 2002;9(5):219-23

[177] Kowalewski M, Urban M, Mroczko B, Szmitkowski M. Pro-inflammatory cytokines (IL-6, TNF-alpha) and cardiac troponin I (cTnI) in serum of young people with ventricular arrhythmias. *Pol Arch Med Wewn* 2002 Jul;108(1):647-51

[178] Riboldi P, Gerosa M, Luzzana C, Catelli L. Cardiac involvement in systemic autoimmune diseases. *Clin Rev Allergy Immunol* 2002 Dec;23(3):247-61

[179] Koenig W. Insulin resistance, heart disease and inflammation. Identifying the 'at-risk' patient: the earlier the better? The role of inflammatory markers. *Int J Clin Pract Suppl* 2002 Oct;(132):23-30

[180] Park A. Beyond cholesterol. Inflammation is emerging as a major risk factor—and not just in heart disease. *Time* 2002 Nov 25;160(22):74-5

[181] Sewter CP, Digby JE, Blows F, Prins JB & O'Rahilly S (1999) Regulation of tumour necrosis factor-alpha release from human adipose tissue *in vitro. Journal of Endocrinology* 163, 33-38.

[182] Hotamisligil GS, Arner P, Caro JF, Atkinson RL & Speigelman BaM (1995) Increased adipose tissue expression of tumor necrosis factor-x in human obesity and insulin resistance. *Journal of Clinical Investigation* 95, 2409-2415.

[183] Hotamisligil GS, (1999) The role of TNFx and TNF receptors in obesity and insulin resistance. *Journal of Internal Medicine* 245, 612-625.

[184] Coppack SW. Pro-inflammatory cytokines and adipose tissue. *Nutrition Society*(2001), 60, 349-356.

[185] Stephens JM & Pakala PH (1991) Transcriptional regression of the GLUT4 and C/EBP genes in 3T3-L1 adipocytes by tumor necrosis factor-alpha.

[186] Mohamed-Ali V, Pinkney JH & Coppack SW (1998) Adipose tissueas an endocrine and paracrine organ. *International Journal of Obesity and Related Metabolic Disorders* 22, 1145-1158.

[187] Plata-Salaman CR (1999) Central nervous system mechanisms contributing to the cachexia-anorexia syndrome. *Nutrition* 16, 1009-1012.

[188] Konstantinides S, Schafer K, Koschnick S, Loskutoff DJ. Leptin-dependent platelet aggregation and arterial thrombois suggests a mechanism for atherothrombotic disease in obesity. *J Clin Invest* 2001 Nov;108(10):1533-40.

[189] Monk TH, Reynolds CF 3rd, Kupfer DJ, Hoch CC, Carrier J, Houck PR. Differences over the life span in daily life-style regularity. *Chronobiol Int* 1997 May;14(3):295-306

[190] Wang Q, Chen M, Hu R, Tang J, Li F, Luo B. The effects of glucocorticoids and insulin on serum leptin level and its diurnal rhythmicity *Zhonghua Nei Ke Za Zhi* 2002 Feb;41(2):104-8

[191] Szucs N, Varga I, Jakab C, Patocs A, Glaz E, Toth M, Kiss R, Racz K. Leptin inhibits cortisol and corticosterone secretion in pathologic human adrenocortical cells. *Pituitary* 2001 Jan-Apr;4(1-2):71-7

[192] Wang Q, Chen M, Hu R, Tang J, Li F, Luo B. The effects of glucocorticoids and insulin on serum leptin level and its diurnal rhythmicity *Zhonghua Nei Ke Za Zhi* 2002 Feb;41(2):104-8

[193] Gualillo O, Eiras S, Lago F, Dieguez C, Casanueva FF. Elevated serum leptin concentrations induced by experimental acute inflammation. *Life Sci* 2000 Oct 6;67(20):2433-41

[194] Fantuzzi G, Faggioni R. Leptin in the regulation of immunity, inflammation, and hematopoiesis. *J Leukoc Biol* 2000 Oct;68(4):437-46

[195] Maruna P, Gurlich R, Frasko R. Leptin—a new acute phase reactant *Vnitr Lek* 2001 Jul;47(7):478-83

[196] Finck BN, Johnson RW. Tumor necrosis factor-alpha regulates secretion of the adipocyte-derived cytokine, leptin. *Microsc Res Tech* 2000 Aug 1;50(3):209-15

[197] Gerhardt CC, Romero IA, Cancello R, Camoin L, Strosberg AD. Chemokines control fat accumulation and leptin secretion by cultured human adipocytes. *Mol Cell Endocrinol* 2001 Apr 25;175(1-2):81-92

[198] Voegeling S, Fantuzzi G. Regulation of free and bound leptin and soluble leptin receptors during inflammation in mice. *Cytokine* 2001 Apr 21;14(2):97-103

[199] Das UN. Is obesity an inflammatory condition? *Nutrition* 2001 Nov-Dec;17(11-12):953-66

[200] Chiellini C, Bertacca A, Novelli SE, Gorgun CZ, Ciccarone A, Giordano A, Xu H, Soukas A, Costa M, Gandini D, Dimitri R, Bottone P, Cecchetti V Increased leptin concentrations correlate with increased concentrations of inflammatory markers in morbidly obese individuals. *Int J Obes Relat Metab Disord* 2001 Dec;25(12):1759-66

[201] P, Pardini E, Perego L, Navalesi R, Folli F, Benzi L, Cinti S, Friedman JM, Hotamisligil GS, Maffei M. Obesity modulates the expression of haptoglobin in the white adipose tissue via TNFalpha. *J Cell Physiol* 2002 Feb;190(2):251-8

[202] Joussen AM, Poulaki V, Mitsiades N, Kirchhof B, Koizumi K, Dohmen S, Adamis AP. Nonsteroidal anti-inflammatory drugs prevent early diabetic retinopathy via TNF-alpha suppression. *FASEB J* 2002 Mar;16(3):438-40

[203] Nishiyama M, Makino S, Suemaru S, Nanamiya W, Asaba K, Kaneda T, Mimoto T, Nishioka T, Takao T, Hashimoto K. Glucocorticoid effects on the diurnal rhythm of circulating leptin levels. *Horm Res* 2000;54(2):69-73

[204] Leal-Cerro A, Soto A, Martinez MA, Dieguez C, Casanueva FF. Influence of cortisol status on leptin secretion. *Pituitary* 2001 Jan-Apr;4(1-2):111-6

[205] Fruhbeck G, Gomez-Ambrosi J. Depot-specific differences in the lipolytic effect of leptin on isolated white adipocytes. *Med Sci Monit* 2002 Feb;8(2):BR47-55

[206] Bjorntorp P. Do stress reactions cause abdominal obesity and comorbidities? *Obes Rev* 2001 May;2(2):73-86

[207] Bjorntorp P, Rossner S, Udden J. "Consolatory eating" is not a myth. Stress-induced increased cortisol levels result in leptin-resistant obesity *Lakartidningen* 2001 Nov 28;98(48):5458-61

[208] Gabriely I, Ma XH, Yang XM, Atzmon G, Rajala MW, Berg AH, Scherer P, Rossetti L, Barzilai N. Removal of visceral fat prevents insulin resistance and glucose intolerance of aging: an adipokine-mediated process? *Diabetes* 2002 Oct;51(10):2951-8

[209] Atkinson LL, Fischer MA, Lopaschuk GD. Leptin activates cardiac fatty acid oxidation independent of changes in the AMP-activated protein kinase - acetyl-CoA carboxylase - malonyl-CoA Axis. *J Biol Chem* 2002 Jun 10

[210] Lopes IM, Forga L, Martinez JA. Effects of leptin resistance on acute fuel metabolism after a high carbohydrate load in lean and overweight young men. *J Am Coll Nutr* 2001 Dec;20(6):643-8

[211] Ukropec J, Sebokova E, Klimes I. Nutrient sensing, leptin and insulin action. *Arch Physiol Biochem* 2001 Feb;109(1):38-51

[212] Fletcher RH, Fairchild KM Vitamins for chronic disease prevention in adults:clinical applications. *JAMA* June 19, 2002;287:3217-3219

[213] Nisoli E, Carruba MO, Tonello C, Macor C, Federspil G & Vettor R (2000b) Induction of fatty acid translocase/CD36, peroxisome proliferators-activated

receptor, leptin, uncoupling proteins 2 and 3, and tumor necrosis factor-x gene expression in human sub-cutaneous fat by lipid infusion. *Diabetes* 49, 319-324.

[214] Simopoulos AP. Omega-3 Fatty acids in inflammation and autoimmune diseases. *J Am Coll Nutr* 2002 Dec;21(6):495-505

[215] James MJ, Gibson RA, Cleland LG. Dietary polyunsaturated fatty acids and inflammatory mediator production. Am J Clin Nutr 2000 Jan;71(1 Suppl):343S-8S

[216] Storlien LH, Higgins JA, Thomas TC, et al. Diet composition and insulin action in animal models. *Br J Nutr* 2000;83:S85-S90.

[217] Storlien LH, Kraegen EW, Chrisholm DJ, et al. Fish oil prevents insulin resistance induced by high-fat feeding in rats. *Science* 1987;237:885-888.

[218] Storlien LH, Jenkins AB, Chrisholm DJ, et al. Influence of dietary fat composition on development of insulin resistance in rats. Relationship to muscle triglyceride and omega-3 fatty acids in muscle phospholipids. *Diabetes* 1991;40:280-289.

[219] Wellhoener P, Fruehwald-Schultes B, Kern W, Dantz D, Kerner W, Bom J, Fehm HL, Peters A. Glucose metabolism rather than insulin is a main determinant of leptin secretion in humans. *J Clin Endocrinol Metab* 85:1267-1271, 2000.

[220] Thies F, Nebe-von-Caron G, Powell JR, Yaqoob P, Newsholme EA, Calder PC. Dietary supplementation with gamma-linolenic acid or fish oil decreases T lymphocyte proliferation in healthy older humans. *J Nutr* 2001 Jul;131(7):1928-27.

[221] Prasad K. Dietary flax seed in prevention of hypercholesterolemic atherosclerosis. *Atherosclerosis* 1997 Jul 11;132(1):69-76.

[222] Gaddi A, Descovich GC, Noseda G, et al. Controlled evaluation of pantethine, a natural hypolipidemic compound, in patients with different forms of hyperlipoproteinemia. *Atherosclerosis* 1984;50:73-83.

[223] Murai A, Miyahara T, Tanaka T, Sako Y, Nishimura N, Kameyama M. The effects of pantethine on lipid and lipoprotein abnormalities in survivors of cerebral infarction. *Artery* 1985;12(4):234-43

[224] Hiramtsu K, Nozaki H, Arimori S. Influence of pantethine on platelet volume, microviscosity, lipid composition and functions in diabetes mellitus with hyperlipdimia. *Tokai J Exp Clin Med* 1981 Jan;6(1):49-57.

[225] Gensini GF, Prisco D, Rogasi PG, Matucci M, Neri Serneri GG. Changes in fatty acid composition of the single platelet phospholipids induced by pantethine treatment. *Int J Clin Pharmacol Res* 1985;5(5):309-18

[226] Arsenio L, Bodria P, Magnati G, Strata A, Trovato R. Effectiveness of long-term treatment with pantethine in patients with dyslipidemia. *Clin Ther* 1986;8(5):537-45

[227] Donati C, Bertieri RS, Barbi G. [Pantethine, diabetes mellitus and atherosclerosis. Clinical study of 1045 patients] *Clin Ter* 1989 Mar 31;128(6):411-22.

[228] Prisco D, Rogasi PG, Matucci M, Paniccia R, Abbate R, Gensini GF, Neri Serneri GG. Effect of oral treatment with pantethine on platelet and plasma phospholipids in IIa hyperlipoproteinemia. *Angiology* 1987 Mar;38(3):241-7

[229] Noma A, Kita M, Okamiya T. Effect of pantethine on post-heparin plasma lipolytic activities and adipose tissue lipoprotein lipase in rats. *Horm Metab Res* 1984 May;16(5):233-6.

[230] Osono Y, Hirose N, Nakajima K, Hata Y. The effects of pantethine on fatty liver and fat distribution. *J Atheroscler Thromb* 2000;7(1):55-8

[231] Katsuki A, Sumida Y, Gabazza EC, Murashima S, Tanaka T, Furuta M, Araki-Sasaki R, Hori Y, Nakatani K, Yano Y, Adachi Y. Plasma levels of agouti-related

protein are increased in obese men. *J Clin Endocrinol Metab* 2001 May;86(5):1921-4

[232] Weimann E. Gender-related differences in elite gymnasts: the female athlete triad. *J Appl Physiol* 2002 May;92(5):2146-52

[233] Nandi J, Meguid MM, Inui A, Xu Y, Makarenko IG, Tada T, Chen C. Central mechanisms involved with catabolism. *Curr Opin Clin Nutr Metab Care* 2002 Jul;5(4):407-18

[234] Saris WH. The concept of energy homeostasis for optimum health during training. *Can J Appl Physiol* 2001;26 Suppl:S167-75

[235] Nandi J, Meguid MM, Inui A, Xu Y, Makarenko IG, Tada T, Chen C. Central mechanisms involved with catabolism. *Curr Opin Clin Nutr Metab Care* 2002 Jul;5(4):407-18

[236] Monteleone P, Martiadis V, Colurcio B, Maj M. Leptin secretion is related to chronicity and severity of the illness in bulimia nervosa. *Psychosom Med* 2002 Nov-Dec;64(6):874-9

[237] Kraus T, Haack M, Schuld A, Hinze-Selch D, Pollmacher T. Low leptin levels but normal body mass indices in patients with depression or schizophrenia. *Neuroendocrinology* 2001 Apr;73(4):243-7

[238] Charnay Y, Cusin I, Vallet PG, Muzzin P, Rohner-Jeanrenaud F, Bouras C. Intracerebroventricular infusion of leptin decreases serotonin transporter binding sites in the frontal cortex of the rat. *Neurosci Lett* 2000 Apr 7;283(2):89-92

[239] Barker ME, Blumsohn A. Is weight loss in obese pre-menopausal women associated with a decline in bone mass? *J Bone Miner Res* 2002 Apr;17(4):746-9

[240] Morley JE. Anorexia, body composition, and ageing. *Curr Opin Clin Nutr Metab Care* 2001 Jan;4(1):9-13

[241] Diehl AM. Nonalcoholic steatosis and steatohepatitis IV. Nonalcoholic fatty liver disease abnormalities in macrophage function and cytokines. *Am J Physiol Gastrointest Liver Physiol* 2002 Jan;282(1):G1-5

[242] Andrico S, Gambera A, Specchia C, Pellegrini C, Falsetti L, Sartori E. Leptin in functional hypothalamic amenorrhoea. *Hum Reprod* 2002 Aug;17(8):2043-8

[243] Unkila-Kallio L, Andersson S, Koistinen HA, Karonen SL, Ylikorkala O, Tiitinen A. Leptin during assisted reproductive cycles: the effect of ovarian stimulation and of very early pregnancy. *Hum Reprod* 2001 Apr;16(4):657-62

[244] Barton BE. IL-6-like cytokines and cancer cachexia: consequences of chronic inflammation. *Immunol Res* 2001;23(1):41-58

[245] Nowicki M, Bryc W, Kokot F. Hormonal regulation of appetite and body mass in patients with advanced prostate cancer treated with combined androgen blockade. *J Endocrinol Invest* 2001 Jan;24(1):31-6

[246] Schols AM, Creutzberg EC, Buurman WA, Campfield LA, Saris WH, Wouters EF. Plasma leptin is related to pro-inflammatory status and dietary intake in patients with chronic obstructive pulmonary disease. *Am J Respir Crit Care Med* 1999 Oct;160(4):1220-6

[247] Marti A, Marcos A, Martinez JA. Obesity and immune function relationships. *Obes Rev* 2001 May;2(2):131-40

[248] Fantuzzi G, Faggioni R. Leptin in the regulation of immunity, inflammation, and hematopoiesis. *J Leukoc Biol* 2000 Oct;68(4):437-46

[249] Faggioni R, Feingold KR, Grunfeld C. Leptin regulation of the immune response and the immunodeficiency of malnutrition. *FASEB J* 2001 Dec;15(14):2565-71

[250] Mancuso P, Gottschalk A, Phare SM, Peters-Golden M, Lukacs NW, Huffnagle GB. Leptin-deficient mice exhibit impaired host defense in Gram-negative pneumonia. *J Immunol* 2002 Apr 15;168(8):4018-24

[251] Busso N, So A, Chobaz-Peclat V, Morard C, Martinez-Soria E, Talabot-Ayer D, Gabay C. Leptin signaling deficiency impairs humoral and cellular immune responses and attenuates experimental arthritis. *J Immunol* 2002 Jan 15;168(2):875-82

[252] Savino W. The thymus gland is a target in malnutrition. *Eur J Clin Nutr* 2002 Aug;56 Suppl 3:S46-9

[253] Matarese G, La Cava A, Sanna V, Lord GM, Lechler RI, Fontana S, Zappacosta S. Balancing susceptibility to infection and autoimmunity: a role for leptin? *Trends Immunol* 2002 Apr 1;23(4):182-7

[254] Matarese G, Sanna V, Di Giacomo A, Lord GM, Howard JK, Bloom SR, Lechler RI, Fontana S, Zappacosta S. Leptin potentiates experimental autoimmune encephalomyelitis in SJL female mice and confers susceptibility to males. *Eur J Immunol* 2001 May;31(5):1324-32

[255] Heer M, Mika C, Grzella I, Drummer C, Herpertz-Dahlmann B. Changes in bone turnover in patients with anorexia nervosa during eleven weeks of inpatient dietary treatment. JW.1: Clin Chem 2002 May;48(5):754-60

[256] Barber MD, Fearon KC, Tisdale MJ, McMillan DC, Ross JA. Effect of a fish oil-enriched nutritional supplement on metabolic mediators in patients with pancreatic cancer cachexia. *Nutr Cancer* 2001;40(2):118-24

[257] Tannhauser PP. Anorexia nervosa: a multifactorial disease of nutritional origin? Int J Adolesc Med Health 2002 Jul-Sep;14(3):185-91

[258] Patrick L. Eating disorders: a review of the literature with emphasis on medical complications and clinical nutrition. *Altern Med Rev* 2002 Jun;7(3):184-202

[259] Su JC, Birmingham CL. Zinc supplementation in the treatment of anorexia nervosa. *Eat Weight Disord* 2002 Mar;7(1):20-2

[260] Koivisto VA, Yki-Jarvinen H, DeFronzo RA. Physical training and insulin sensitivity. *Diabetes Metab Rev* 1986;1:445-481

[261] Henriksen EJ. Invited Review: Effects of acute exercise and exercise training on insulin resistance. *J Appl Physiol* 2002 Aug;93(2):788-96

[262] Bogardus C, Ravussin E, Robbins DC, et al. Effects of physical training and diet therapy on carbohydrate metabolism in patients with glucose intolerance and non-insulin dependent diabetes. *Diabetes* 1984;33:311-318

[263] Wasserman DH, Lacy DB, Goldstein RE, Williams PE, Cherington AD. Exercise-induced fall in insulin and the increase in fat metabolism during prolonged exercise. Diabetes 1989;38:484-490

[264] Baba T, Kanda T, Yoshida A, Tsukui S, Nara M, Inukai T, Umeda T, Tamura J, Kobayashi I. Reciprocal changes in leptin and tumor necrosis factor-alpha with exercise in insulin resistant rats. *Res Commun Mol Pathol Pharmacol* 2000 Jul-Aug;108(1-2):133-43

[265] Kahara T, Takamura T, Hayakawa T, Nagai Y, Yamaguchi H, Katsuki T, Katsuki K, Katsuki M, Kobayashi K. Prediction of exercise-mediated changes in metabolic markers by gene polymorphism. *Diabetes Res Clin Pract* 2002 Aug;57(2):105-10

[266] Rozzano, MI. Arrhythmia risk stratification in patients with heart failure according to drug treatment and its effects *Ital Heart J* 2001 Dec;2(12 Suppl):1278-83

[267] Adigun AQ, Asiyanbola B, Ajayi AA. Cardiac autonomic function in Blacks with congestive heart failure: vagomimetic action, alteration in sympathovagal balance, and the effect of ACE inhibition on central and peripheral vagal tone. *Cell Mol Biol* (Noisy-le-gland) 2001 Sep;47(6):1063-7.

[268] Billman GE. Aerobic exercise conditioning: a nonpharmacological antiarrhythmic intervention. *J Appl Physiol* 2002 Feb;92(2):446-54.

[269] Ito H, Ohshima A, Tsuzuki M, Ohto N, Yanagawa M, Maruyama T, Kaji Y, Kanaya S, Nishioka K. Effects of increased physical activity and mild calorie restriction on heart rate variability in obese women. *Jpn Heart J* 2001 Jul;42(4):459-69.

[270] Matsushita T, Tanaka Y, Horinouchi O, Sonoda M, Arima T. Heart rate decline after exercise in patients with hypertrophic cardiomyopathy. *J Electrocardiol* 2001 Apr;34(2(:141-6.

[271] Rosenwinkel ET, Bloomfield DM, Arwady MA, Goldsmith RL. Exercise and autonomic function in health and cardiovascular disease. *Cardiol Clin* 2001 Aug;19(3):369-87.

[272] Goldsmith RL, Bloomfield DM, Rosenwinkel ET. Exercise and autonomic function. *Coron Artery Dis* 2000 Mar;11(2):129-35.

[273] Sartorio A, Narici MV, Fumagalli E, Faglia G, Lafortuna CL. Aerobic and anaerobic performance before and after a short-term body mass reduction program in obese subjects. *Diabetes Nutr Metab* 2001 Feb;14(1):51-7.

[274] Iwane M, Arita M, Tomimoto S, Satani O, Matsumoto M, Miyashita K, Nishio I. Walking 10,000 steps/day or more reduces blood pressure and sympathetic nerve activity in mild essential hypertension. *Hypertens Res* 2000 Nov;23(6):573-80.

[275] Amano M, Kanda T, Ue H, Moritani T. Exercise training and autonomic nervous system activity in obese individuals. *Med Sci Sports Exerc* 2001 Aug;33(8):1287-91.

[276] Collins HL, Rodenbaugh DW, Dicarlo SE. Dialy exercise attenuated the sympathetic component of the spontaneous arterial baroreflex control of heart rate in hypertensive rats. *Clin Exp Hypertens* 2000 Aug;22(6):607-22.

[277] Gutin B, Barbeau P, Litaker MS, Ferguson M, Owens S. Heart rate variability in obese children: relations to total body and visceral adiposity, and changes with physical training and detraining. *Obes Res* 2000 Jan;8(1):12-9.

[278] Nindl BC, Kraemer WJ, Arciero PJ, Samatallee N, Leone CD, Mayo MF, Hafeman DL. Leptin concentrations experience a delayed reduction after resistance exercise in men. *Med Sci Sports Exerc* 2002 Apr;34(4):608-13

[279] Kanaley JA, Fenicchia LM, Miller CS, Ploutz-Synder LL, Weinstock RS, Carhart R, Azevedo JL Jr. Resting leptin responses to acute and chronic resistance training in type 2 diabetic men and women. *Int J Obes Relat Metab Disord* 2001 Oct;25(10):1474-80

[280] Gippini A, Mato A, Pazos R, Suarez B, Vila B, Gayoso P, Lage M, Casanueva FF. Effect of long-term strength training on glucose metabolism. Implications for individual impact of high lean mass and high fat mass on relationship between BMI and insulin sensitivity. *J Endocrinol Invest* 2002 Jun;25(6):520-5

[281] Hayase H, Nomura S, Abe T, Izawa T. Relation between fat distributions and several plasma adipocytokines after exercise training in pre-menopausal and postmenopausal women. *J Physiol Anthropol Appl Human Sci* 2002 Mar;21(2):105-13

[282] Van Someren EJ. More than a marker: interaction between the circadian regulation of temperature and sleep, age-related changes, and treatment possibilities. *Chronobiol Int* 2000 May;17(3):313-54

[283] Krauchi K, Wirz-Justice A. Circadian clues to sleep onset mechanisms. *Neuropsychopharmacology* 2001 Nov;25(5 Suppl):S92-6

[284] Carrier J, Paquet J, Morettini J, Touchette E. Phase advance of sleep and temperature circadian rhythms in the middle years of life in humans. *Neurosci Lett* 2002 Mar 1;320(1-2):1-4

[285] Baydas G, Gursu F, Canpolat S, Konar V, Yasar A, Canatan H, Kelestimur H. Effects of pinealectomy on the circadian release pattern of leptin in male rat. *Neuroendocrinol Lett* 2001 Dec;22(6):449-52

[286] Canpolat S, Sandal S, Yilmaz B, Yasar A, Kutlu S, Baydas G, Kelestimur H. Effects of pinealectomy and exogenous melatonin on serum leptin levels in male rat. *Eur J Pharmacol* 2001 Sep 28;428(1):145-8

[287] Wolden-Hanson T, Mitton DR, McCants RL, Yellon SM, Wilkinson CW, Matsumoto AM, Rasmussen DD. Daily melatonin administration to middle-aged male rats suppresses body weight, intraabdominal adiposity, and plasma leptin and insulin independent of food intake and total body fat. *Endocrinology* 2000 Feb;141(2):487-97

[288] Nishida S, Segawa T, Murai I, Nakagawa S. Long-term melatonin administration reduces hyperinsulinemia and improves the altered fatty-acid compositions in type 2 diabetic rats via the restoration of Delta-5 desaturase activity. *J Pineal Res* 2002 Jan;32(1):26-33

[289] Kraus T, Haack M, Schuld A, Hinze-Selch D, Pollmacher T. Low leptin levels but normal body mass indices in patients with depression or schizophrenia. *Neuroendocrinology* 2001 Apr;73(4):243-7

[290] Charnay Y, Cusin I, Vallet PG, Muzzin P, Rohner-Jeanrenaud F, Bouras C. Intracerebroventricular infusion of leptin decreases serotonin transporter binding sites in the frontal cortex of the rat. *Neurosci Lett* 2000 Apr 7;283(2):89-92

[291] Nedvidkova J, Papezova H, Haluzik M, Schreiber V. Interaction between serum leptin levels and hypothalamo-hypophyseal-thyroid axis in patients with anorexia nervosa. *Endocr Res* 2000 May;26(2):219-30

[292] Sasaki M, Jordan P, Joh T, Itoh M, Jenkins M, Pavlick K, Minagar A, Alexander SJ. Melatonin reduces TNF-a induced expression of MAdCAM-1 via inhibition of NF kappaB. *BMC Gastroenterol* 2002 Apr 24;2(1):9

[293] Nava M, Quiroz Y, Vaziri ND, Rodriguez-Iturbe B. MELATONIN REDUCES RENAL INTERSTITIAL INFLAMMATION AND IMPROVES HYPERTENSION IN SPONTANEOUSLY HYPERTENSIVE RATS. *Am J Physiol Renal Physiol* 2002 Nov 19;

[294] Clasey JL, Weltman A, Patrie J, Weltman JY, Pezzoli S, Bouchard C, Thorner MO,Hartman ML. Abdominal visceral fat and fasting insulin are important predictors of 24-hour GH release independent of age, gender, and other physiological factors. *J Clin Endocrinol Metab* 2001 Aug;86(8):3845-52

[295] McCallum RW, Petrie JR, Dominiczak AF, Connell JM. Growth hormone deficiency and vascular risk. *Clin Endocrinol (Oxf)* 2002 Jul;57(1):11-24

[296] Moretti C, Mencacci C, Frajese GV, Cerilli M, Frajese G. Growth hormone-releasing hormone and pituitary adenylate cyclase-activating polypeptide in the reproductive system. *Trends Endocrinol Metab* 2002 Dec;13(10):428-35

[297] Monzavi R, Cohen P. IGFs and IGFBPs: role in health and disease. *Best Pract Res Clin Endocrinol Metab* 2002 Sep;16(3):433-47

[298] Furstenberger G, Senn HJ. Insulin-like growth factors and cancer. *Lancet Oncol* 2002 May;3(5):298-302

[299] van Garderen E, Schalken JA. Morphogenic and tumorigenic potentials of the mammary growth hormone/growth hormone receptor system. *Mol Cell Endocrinol* 2002 Nov 29;197(1-2):153-65

[300] Sandhu MS, Dunger DB, Giovannucci EL. Insulin, insulin-like growth factor-I (IGF-I), IGF binding proteins, their biologic interactions, and colorectal cancer. *J Natl Cancer Inst* 2002 Jul 3;94(13):972-80

[301] Chatzistamou I, Schally AV, Pafiti A, Kiaris H, Koutselini H. Expression of growth hormone-releasing hormone in human primary endometrial carcinomas. *Eur J Endocrinol* 2002 Sep;147(3):381-6

[302] Moretti C, Mencacci C, Frajese GV, Cerilli M, Frajese G. Growth hormone-releasing hormone and pituitary adenylate cyclase-activating polypeptide in the reproductive system. *Trends Endocrinol Metab* 2002 Dec;13(10):428-35

[303] Laban C, Bustin SA, Jenkins PJ. The GH-IGF-I axis and breast cancer. *Trends Endocrinol Metab* 2002 Dec;14(1):28-34

[304] Zeitler P, Siriwardana G. Antagonism of endogenous growth hormone-releasing hormone (GHRH) leads to reduced proliferation and apoptosis in MDA231 breast cancer cells. *Endocrine* 2002 Jun;18(1):85-90

[305] Halmos G, Schally AV, Czompoly T, Krupa M, Varga JL, Rekasi Z. Expression of growth hormone-releasing hormone and its receptor splice variants in human prostate cancer. *J Clin Endocrinol Metab* 2002 Oct;87(10):4707-14

[306] Chopin LK, Veveris-Lowe TL, Philipps AF, Herington AC. Co-expression of GH and GHR isoforms in prostate cancer cell lines. *Growth Horm IGF Res* 2002 Apr;12(2):126-36

[307] Swerdlow AJ, Higgins CD, Adlard P, Preece MA. Risk of cancer in patients treated with human pituitary growth hormone in the UK, 1959-85: a cohort study. *Lancet* 2002 Jul 27;360(9329):273-7 Comment in: Lancet. 2002 Jul 27;360(9329):268-9.

[308] Engelson ES, Glesby MJ, Mendez D, Albu JB, Wang J, Heymsfield SB, Kotler DP. Effect of recombinant human growth hormone in the treatment of visceral fat accumulation in HIV infection. *J Acquir Immune Defic Syndr* 2002 Aug 1;30(4):379-91

[309] Monzavi R, Cohen P. IGFs and IGFBPs: role in health and disease. *Best Pract Res Clin Endocrinol Metab* 2002 Sep;16(3):433-47

[310] Rose DR, Clemmons DR. Growth hormone receptor antagonist improves insulin resistance in acromegaly. *Growth Horm IGF Res* 2002 Dec;12(6):418-24

[311] Gravholt CH, Naeraa RW, Brixen K, Kastrup KW, Mosekilde L, Jorgensen JO, Christiansen JS. Short-term growth hormone treatment in girls with turner syndrome decreases fat mass and insulin sensitivity: a randomized, double-blind, placebo-controlled, crossover study. *Pediatrics* 2002 Nov;110(5):889-96

[312] Van Pareren YK, De Muinck Keizer-Schrama SM, Stijnen T, Sas TC, Drop SL. Effect of Discontinuation of Long-Term Growth Hormone Treatment on Carbohydrate Metabolism and Risk Factors for Cardiovascular Disease in Girls with Turner Syndrome. *J Clin Endocrinol Metab* 2002 Dec 1;87(12):5442-5448

[313] Blackman MR, Sorkin JD, Munzer T, Bellantoni MF, Busby-Whitehead J, Stevens TE, Jayme J, O'Connor KG, Christmas C, Tobin JD, Stewart KJ, Cottrell E, St Clair C, Pabst KM, Harman SM. Growth hormone and sex steroid administration in healthy aged women and men: a randomized controlled trial. *JAMA* 2002 Nov 13;288(18):2282-92

[314] Roelfsema F, Biermasz NR, Veldman RG, Veldhuis JD, Frolich M, Stokvis-Brantsma WH, Wit JM. Growth hormone (GH) secretion in patients with an inactivating defect of the GH-releasing hormone (GHRH) receptor is pulsatile: evidence for a role for non-GHRH inputs into the generation of GH pulses. *J Clin Endocrinol Metab* 2001 Jun;86(6):2459-64

[315] Maheshwari HG, Pezzoli SS, Rahim A, Shalet SM, Thorner MO, Baumann G. Pulsatile growth hormone secretion persists in genetic growth hormone-releasing hormone resistance. *Am J Physiol Endocrinol Metab* 2002 Apr;282(4):E943-51

[316] Pombo M, Pombo CM, Garcia A, Caminos E, Gualillo O, Alvarez CV, Casanueva FF, Dieguez C. Hormonal control of growth hormone secretion. *Horm Res* 2001;55 Suppl 1:11-6

[317] Isozaki O, Tsushima T, Miyakawa M, Demura H, Seki H. Interaction between leptin and growth hormone (GH)/IGF-I axis. *Endocr J* 1999 Mar;46 Suppl:S17-24

[318] Isozaki O, Tsushima T, Miyakawa M, Nozoe Y, Demura H, Seki H. Growth hormone directly inhibits leptin gene expression in visceral fat tissue in fatty Zucker rats. *J Endocrinol* 1999 Jun;161(3):511-6

[319] Lee KN, Jeong IC, Lee SJ, Oh SH, Cho MY. Regulation of leptin gene expression by insulin and growth hormone in mouse adipocytes. *Exp Mol Med* 2001 Dec 31;33(4):234-9

[320] Dunger D, Ahmed L, Ong K. Growth and body composition in type 1 diabetes mellitus. *Horm Res* 2002;58 Suppl 1:66-71

[321] Heptulla R, Smitten A, Teague B, Tamborlane WV, Ma YZ, Caprio S. Temporal patterns of circulating leptin levels in lean and obese adolescents: relationships to insulin, growth hormone, and free fatty acids rhythmicity. *J Clin Endocrinol Metab* 2001 Jan;86(1):90-6

[322] Soderberg S, Ahren B, Eliasson M, Dinesen B, Brismar K, Olsson T. Circulating IGF binding protein-1 is inversely associated with leptin in non-obese men and obese postmenopausal women. *Eur J Endocrinol* 2001 Mar;144(3):283-90

[323] Furuhata Y, Kagaya R, Hirabayashi K, Ikeda A, Chang KT, Nishihara M, Takahashi M. Development of obesity in transgenic rats with low circulating growth hormone levels: involvement of leptin resistance. *Eur J Endocrinol* 2000 Oct;143(4):535-41

[324] Armellini F, Zamboni M, Bosello O. Hormones and body composition in humans: clinical studies. *Int J Obes Relat Metab Disord* 2000 Jun;24 Suppl 2:S18-21

[325] Garcia-Rudaz MC, Ropelato MG, Escobar ME, Veldhuis JD, Barontini M. Amplified and orderly growth hormone secretion characterizes lean adolescents with polycystic ovary syndrome. *Eur J Endocrinol* 2002 Aug;147(2):207-16

[326] Zaczek D, Hammond J, Suen L, Wandji S, Service D, Bartke A, Chandrashekar V, Coschigano K, Kopchick J. Impact of growth hormone resistance on female reproductive function: new insights from growth hormone receptor knockout mice. *Biol Reprod* 2002 Oct;67(4):1115-24

[327] Muller AF, Lamberts SW, Janssen JA, Hofland LJ, Koetsveld PV, Bidlingmaier M, Strasburger CJ, Ghigo E, Van der Lely AJ. Ghrelin drives GH secretion during fasting in man. *Eur J Endocrinol* 2002 Feb;146(2):203-7

[328] Cappiello V, Ronchi C, Morpurgo PS, Epaminonda P, Arosio M, Beck-Peccoz P, Spada A. Circulating ghrelin levels in basal conditions and during glucose tolerance test in acromegalic patients. *Eur J Endocrinol* 2002 Aug;147(2):189-94

[329] Muller EE, Rigamonti AE, Colonna Vde G, Locatelli V, Berti F, Cella SG. GH-related and extra-endocrine actions of GH secretagogues in aging. *Neurobiol Aging* 2002 Sep-Oct;23(5):907

[330] Tschop M, Weyer C, Tataranni PA, Devanarayan V, Ravussin E, Heiman ML. Circulating ghrelin levels are decreased in human obesity. *Diabetes* 2001 Apr;50(4):707-9

[331] English PJ, Ghatei MA, Malik IA, Bloom SR, Wilding JP. Food fails to suppress ghrelin levels in obese humans. *J Clin Endocrinol Metab* 2002 Jun;87(6):2984

[332] Bagnasco M, Kalra PS, Kalra SP. Ghrelin and leptin pulse discharge in fed and fasted rats. *Endocrinology* 2002 Feb;143(2):726-9

[333] Wang P, Li N, Li JS, Li WQ. The role of endotoxin, TNF-alpha, and IL-6 in inducing the state of growth hormone insensitivity. *World J Gastroenterol* 2002 Jun;8(3):531-6

[334] Yumet G, Shumate ML, Bryant P, Lin CM, Lang CH, Cooney RN. Tumor necrosis factor mediates hepatic growth hormone resistance during sepsis. *Am J Physiol Endocrinol Metab* 2002 Sep;283(3):E472-81

[335] Lieskovska J, Guo D, Derman E. IL-6-overexpression brings about growth impairment potentially through a GH receptor defect. *Growth Horm IGF Res* 2002 Dec;12(6):388-98

[336] Landis CA, Lentz MJ, Rothermel J, Riffle SC, Chapman D, Buchwald D, Shaver JL. Decreased nocturnal levels of prolactin and growth hormone in women with fibromyalgia. *J Clin Endocrinol Metab* 2001 Apr;86(4):1672-8

[337] Crown AL, Cottle K, Lightman SL, Falk S, Mohamed-Ali V, Armstrong L, Millar AB, Holly JM. What is the role of the insulin-like growth factor system in the pathophysiology of cancer cachexia, and how is it regulated? *Clin Endocrinol* (Oxf) 2002 Jun;56(6):723-33

[338] Belury MA. DIETARY CONJUGATED LINOLEIC ACID IN HEALTH: Physiological Effects and Mechanisms of Action. *Annu Rev Nutr* 2002;22:505-31

[339] Sugano M, Akahoshi A, Koba K, Tanaka K, Okumura T, Matsuyama H, Goto Y, Miyazaki T, Murao K, Yamasaki M, Nonaka M, Yamada K. Dietary manipulations of body fat-reducing potential of conjugated linoleic acid in rats. *Biosci Biotechnol Biochem* 2001 Nov;65(11):2535-41

[340] DeLany JP, Blohm F, Truett AA, Scimeca JA, West DB. Conjugated linoleic acid rapidly reduces body fat content in mice without affecting energy intake. *Am J Physiol* 1999 Apr;276(4 Pt 2):R1172-9

[341] Ryder JW, Portocarrero CP, Song XM, Cui L, Yu M, Combatsiaris T, Galuska D, Bauman DE, Barbano DM, Charron MJ, Zierath JR, Houseknecht KL. Isomer-specific antidiabetic properties of conjugated linoleic acid. Improved glucose tolerance, skeletal muscle insulin action, and UCP-2 gene expression. *Diabetes* 2001 May;50(5):1149-57

[342] McCarty MF. Hepatothermic therapy of obesity: rationale and an inventory of resources. *Med Hypotheses* 2001 Sep;57(3):324-36

[343] Kang K, Pariza MW. trans-10,cis-12-Conjugated linoleic acid reduces leptin secretion from 3T3-L1 adipocytes. *Biochem Biophys Res Commun* 2001 Sep 21;287(2):377-82

[344] Rahman SM, Wang Y, Yotsumoto H, Cha J, Han S, Inoue S, Yanagita T. Effects of conjugated linoleic acid on serum leptin concentration, body-fat accumulation, and beta-oxidation of fatty acid in OLETF rats. *Nutrition* 2001 May;17(5):385-90

[345] Akahoshi A, Goto Y, Murao K, Miyazaki T, Yamasaki M, Nonaka M, Yamada K, Sugano M. Conjugated linoleic acid reduces body fats and cytokine levels of mice. *Biosci Biotechnol Biochem* 2002 Apr;66(4):916-20

[346] Akahoshi A, Goto Y, Murao K, Miyazaki T, Yamasaki M, Nonaka M, Yamada K, Sugano M. Conjugated linoleic acid reduces body fats and cytokine levels of mice. *Biosci Biotechnol Biochem* 2002 Apr;66(4):916-20

[347] Van Cauter EV, Polonsky KS, Blackman JD, Roland D, Sturis J, Byrne MM, Scheen AJ. Abnormal temporal patterns of glucose tolerance in obesity: relationship to sleep-related growth hormone secretion and circadian cortisol rhythmicity. *J Clin Endocrinol Metab* 1994 Dec;79(6):1797-805

[348] Van Cauter EV, Polonsky KS, Blackman JD, Roland D, Sturis J, Byrne MM, Scheen AJ. Abnormal temporal patterns of glucose tolerance in obesity: relationship to sleep-related growth hormone secretion and circadian cortisol rhythmicity. *J Clin Endocrinol Metab* 1994 Dec;79(6):1797-805

[349] Parr TB. A new technique to elevate night time growth hormone release and potential growth hormone feedback control loop. *Med Hypotheses* 2001 May;56(5):610-3.

[350] Bidzinska B, Petraglia F, Angioni S, Genazzani AD, Criscuolo M, Ficarra G, Gallinelli A, Trentini GP, Genazzani AR. Effect of differenct chronic intermittent stressors and acetyl-l-carnitine on hypothalamic beta-endorphin and GnRH and on plasma testosterone levels in male rats. *Neuroendocrinology* 1993 Jun;57(6):985-90.

[351] Iossa S, Mollica MP, Lionetti L, Crescenzo R, Botta M, Barletta A, Liverini G. Acetyl-L-carnitine supplementation differently influences nutrient partitioning, serum leptin concentration and skeletal muscle mitochondrial respiration in young and old rats. *J Nutr* 2002 Apr;132(4):636-42

[352] Spagnoli A, et al. Long-term acetyl-L-carnitine treatment in Alzheimer's disease. *Neurology* 41:1726-1732; 1991.

[353] Calvani M, et al. Action of acetyl-L-carnitine in neurodegeneration and Alzheimer's disease. *Ann NY Acad Sci* 663:483-486; 1992.

[354] Carta A, et al. Acetyl-L-carnitine and Alzheimer's disease: pharmacological considerations beyond the cholinergic sphere. *Ann NY Acad Sci* 695:324-326; 1993.

[355] Parnetti L, et al. Milticentre atudy of l-alpha-glyceryl-phosphorylcholine vs ST200 among patients with probable senile dementia of Alzheimer's type. *Drugs Aging* 3:159-164; 1993.

[356] Guarnascheiil C, Fugazza G, Pistarini C. Pathological brain ageing: evaluation of the efficacy of a pharmacological aid. *Drugs Exp Clin Res* 14:715-718; 1998.

[357] Rai G, et al. Doulbe-blind, placebo-controlled study of acetyl-L-carnitine in patients with Alzheimer's dementia. *Curr Med Res Opin* 11:638-647; 1990.

[358] Bella R, Biondi R, Raffaele R, Pennisi G. Effect of acetyl-L-carnitine on generic patients suffering from dysthymic disorders. *Int J Clin Pharmacol Res* 10:355-360; 1990.

[359] Gecele M, Francesetti G, Meluzzi A. Acetyl-L-carnitine in aged subjects with major depression: clinical efficacy and effects on the circadian rhythm of cortisol. *Dementia* 2:333-337; 1991.

[360] Tempesta E, et al. L-acetylcarnitine in depressed elderly subjects. A cross-over study vs placebo. *Drugs Exp Clin Res* 13:417-423; 1987.

[361] Carta A, et al. Acetyl-L-carnitine and Alzheimer's disease: pharmacological considerations beyond the cholinergic sphere. *Ann NY Acad Sci* 695:324-326; 1993.

[362] Aureli T, Puccetti C, Di Cocco ME, Arduini A, Ricciolini R, Scalibastri M, Manetti C, Conti F. entry of [(1,2-13C2)acetyl]-L-carnitine in liver tricarboxylic acid cycle and lipogenesis: a study by 13C NMR spectroscopy in conscious, freely moving rats. *Eur J Biochem* 1999 Jul;263(1):287-93.

[363] Aureli T, Di Cocco ME, Capuani G, Ricciolini R, Manetti C, Miccheli A, Conti F. Effect of long-term feeding with acetyl-L-carnitine on the age-related changes in rat brain lipid composition: a study by 31P NMR spectroscopy. *Neurochem Res* 2000 Mar;25(3):395-9

[364] Aureli T, Di Cocco ME, Puccetti C, Ricciolini R, Scalibastri M, Miccheli A, Manetti C, Conti F. Acetyl-L-carnitine modulates glucose metabolism and stimulates glycogen syntheis in rat brain. *Brain Res* 1998 Jun 15;796(1-2):75-81.

[365] Soneru IL, Khan T, Orfalian Z, Abraira C. Acetyl-L-Carnitine effects on nerve conduction and glycemic regulation in experimental diabetes. *Endocr Res* 1997 Feb-May;23(1-2):27-36.

[366] Kano M, Kawakami T, Hori H, Hashimoto Y, Tao Y, Ishikawa Y, Takenaka T. Effects of ALCAR on the fast axoplasmic transport in cultured sensory neurons of streptozotocin-induced diabetic rats. *Neurosci Res* 1999 Mar;33(3):207-13.

[367] Wideman L, Weltman JY, Hartman ML, Veldhuis JD, Weltman A. Growth hormone release during acute and chronic aerobic and resistance exercise: recent findings. *Sports Med* 2002;32(15):987-1004

[368] Deschenes MR, Kraemer WJ. Performance and physiologic adaptations to resistance training. *Am J Phys Med Rehabil* 2002 Nov;81(11 Suppl):S3-16

[369] Werlang Coelho C, Rebello Velloso C, Resende de Lima Oliveira Brasil R, Vaisman M, Gil Soares de Araujo C. Muscle power increases after resistance

training in growth-hormone-deficient adults. *Med Sci Sports Exerc* 2002 Oct;34(10):1577-81

370 Hakkinen K, Kraemer WJ, Pakarinen A, Triplett-McBride T, McBride JM, Hakkinen A, Alen M, McGuigan MR, Bronks R, Newton RU. Effects of heavy resistance/power training on maximal strength, muscle morphology, and hormonal response patterns in 60-75-year-old men and women. *Can J Appl Physiol* 2002 Jun;27(3):213-31

371 Heaton JP, Morales A. Andropause—a multisystem disease. *Can J Urol* 2001 Apr;8(2):1213-22

372 Zmuda J, Cauley, J, Kriska, A, Glynn, N, Gutai, J, Kuller, L. Longitudinal relation between endogenous testosterone and cardiovascular disease risk factors in middle-aged men. *Am J Epidemiol.* 1997: 146:609-617.

373 Edwards, E, Hamilton, J, Duntley, S. Testosterone propionate as a therapeutic agent in patients with organic disease of the peripheral vessels. *N Engl J Med.* 1939; 220 :865.

374 Jaffee, M. Effect of testosterone cypionate on post-exercise St segment depression. *Br Heart J.* 1977; 39:1217-1222.

375 Wu SZ, Weng XZ. Therapeutic effects of an androgenic preparation on myocardial ischemia and cardiac function in 62 elderly male coronary heart disease patients. *Chin Med J* (Engl). 1993; 106:415-418.

376 Phillips, GB, Pinkernell, BH, Jing TY. The association of hypotestosteronemia with coronary artery disease in men. *Arterioscler Thromb.* 1994; 14:701-706.

377 Barrett-Connor, EL. Testosterone and risk factors for cardiovascular disease in men. *Diabete Metab.* 1995: 21:156-161.

378 Tenover, JL. Testosterone and the aging male. *J Androl.* 1997: 18:103-106.

379 Rolf C, von Eckardstein S, Koken U, Nieschlag E. Testosterone substitution of hypogonadal men prevents the age-dependent increases in body mass index, body fat and leptin seen in healthy ageing men: results of a cross-sectional study. *Eur J Endocrinol* 2002 Apr;146(4):505-11

380 Soderberg S, Olsson T, Eliasson M, Johnson O, Brismar K, Carlstrom K, Ahren B. A strong association between biologically active testosterone and leptin in non-obese men and women is lost with increasing (central) adiposity. *Int J Obes Relat Metab Disord* 2001 Jan;25(1):98-105

381 Ogura T, Tobe K, Mimura Y, Otsuka F, Yamauchi T, Imai A, Tsukamoto C, Iwasaki Y, Matsuura K. Testosterone modulates serum leptin concentrations in a male patient with hypothalamic hypogonadism. *J Endocrinol Invest* 2000 Apr;23(4):246-50

382 Tena-Sempere M, Barreiro ML. Leptin in male reproduction: the testis paradigm. *Mol Cell Endocrinol* 2002 Feb 25;188(1-2):9-13

383 Casabiell X, Pineiro V, Vega F, De La Cruz LF, Dieguez C, Casanueva FF. Leptin, reproduction and sex steroids. *Pituitary* 2001 Jan-Apr;4(1-2):93-9

384 Sih R, Morley JE, Kaiser FE, Perry HM 3rd, Patrick P, Ross C. Testosterone replacement in older hypogonadal men: a 12-month randomized controlled trial. *J Clin Endocrinol Metab* 1997 Jun;82(6):1661-7

385 Glander HJ, Lammert A, Paasch U, Glasow A, Kratzsch J. Leptin exists in tubuli seminiferi and in seminal plasma. *Andrologia* 2002 Sep;34(4):227-33

386 Abate N, Haffner SM, Garg A, Peshock RM, Grundy SM. Sex steroid hormones, upper body obesity, and insulin resistance. *J Clin Endocrinol Metab* 2002 Oct;87(10):4522-7

387 Jansson PA, Eliasson B, Lindmark S, Eriksson JW. Endocrine abnormalities in healthy first-degree relatives of type 2 diabetes patients—potential role of steroid hormones and leptin in the development of insulin resistance. *Eur J Clin Invest* 2002 Mar;32(3):172-8

[388] Chan JL, Bluher S, Yiannakouris N, Suchard MA, Kratzsch J, Mantzoros CS. Regulation of circulating soluble leptin receptor levels by gender, adiposity, sex steroids, and leptin: observational and interventional studies in humans. *Diabetes* 2002 Jul;51(7):2105-12

[389] Prasad A. Zinc in growth and development and spectrum of human zinc deficiency. *J Am Coll Nutr* 7 377-384, 1988.

[390] Netter A, et al. Effects of zinc administration on plasma testosterone, dihydrotestosterone and sperm count. *Arch Androl* 7 69-73, 1981.

[391] Xu Z, Kawai M, Bandiera SM, Chang TK. Influence of dietary zinc deficiency during development on hepatic CYP2C11, CYP2C12, CYP3A2, CYP3A9, and CYP3A18 expression in postpubertal male rats. *Biochem Pharmacol* 2001 Nov 1;62(9):1283-91

[392] Gauthaman K, Adaikan PG, Prasad RN. Aphrodisiac properties of Tribulus Terrestris extract (Protodioscin) in normal and castrated rats. *Life Sci* 2002 Aug 9;71(12):1385-96

[393] Dimitrov, M, Gerogiev, P, Vitanov, S. Use of tribestan on rams with sexual disorders. *Vet Med Nauki.* 1987; 24(5): 102-110.

[394] Zarkova, S. Steroid saponins of Tribulus terrestris L. have a stimulant effect on the sexual function. *Rev Port Ciencias Vet* 1984; 79 (470): 117-126.

[395] Protich, M, Twvetkov, D, nalbanski, B, et al. Clinical trial of a preparation Tribestan in infertile men. *Akush Ginekol.* 1983; 22(4): 326-329. (in Bulgarian)

[396] Coleman, DL, Schwizer, RW, Leiter, EH. DHEA's Effects on Weight. *Diabetes.* Jan 1984; 33(1): 26-32.

[397] Regulation of the immune response by dehydroepiandrosterone and its metabolites. *Journal of Endocrinology (United Kingdom).* 1996;150/Suppl. S209-S220.

[398] Yen, SS, Morales, AJ, Khorram, O. Replacement of DHEA in aging men and women – Potential remedial effects. *Ann NY Acad Sci (U.S.)* . 1995; 774: 128-142.

[399] Brown GA, Vukovich MD, Martini ER, Kohut ML, Franke WD, Jackson DA, King DS. Effects of androstenedione-herbal supplementation on serum sex hormone concentrations in 30- to 59-year-old men. *Int J Vitam Nutr Res* 2001 Sep;71(5):293-301

[400] Kochakian, CD. Metabolites of testosterone, significance in the vital economy. *Steroids.* 1990; 55: 92-97.

[401] Mahesh, VB, Greenblatt, RB. The in-vivo conversion of dehydroepiandrosterone and androstenedione to testosterone in the human. Acta Endocrinol. 1962; 41: 400-406.

[402] Scordalakes EM, Imwalle DB, Rissman EF. Oestrogen's masculine side: mediation of mating in male mice. *Reproduction* 2002 Sep;124(3):331-8

[403] Cohen PG. Aromatase, adiposity, aging and disease. The hypogonadal-metabolic-atherogenic-disease and aging connection. *Med Hypotheses* 2001 Jun;56(6):702-8

[404] Machinal-Quelin F, Dieudonne MN, Pecquery R, Leneveu MC, Giudicelli Y. Direct in vitro effects of androgens and estrogens on ob gene expression and leptin secretion in human adipose tissue. *Endocrine* 2002 Jul;18(2):179-84

[405] Dhawan K, Sharma A. Prevention of chronic alcohol and nicotine-induced azospermia, sterility and decreased libido, by a novel tri-substituted benzoflavone moiety from Passiflora incarnata Linneaus in healthy male rats. *Life Sci* 2002 Nov 15;71(26):3059-69

[406] Bakker J, Honda S, Harada N, Balthazart J. Sexual partner preference requires a functional aromatase (cyp19) gene in male mice. *Horm Behav* 2002 Sep;42(2):158-71

[407] Li X, Warri A, Makela S, Ahonen T, Streng T, Santti R, Poutanen M. Mammary gland development in transgenic male mice expressing human P450 aromatase. *Endocrinology* 2002 Oct;143(10):4074-83

[408] Vermeulen A, Kaufman JM, Goemaere S, van Pottelberg I. Estradiol in elderly men. *Aging Male* 2002 Jun;5(2):98-102

[409] Satoh K, Sakamoto Y, Ogata A, Nagai F, Mikuriya H, Numazawa M, Yamada K, Aoki N. Inhibition of aromatase activity by green tea extract catechins and their endocrinological effects of oral administration in rats. *Food Chem Toxicol* 2002 Jul;40(7):925-33

[410] Atrazine is the most commonly used herbicide in the U.S. and probably the world.

[411] Kato S, Mano T, Kobayashi T, Yamazaki N, Himeno Y, Yamamoto K, Itoh M, Harada N, Nagasaka A. A calcium-deficient diet caused decreased bone mineral density and secondary elevation of estrogen in aged male rats-effect of menatetrenone and elcatonin. *Metabolism* 2002 Oct;51(10):1230-4

[412] Martin WJ, McGowan E, Cashen DE, Gantert LT, Drisko JE, Hom GJ, Nargund R, Sebhat I, Howard AD, Van der Ploeg LH, MacIntyre DE. Activation of melanocortin MC(4) receptors increases erectile activity in rats ex copula. *Eur J Pharmacol* 2002 Nov 1;454(1):71-9

[413] Sainsbury A, Schwarzer C, Couzens M, Jenkins A, Oakes SR, Ormandy CJ, Herzog H. Y4 receptor knockout rescues fertility in ob/ob mice. *Genes Dev* 2002 May 1;16(9):1077-88

[414] Martin LJ, Mahaney MC, Almasy L, MacCluer JW, Blangero J, Jaquish CE, Comuzzie AG. Leptin's sexual dimorphism results from genotype by sex interactions mediated by testosterone. *Obes Res* 2002 Jan;10(1):14-21

[415] Casabiell X, Pineiro V, Vega F, De La Cruz LF, Dieguez C, Casanueva FF. Leptin, reproduction and sex steroids. *Pituitary* 2001 Jan-Apr;4(1-2):93-9

[416] Cizza G, Dorn LD, Lotsikas A, Sereika S, Rotenstein D, Chrousos GP. Circulating plasma leptin and IGF-1 levels in girls with premature adrenarche: potential implications of a preliminary study. *Horm Metab Res* 2001 Mar;33(3):138-43

[417] Tanaka M, Nakaya S, Kumai T, Watanabe M, Tateishi T, Shimizu H, Kobayashi S. Effects of estrogen on serum leptin levels and leptin mRNA expression in adipose tissue in rats. *Horm Res* 2001;56(3-4):98-104

[418] Fedorcsak P, Storeng R, Dale PO, Tanbo T, Torjesen P, Urbancsek J, Abyholm T. Leptin and leptin binding activity in the preovulatory follicle of polycystic ovary syndrome patients. *Scand J Clin Lab Invest* 2000 Dec;60(8):649-55

[419] Spritzer PM, Poy M, Wiltgen D, Mylius LS, Capp E. Leptin concentrations in hirsute women with polycystic ovary syndrome or idiopathic hirsutism: influence on LH and relationship with hormonal, metabolic, and anthropometric measurements. *Hum Reprod* 2001 Jul;16(7):1340-6

[420] Gambineri A, Pelusi C, Vicennati V, Pagotto U, Pasquali R. Obesity and the polycystic ovary syndrome. *Int J Obes Relat Metab Disord* 2002 Jul;26(7):883-96

[421] Veldhuis JD, Pincus SM, Garcia-Rudaz MC, Ropelato MG, Escobar ME, Barontini M. Disruption of the synchronous secretion of leptin, LH, and ovarian androgens in nonobese adolescents with the polycystic ovarian syndrome. *J Clin Endocrinol Metab* 2001 Aug;86(8):3772-8

[422] Schofl C, Horn R, Schill T, Schlosser HW, Muller MJ, Brabant G. Circulating ghrelin levels in patients with polycystic ovary syndrome. *J Clin Endocrinol Metab* 2002 Oct;87(10):4607-10

[423] Villa P, Soranna L, Mancini A, De Marinis L, Valle D, Mancuso S, Lanzone A. Effect of feeding on growth hormone response to growth hormone-releasing

hormone in polycystic ovarian syndrome: relation with body weight and hyperinsulinism. *Hum Reprod* 2001 Mar;16(3):430-4

[424] Van Dam EW, Roelfsema F, Helmerhorst FH, Frolich M, Meinders AE, Veldhuis JD,Pijl H. Low amplitude and disorderly spontaneous growth hormone release in obese women with or without polycystic ovary syndrome. *J Clin Endocrinol Metab* 2002 Sep;87(9):4225-30

[425] Garcia-Rudaz MC, Ropelato MG, Escobar ME, Veldhuis JD, Barontini M. Amplified and orderly growth hormone secretion characterizes lean adolescents with polycystic ovary syndrome. *Eur J Endocrinol* 2002 Aug;147(2):207-16

[426] Wu X, Sallinen K, Zhou S, Su Y, Pollanen P, Erkkola R. Androgen excess contributes to altered growth hormone/insulin-like growth factor-1 axis in nonobese women with polycystic ovary syndrome. *Fertil Steril* 2000 Apr;73(4):730-4

[427] Anim-Nyame N, Domoney C, Panay N, Jones J, Alaghband-Zadeh J, Studd JW. Plasma leptin concentrations are increased in women with premenstrual syndrome. *Hum Reprod* 2000 Nov;15(11):2329-32

[428] Messinis IE, Papageorgiou I, Milingos S, Asprodini E, Kollios G, Seferiadis K. Oestradiol plus progesterone treatment increases serum leptin concentrations in normal women. *Hum Reprod* 2001 Sep;16(9):1827-32

[429] Maruyama S, Minami S, Kaseki H, Ishihara K, Araki S, Suzue R. A comparison of serum leptin concentrations in obese and normal weight Japanese women with regular menstrual cycle. *J Nutr Sci Vitaminol* (Tokyo) 2001 Feb;47(1):87-9

[430] Poston L. Leptin and preeclampsia. *Semin Reprod Med* 2002;20(2):131-8

[431] Kirwan JP, Hauguel-De Mouzon S, Lepercq J, Challier JC, Huston-Presley L, Friedman JE, Kalhan SC, Catalano PM. TNF-alpha is a predictor of insulin resistance in human pregnancy. *Diabetes* 2002 Jul;51(7):2207-13

[432] Tsai EM, Yang CH, Chen SC, Liu YH, Chen HS, Hsu SC, Lee JN. Leptin affects pregnancy outcome of in vitro fertilization and steroidogenesis of human granulosa cells. *J Assist Reprod Genet* 2002 Apr;19(4):169-76

[433] Gogacz M, Polak G, Jakowicki J, Kotarski J. Peritoneal fluid leptin concentration in infertile patients. *J Reprod Immunol* 2001 Aug;51(2):159-65

[434] Unkila-Kallio L, Andersson S, Koistinen HA, Karonen SL, Ylikorkala O, Tiitinen A. Leptin during assisted reproductive cycles: the effect of ovarian stimulation and of very early pregnancy. *Hum Reprod* 2001 Apr;16(4):657-62

[435] Kitawaki J, Koshiba H, Ishihara H, Kusuki I, Tsukamoto K, Honjo H. Expression of leptin receptor in human endometrium and fluctuation during the menstrual cycle. *J Clin Endocrinol Metab* 2000 May;85(5):1946-50

[436] Matarese G, Alviggi C, Sanna V, Howard JK, Lord GM, Carravetta C, Fontana S, Lechler RI, Bloom SR, De Placido G. Increased leptin levels in serum and peritoneal fluid of patients with pelvic endometriosis. *J Clin Endocrinol Metab* 2000 Jul;85(7):2483-7

[437] Wu MH, Chuang PC, Chen HM, Lin CC, Tsai SJ. Increased leptin expression in endometriosis cells is associated with endometrial stromal cell proliferation and leptin gene up-regulation. *Mol Hum Reprod* 2002 May;8(5):456-64

[438] Lebovic DI, Chao VA, Martini JF, Taylor RN. IL-1beta induction of RANTES (regulated upon activation, normal T cell expressed and secreted) chemokine gene expression in endometriotic stromal cells depends on a nuclear factor-kappaB site in the proximal promoter. *J Clin Endocrinol Metab* 2001 Oct;86(10):4759-64

[439] Bidzinska B, Petraglia F, Angioni S, Genazzani AD, Criscuolo M, Ficarra G, Gallinelli A, Trentini GP, Genazzani AR. Effect of different chronic intermittent stressors and acetyl-l-carnitine on hypothalamic beta-endorphin and GnRH and

on plasma testosterone levels in male rats. *Neuroendocrinology* 1993 Jun;57(6):985-90.

440 Genazzani AD, Petraglia F, Algeri I, Gastaldi M, Calvani M, Botticelli G, Genazzani AR. Acetyl-l-carnitine as possible drug in the treatment of hypothalamic amenorrhea. *Acta Obstet Gynecol Scand* 1991;70(6):487-92.

441 Iossa S, Mollica MP, Lionetti L, Crescenzo R, Botta M, Barletta A, Liverini G. Acetyl-L-carnitine supplementation differently influences nutrient partitioning, serum leptin concentration and skeletal muscle mitochondrial respiration in young and old rats. *J Nutr* 2002 Apr;132(4):636-42

442 Pearlstein T. Selective serotonin reuptake inhibitors for premenstrual dysphoric disorder: the emerging gold standard? *Drugs* 2002;62(13):1869-85

443 Van Ameringen M, Mancini C, Pipe B, Campbell M, Oakman J. Topiramate treatment for SSRI-induced weight gain in anxiety disorders. *J Clin Psychiatry* 2002 Nov;63(11):981-4

444 Masand PS, Gupta S. Selective serotonin-reuptake inhibitors: an update. *Harv Rev Psychiatry* 1999 Jul-Aug;7(2):69-84

445 Silvestri R, Pace-Schott EF, Gersh T, Stickgold R, Salzman C, Hobson JA. Effects of fluvoxamine and paroxetine on sleep structure in normal subjects: a home-based Nightcap evaluation during drug administration and withdrawal. *J Clin Psychiatry* 2001 Aug;62(8):642-52

446 Dagan Y. Circadian Rhythm Sleep Disorders (CRSD) in psychiatry—a review. *Isr J Psychiatry Relat Sci* 2002;39(1):19-27

447 Writing Group for the Women's Health Initiative Investigators. Risks and benefits of estrogen plus progestin in healthy postmenopausal women: principal results From the Women's Health Initiative randomized controlled trial. *JAMA* 2002 Jul 17;288(3):321-33

448 A. H. Follingstad M.D. Estriol, the forgotten estrogen. *JAMA*, Jan. 2 1978 Vol 239 No.1

449 Lemon H, Wotiz H, Parsons L, Mozden P. Reduced Estriol secretion in patients with breast cancer prior to endocrine therapy. *JAMA* 1966; 196;112-120.

450 Reyes-Romero MA. The physiological role of estriol during human fetal development is to act as antioxidant at lipophilic milieus of the central nervous system. *Med Hypotheses* 2001 Jan;56(1):107-9

451 O'Hara MW, Schlechte JA, Lewis DA, Wright EJ. Prospective study of postpartum blues. Biologic and psychosocial factors. *Arch Gen Psychiatry* 1991 Sep;48(9):801-6

452 Zeisler H, Jirecek S, Hohlagschwandtner M, Knofler M, Tempfer C, Livingston JC. Concentrations of estrogens in patients with preeclampsia. *Wien Klin Wochenschr* 2002 Jun 28;114(12):458-61

453 Voskuhl RR, Palaszynski K. Sex hormones in experimental autoimmune encephalomyelitis: implications for multiple sclerosis. Neuroscientist 2001 Jun;7(3):258-70

454 Sicotte NL, Liva SM, Klutch R, Pfeiffer P, Bouvier S, Odesa S, Wu TC, Voskuhl RR. Treatment of multiple sclerosis with the pregnancy hormone estriol. *Ann Neurol* 2002 Oct;52(4):421-8

455 Buntner B, Rosciszewska D. Urinary excretion of estrogen fractions, alpha and beta pregnanediol and pregnanetriol in women with epileptic seizures during the premenstrual period. *urol Neurochir Pol* 1975 May-Jun;9(3):311-7

456 Zemlyak I, Brooke SM, Sapolsky RM. Protection against gp120-induced neurotoxicity by an array of estrogenic steroids. *Brain Res* 2002 Dec 27;958(2):272-6

[457] Kajta M, Budziszewska B, Marszal M, Lason W. Effects of 17-beta estradiol and estriol on NMDA-induced toxicity and apoptosis in primary cultures of rat cortical neurons. *J Physiol Pharmacol* 2001 Sep;52(3):437-46

[458] Plaino L, Stomati M, Casarosa E, Artini PG, Santuz M, D'Ambrogio G, Cobellis L, Luisi M, Genazzani AR, Petraglia F. Ovarian follicular fluid contains immunoreactive estriol: lack of correlation with estradiol concentrations. *Gynecol Endocrinol* 2000 Aug;14(4):231-5

[459] Ghosh S, Kabir SN, Pakrashi A, Chatterjee S, Chakravarty B. Subclinical hypothyroidism: a determinant of polycystic ovary syndrome. *Horm Res* 1993;39(1-2):61-6 Comment in: Horm Res. 1994;41(1):43-4.

[460] Lee JR. *What Your Doctor May Not Tell You About Menopasue.* New York. Warner Books, 1996

[461] Moen MH, Buajordet M, Leirstrand T. Progesterone cream—efficient in premenstrual syndrome and climacteric problems? Tidsskr Nor Laegeforen 2002 Jun 10;122(15):1477-8

[462] Triezenberg DJ, Ang J. Are progesterone or progestogens effective in managing premenstrual syndrome (PMS) symptoms? *J Fam Pract* 2002 Feb;51(2):109

[463] Wyatt K, Dimmock P, Jones P, Obhrai M, O'Brien S. Efficacy of progesterone and progestogens in management of premenstrual syndrome: systematic review. *BMJ* 2001 Oct 6;323(7316):776-80

[464] O'Sullivan AJ, Martin A, Brown MA. Efficient fat storage in pre-menopausal women and in early pregnancy: a role for estrogen. *J Clin Endocrinol Metab* 2001 Oct;86(10):4951-6

[465] Li WL, Guo XY, Zhang JY, Peng P, Zhang YL. Serum leptin levels of menopausal women before and after hormone replacement therapy. Di Yi Jun Yi Da Xue Xue Bao 2002 Jul;22(7):635-6

[466] Ainslie DA, Morris MJ, Wittert G, Turnbull H, Proietto J, Thorburn AW. Estrogen deficiency causes central leptin insensitivity and increased hypothalamic neuropeptide Y. *Int J Obes Relat Metab Disord* 2001 Nov;25(11):1680-8

[467] Wyon YA, Spetz AC, Theodorsson GE, Hammar ML. Concentrations of calcitonin gene-related peptide and neuropeptide Y in plasma increase during flushes in postmenopausal women. *Menopause* 2000 Jan-Feb;7(1):25-30

[468] Kanaley JA, Sames C, Swisher L, Swick AG, Ploutz-Snyder LL, Steppan CM, Sagendorf KS, Feiglin D, Jaynes EB, Meyer RA, Weinstock RS. Abdominal fat distribution in pre- and postmenopausal women: The impact of physical activity, age, and menopausal status. *Metabolism* 2001 Aug;50(8):976-82

[469] Isidori AM, Strollo F, More M, Caprio M, Aversa A, Moretti C, Frajese G, Riondino G, Fabbri A. Leptin and aging: correlation with endocrine changes in male and female healthy adult populations of different body weights. *J Clin Endocrinol Metab* 2000 May;85(5):1954-62

[470] Martini G, Valenti R, Giovani S, Campagna S, Franci B, Nuti R. Leptin and body composition in healthy postmenopausal women. *Panminerva Med* 2001 Sep;43(3):149-54

[471] Cioffi M, Esposito K, Vietri MT, Gazzerro P, D'Auria A, Ardovino I, Puca GA,Molinari AM. Cytokine pattern in postmenopause. *Maturitas* 2002 Mar 25;41(3):187-92

[472] Schurman L, Sedlinsky C, Mangano A, Sen L, Leiderman S, Fernandez G, Theas S, Damilano S, Gurfinkel M, Seilicovich A. Estrogenic status influences nitric oxide-regulated TNF-alpha release from human peripheral blood monocytes. *Exp Clin Endocrinol Diabetes* 2001;109(6):340-4

[473] Sites CK, Toth MJ, Cushman M, L'Hommedieu GD, Tchernof A, Tracy RP, Poehlman ET. Menopause-related differences in inflammation markers and their

relationship to body fat distribution and insulin-stimulated glucose disposal. *Fertil Steril* 2002 Jan;77(1):128-35

[474] Kano H, Hayashi T, Sumi D, Matusi-Hirai H, Tsunekawa T, Endo H, Iguchi A. Estriol retards and stabilizes atherosclerosis through an NO-mediated system. Life Sci 2002 May 24;71(1):31-42

[475] Ohata S, Ishibashi Y, Hirano Y, Sakane T, Takahashi N, Sugamori T, Inoue S, Katoh H, Ochiai K, Sano K, Murakami Y, Shimada T. Relationship between endothelial function and female hormone level in very old females: evaluation from ischemic reactive hyperemic response in forearm vessels *J Cardiol* 2000 Jun;35(6):417-24

[476] Itoi H, Minakami H, Iwasaki R, Sato I. Comparison of the long-term effects of oral estriol with the effects of conjugated estrogen on serum lipid profile in early menopausal women. *Maturitas* 2000 Oct 31;36(3):217-22

[477] Hayashi T, Ito I, Kano H, Endo H, Iguchi A. Estriol (E3) replacement improves endothelial function and bone mineral density in very elderly women. *J Gerontol A Biol Sci Med Sci* 2000 Apr;55(4):B183-90; discussion B191-3

[478] Manonai J, Theppisai U. Effect of oral estriol on urogenital symptoms, vaginal cytology, and plasma hormone level in postmenopausal women. *J Med Assoc Thai* 2001 Apr;84(4):539-44

[479] Mandigers RJ, Nell T. Treatment of bitches with acquired urinary incontinence with oestriol. *Vet Rec* 2001 Dec 22-29;149(25):764-7

[480] Raz R. Postmenopausal women with recurrent UTI. *Int J Antimicrob Agents* 2001 Apr;17(4):269-71

[481] Yoshimura T, Okamura H. Short term oral estriol treatment restores normal pre-menopausal vaginal flora to elderly women. *Maturitas* 2001 Sep 28;39(3):253-7

[482] Kuczynska K, Wolczynski S, Janucik-Gacuta M, Zbroch T. Influence of hormonal replacement therapy on bacterial vaginosis in the group of peri- and postmenopausal women *Ginekol Pol* 2001 Oct;72(10):816-24

[483] Heimer G. Estriol in the postmenopausal. *Acta Obstet Gynecol Scand.* 1987; Suppl 139;1-23.

[484] Losif C. Effects of protracted administration of Estriol on the lower genito urinary tract in postmenopausal women. *Arch Gynecol Obstet* 1992; 251; 115-120.

[485] Ushiroyama T, Sakai M, Higashiyama T, Ikeda A, Ueki M. Estrogen replacement therapy in postmenopausal women: a study of the efficacy of estriol and changes in plasma gonadotropin levels. Gynecol Endocrinol 2001 Feb;15(1):74-80

[486] Granberg S, Eurenius K, Lindgren R, Wilhelmsson L. The effects of oral estriol on the endometrium in postmenopausal women. *Maturitas* 2002 Jun 25;42(2):149-56

[487] Lundstrom E, Wilczek B, von Palffy Z, Soderqvist G, von Schoultz B. Mammographic breast density during hormone replacement therapy: effects of continuous combination, unopposed transdermal and low-potency estrogen regimens. *Climacteric* 2001 Mar;4(1):42-85.

[488] Takahashi K, Okada M, Ozaki T, Kurioka H, Manabe A, Kanasaki H, Miyazaki K. Safety and efficacy of oestriol for symptoms of natural or surgically induced menopause. *Hum Reprod* 2000 May;15(5):1028-366.

[489] Son DS, Roby KF, Rozman KK, Terranova PF. Estradiol enhances and estriol inhibits the expression of CYP1A1 induced by 2,3,7,8-tetrachlorodibenzo-p-dioxin in a mouse ovarian cancer cell line. Toxicology 2002 Jul 15;176(3):229-43

[490] Lemon H. Oestriol and prevention of breast cancer. Lancet 1973; 546-547.

[491] Lemon H, Kumar P, Peterson C, Rodriguez-Sierra J, Abbo K. Inhibition of radiogenic mammary carcinoma in rats by Estriol or tamoxifen. cancer 1989;63:1685-1692.

[492] Heimer G. Estriol in the postmenopausal. *Acta Obstet Gynecol Scand.* 1987; Suppl 139;1-23.

[493] Zang YC, Halder JB, Hong J, Rivera VM, Zhang JZ. Regulatory effects of estriol on T cell migration and cytokine profile: inhibition of transcription factor NF-kappa

[494] B. J Neuroimmunol 2002 Mar;124(1-2):106-14 8. Pasqualini JR, Gelly C, Nguyen BL, Vella C. Importance of estrogen sulfates in breast cancer. J Steroid Biochem 1989;34(1-6):155-63.

[495] Lauritzen C. Results of a 5-year prospective study of Estriol succinate treatment in patients with climacteric complaints. *Horm Metabol Res.* 1987; 19; 579-584.

[496] Matsubara M, Yoshizawa T, Morioka T, Katayose S. Serum leptin and lipids in patients with thyroid dysfunction. *J Atheroscler Thromb* 2000;7(1):50-4

[497] Wang JL, Chinookoswong N, Yin S, Shi ZQ. Calorigenic actions of leptin are additive to, but not dependent on, those of thyroid hormones. *Am J Physiol Endocrinol Metab* 2000 Dec;279(6):E1278-85

[498] Chen MD, Song YM, Tsou CT, Lin WH, Sheu WH. Leptin concentration and the Zn/Cu ratio in plasma in women with thyroid disorder. *Biol Trace Elem Res* 2000 Summer;75(1-3):99-105

[499] Miyakawa M, Tsushima T, Murakami H, Isozaki O, Takano K. Serum leptin levels and bioelectrical impedance assessment of body composition in patients with Graves' disease and hypothyroidism. *Endocr J* 1999 Oct;46(5):665-73

[500] Tagliaferri M, Berselli ME, Calo G, Minocci A, Savia G, Petroni ML, Viberti GC, Liuzzi A. Subclinical hypothyroidism in obese patients: relation to resting energy expenditure, serum leptin, body composition, and lipid profile. *Obes Res* 2001 Mar;9(3):196-201

[501] Kautzky-Willer A, Ludwig C, Nowotny P, Roden A, Huemer C, Widhalm K, Vierhapper H, Waldhausl W, Roden M. Elevation of plasma leptin concentrations in obese hyperinsulinaemic hypothyroidism before and after treatment. *Eur J Clin Invest* 1999 May;29(5):395-403

[502] Iossa S, Lionetti L, Mollica MP, Crescenzo R, Barletta A, Liverini Fat balance and serum leptin concentrations in normal, hypothyroid, and hyperthyroid rats.G.*Int J Obes Relat Metab Disord* 2001 Mar;25(3):417-25

[503] Rubello D, Sonino N, Casara D, et al. Acute and chronic effects of high glucocorticoid levels on hypothalamic-pituitary-thyroid axis in man. *J Endocrinol Invest* 1992:15:437-441

[504] Bobek S, Sechman A, Niezgoda J, Jacek T. Reverse 3,3',5'-triiodothyronine suppresses increase in free fatty acids in chickens elicited by dexamethasone or adrenaline. *J Vet Med A Physiol Pathol Clin Med* 2002 Apr;49(3):121-4

[505] Silberman DM, Wald M, Genaro AM. Effects of chronic mild stress on lymphocyte proliferative response. Participation of serum thyroid hormones and corticosterone. *Int Immunopharmacol* 2002 Mar;2(4):487-97

[506] Servatius RJ, Natelson BH, Moldow R, Pogach L, Brennan FX, Ottenweller JE. Persistent neuroendocrine changes in multiple hormonal axes after a single or repeated stressor exposures. *Stress* 2000 Nov;3(4):263-74

[507] Stathatos N, Levetan C, Burman KD, Wartofsky L. The controversy of the treatment of critically ill patients with thyroid hormone. *Best Pract Res Clin Endocrinol Metab* 2001 Dec;15(4):465-78

[508] Alink GM, Brouwer A, Heussen GA. Effects of outdoor and indoor airborne particulate matter on thyroid hormone and vitamin A metabolism. *Toxicol Lett* 1994 Jun;72(1-3):73-81

[509] Zaitseva NV, Zemlianova MA, Kir'ianov DA. Identification of specific features of the development of iodine deficiency in children exposed to low-intensity ecological factors (in case of the Perm Region) *Vestn Ross Akad Med Nauk* 2001;(6):39-45

[510] Dodina LG. The clinical functional status of the thyroid and the cortisol level in those living in a region of ecological stress *Med Tr Prom Ekol* 1999;(10):8-10

[511] Langer P, Tajtakova M, Fodor G, Kocan A, Bohov P, Michalek J, Kreze A. Increased thyroid volume and prevalence of thyroid disorders in an area heavily polluted by polychlorinated biphenyls. *Eur J Endocrinol* 1998 Oct;139(4):402-9

[512] Osius N, Karmaus W. Thyroid hormone level in children in the area of a toxic waste incinerator in South Essen *Gesundheitswesen* 1998 Feb;60(2):107-12

[513] Porter WP, Jaeger JW, Carlson IH. Endocrine, immune, and behavioral effects of aldicarb (carbamate), atrazine (triazine) and nitrate (fertilizer) mixtures at groundwater concentrations. *Toxicol Ind Health* 1999 Jan-Mar;15(1-2):133-50

[514] Leatherland JF. Changes in thyroid hormone economy following consumption of environmentally contaminated Great Lakes fish. Toxicol Ind Health 1998 Jan-Apr;14(1-2):41-57

[515] Vladeva S, Gatseva P, Gopina G. Comparative analysis of results from studies of goitre in children from Bulgarian villages with nitrate pollution of drinking water in 1995 and 1998. *Cent Eur J Public Health* 2000 Aug;8(3):179-81

[516] Khmel'nitskii OK, Tret'iakova MS, Kiselev AV, Basinskii VA, Batashova VS, Vasil'ev IuB, Gorbachev AL, Derizhanova IS, Kovalenko VL, Kulaev IA, Konstantinov GS, Murochkin VV, Tararak, TIa, Ashanin BS, Troshin VP, Khodasevich LS, Maliavskii IIu. Morpho-ecological characteristics of thyroid diseases in various regions of Russia and Belorussia from surgical data *Arkh Patol* 2000 Jul-Aug;62(4):19-27

[517] Gasparoni A, Autelli M, Ravagni-Probizer MF, Bartoli A, Regazzi-Bonora M, Chirico G, Rondini G. Effect of passive smoking on thyroid function in infants. *Eur J Endocrinol* 1998 Apr;138(4):379-82

[518] Wade MG, Parent S, Finnson KW, Foster W, Younglai E, McMahon A, Cyr DG, Hughes C. Thyroid toxicity due to subchronic exposure to a complex mixture of 16 organochlorines, lead, and cadmium. *Toxicol Sci* 2002 Jun;67(2):207-18

[519] Schantz SL, Widholm JJ. Cognitive effects of endocrine-disrupting chemicals in animals. *Environ Health Perspect* 2001 Dec;109(12):1197-206

[520] Saxena NK, Ikeda K, Rockey DC, Friedman SL, Anania FA. Leptin in hepatic fibrosis: evidence for increased collagen production in stellate cells and lean littermates of ob/ob mice. *Hepatology* 2002 Apr;35(4):762-71

[521] Ikejima K, Honda H, Yoshikawa M, Hirose M, Kitamura T, Takei Y, Sato N. Leptin augments inflammatory and profibrogenic responses in the murine liver induced by hepatotoxic chemicals. *Hepatology* 2001 Aug;34(2):288-97

[522] Nicassio PM, Moxham EG, Schuman CE, Gevirtz RN. The contribution of pain, reported sleep quality, and depressive symptoms to fatigue in fibromyalgia. *Pain* 2002 Dec;100(3):271-9

[523] Lawson K. Tricyclic antidepressants and fibromyalgia: what is the mechanism of action? *Expert Opin Investig Drugs* 2002 Oct;11(10):1437-45

[524] Moldofsky H. Management of sleep disorders in fibromyalgia. *Rheum Dis Clin North Am* 2002 May;28(2):353-65

[525] Paulson M, Norberg A, Danielson E. Men living with fibromyalgia-type pain: experiences as patients in the Swedish health care system. *J Adv Nurs* 2002 Oct;40(1):87-95

[526] Schlienger JL, Perrin AE, Grunenberger F, Goichot B. Hormonal perturbations in fibromyalgia. *Ann Endocrinol* (Paris) 2001 Dec;62(6):542-8

[527] Tsigos C, Chrousos GP. Hypothalamic-pituitary-adrenal axis, neuroendocrine factors and stress. *J Psychosom Res* 2002 Oct;53(4):865-71

[528] Okifuji A, Turk DC. Stress and psychophysiological dysregulation in patients with fibromyalgia syndrome. *Appl Psychophysiol Biofeedback* 2002 Jun;27(2):129-41

[529] Geenen R, Jacobs JW, Bijlsma JW. Evaluation and management of endocrine dysfunction in fibromyalgia. *Rheum Dis Clin North Am* 2002 May;28(2):389-404

[530] Geenen R, Jacobs JW, Bijlsma JW. Evaluation and management of endocrine dysfunction in fibromyalgia. *Rheum Dis Clin North Am* 2002 May;28(2):389-404

[531] Bennett RM. Adult growth hormone deficiency in patients with fibromyalgia. *Curr Rheumatol Rep* 2002 Aug;4(4):306-12

[532] Paiva ES, Deodhar A, Jones KD, Bennett R. Impaired growth hormone secretion in fibromyalgia patients: evidence for augmented hypothalamic somatostatin tone. *Arthritis Rheum* 2002 May;46(5):1344-50

[533] Riedel W, Schlapp U, Leck S, Netter P, Neeck G Blunted ACTH and cortisol responses to systemic injection of corticotropin-releasing hormone (CRH) in fibromyalgia: role of somatostatin and CRH-binding protein. *Ann N Y Acad Sci* 2002 Jun;966:483-90

[534] Hein G, Franke S Are advanced glycation end-product-modified proteins of pathogenetic importance in fibromyalgia? *Rheumatology* (Oxford) 2002 Oct;41(10):1163-7

[535] Tsigos C, Chrousos GP. Hypothalamic-pituitary-adrenal axis, neuroendocrine factors and stress. *J Psychosom Res* 2002 Oct;53(4):865-71

[536] Rohr UD, Herold J. Melatonin deficiencies in women. *Maturitas* 2002 Apr 15;41 Suppl 1:S85-104

[537] Kelly GS. Larch arabinogalactan: clinical relevance of a novel immune-enhancing polysaccharide. *Altern Med Rev* 1999 Apr;4(2):96-103

[538] Hein G, Franke S Are advanced glycation end-product-modified proteins of pathogenetic importance in fibromyalgia? *Rheumatology* (Oxford) 2002 Oct;41(10):1163-7

[539] Bierhaus A, Chevion S, Chevion M, Hofmann M, Quehenberger P, Illmer T, Luther T, Berentshtein E, Tritschler H, Muller M, Wahl P, Ziegler R, Nawroth PP. Advanced glycation end product-induced activation of NF kappaB is suppressed by alpha-lipoic acid in cultured endothelial cells. *Diabetes* 1997 Sep;46(9):1481-90

[540] Suzuki YJ, Aggarwal BB, Packer L. Alpha-lipoic acid is a potent inhibitor of NF-kappa B activation in human T cells. *Biochem Biophys Res Commun* 1992 Dec 30;189(3):1709-15

[541] Zhang WJ, Frei B. Alpha-lipoic acid inhibits TNF-alpha-induced NF kappaB activation and adhesion molecule expression in human aortic endothelial cells. *FASEB J* 2001 Nov;15(13):2423-32

[542] Lee HA, Hughes DA. Alpha-lipoic acid modulates NF kappaB activity in human monocytic cells by direct interaction with DNA. *Exp Gerontol* 2002 Jan-Mar;37(2-3):401-10

[543] Nagamatsu M, Nickander K, et al. Lipoic acid improves nerve blood flow, reduces oxidative stress, and improves distal nerve conduction in experimental diabetic neuropathy. *Diabetes Care* 18:1160, 1995.

[544] Ziegler D, and Gries F. Alpha-lipoic acid in the treatment of Diabetic Peripheral and Cardiac Autonomic Neuropathy. *Diabetes* 46(2):S62-S66, 1997.

[545] Christie, R.B. The medical uses of proteolytic enzymes, in Topics in Enzyme and Fermentation Biotechnology, Vol. 4, Wiseman, A., Ed., Ellis Horwood Ltd., Chichester, 1980, 25

[546] Taussig SJ, Batkin S. Bromelain, the enzyme complex of pineapple (Ananas comosus) and its clinical application. An update. *J Ethnopharmacol* 1988 Feb-Mar;22(2):191-203

[547] Wadsworth TL, McDonald TL, Koop DR. *Biochem Pharmacol* Effects of Ginkgo biloba extract (EGb 761) and quercetin on lipopolysaccharide-induced signaling pathways involved in the release of tumor necrosis factor-alpha. 2001 Oct 1;62(7):963-74

[548] Surh YJ, Chun KS, Cha HH, Han SS, Keum YS, Park KK, Lee SS. Molecular mechanisms underlying chemopreventive activities of anti-inflammatory phytochemicals: down-regulation of COX-2 and iNOS through suppression of NF-kappa B activation. *Mutat Res* 2001 Sep 1;480-481:243-68

[549] Chuang SE, Yeh PY, Lu YS, Lai GM, Liao CM, Gao M, Cheng AL. Basal levels and patterns of anticancer drug-induced activation of nuclear factor-kappaB (NF kappaB), and its attenuation by tamoxifen, dexamethasone, and curcumin in carcinoma cells. *Biochem Pharmacol* 2002 May 1;63(9):1709-16

[550] W.Y. John Chen, Ph.D; Giovanni Abetangelo, MD, Ph.D: Functions of hyaluronan in wound repair. *WOUND REP REG* 1999; 7:79-89

[551] Hakkinen K, Pakarinen A, Hannonen P, Hakkinen A, Airaksinen O, Valkeinen H, Alen M. Effects of strength training on muscle strength, cross-sectional area, maximal electromyographic activity, and serum hormones in pre-menopausal women with fibromyalgia. *J Rheumatol* 2002 Jun;29(6):1287-95

[552] Kang K, Pariza MW. trans-10,cis-12-Conjugated linoleic acid reduces leptin secretion from 3T3-L1 adipocytes. *Biochem Biophys Res Commun* 2001 Sep 21;287(2):377-82

[553] Rahman SM, Wang Y, Yotsumoto H, Cha J, Han S, Inoue S, Yanagita T. Effects of conjugated linoleic acid on serum leptin concentration, body-fat accumulation, and beta-oxidation of fatty acid in OLETF rats. *Nutrition* 2001 May;17(5):385-90

[554] Akahoshi A, Goto Y, Murao K, Miyazaki T, Yamasaki M, Nonaka M, Yamada K, Sugano M. Conjugated linoleic acid reduces body fats and cytokine levels of mice. *Biosci Biotechnol Biochem* 2002 Apr;66(4):916-20

[555] Douyon L, Schteingart DE. Effect of obesity and starvation on thyroid hormone, growth hormone, and cortisol secretion. *Endocrinol Metab Clin North Am* 2002 Mar;31(1):173-89

[556] van der Poll T, Romijn JA, Wiersinga WM, Sauerwein HP. Tumor necrosis factor: a putative mediator of the sick euthyroid syndrome in man. *J Clin Endocrinol Metab* 1990 Dec;71(6):1567-72

[557] Boelen A, Maas MA, Lowik CW, Platvoet MC, Wiersinga WM. Induced illness in interleukin-6 (IL-6) knock-out mice: a causal role of IL-6 in the development of the low 3,5,3'-triiodothyronine syndrome. *Endocrinology* 1996 Dec;137(12):5250-4

[558] Chopra IJ, Solomon DH, Hepner GW, Morgenstein AA. Misleadingly low free thyroxine index and usefulness of reverse triiodothyronine measurement in nonthyroidal illnesses. *Ann Intern Med* 1979 Jun;90(6):905-12

[559] Michalaki M, Vagenakis AG, Makri M, Kalfarentzos F, Kyriazopoulou V. Dissociation of the early decline in serum T(3) concentration and serum IL-6 rise and TNFalpha in nonthyroidal illness syndrome induced by abdominal surgery. *J Clin Endocrinol Metab* 2001 Sep;86(9):4198-205

[560] Friberg L, Drvota V, Bjelak AH, Eggertsen G, Ahnve S. Association between increased levels of reverse triiodothyronine and mortality after acute myocardial infarction. *Am J Med* 2001 Dec 15;111(9):699-703

[561] Pavlou HN, Kliridis PA, Panagiotopoulos AA, Goritsas CP, Vassilakos PJ. Euthyroid sick syndrome in acute ischemic syndromes. *Angiology* 2002 Nov-Dec;53(6):699-707

[562] Schulte C, Reinhardt W, Beelen D, Mann K, Schaefer U. Low T3-syndrome and nutritional status as prognostic factors in patients undergoing bone marrow transplantation. *Bone Marrow Transplant* 1998 Dec;22(12):1171-8

[563] Herrmann F, Hambsch K, Sorger D, Hantzschel H, Muller P, Nagel I. Low T3 syndrome and chronic inflammatory rheumatism *Z Gesamte Inn Med* 1989 Sep 1;44(17):513-8

[564] Goichot B, Schlienger JL, Grunenberger F, Pradignac A, Sapin R. Thyroid hormone status and nutrient intake in the free-living elderly. Interest of reverse triiodothyronine assessment. *Eur J Endocrinol* 1994 Mar;130(3):244-52

[565] Kranjcec D, Pinter A, Birtic T, Cabrijan T, Halle J, Tomicic D, Halle Z, Pintaric H, Radacic M, Novak N. Metabolic syndrome X—high risk factor for acute myocardial infarction and its complications. *Coll Antropol* 2002 Jun;26(1):23-9

[566] Quentmeier H, Dirks WG, Fleckenstein D, Zaborski M, Drexler HG. Tumor necrosis factor-alpha-induced proliferation requires synthesis of granulocyte-macrophage colony-stimulating factor. *Exp Hematol* 2000 Sep;28(9):1008-15

[567] Karin M, Lin A. NF kappaB at the crossroads of life and death. *Nat Immunol* 2002 Mar;3(3):221-7

[568] Yamamoto Y, Gaynor R B. Role of the NF kappaB pathway in the pathogenesis of human disease states. *Curr Mol Med* 2001 Jul;1(3):287-96

[569] Kasof GM, Lu JJ, Liu D, Speer B, Mongan KN, Gomes BC, Lorenzi MV. Tumor necrosis factor-alpha induces the expression of DR6, a member of the TNF receptor family, through activation of NF kappaB. *Oncogene* 2001 Nov 29;20(55):7965-75

[570] Chen S, Fribley A, Wang CY. Potentiation of tumor necrosis factor-mediated apoptosis of oral squamous cell carcinoma cells by adenovirus-mediated gene transfer of NF kappaB inhibitor. *J Dent Res* 2002 Feb;81(2):98-102

[571] Staudt LM. Gene expression profiling of lymphoid malignancies. *Annu Rev Med* 2002;53:303-18

[572] Delhalle S, Deregowski V, Benoit V, Merville MP, Bours V. NF kappaB-dependent MnSOD expression protects adenocarcinoma cells from TNF-alpha-induced apoptosis. *Oncogene* 2002 May 30;21(24):3917-24

[573] Javelaud D, Poupon MF, Wietzerbin J, Besancon F. Inhibition of constitutive NF-kappa B activity suppresses tumorigenicity of Ewing sarcoma EW7 cells. *Int J Cancer* 2002 Mar 10;98(2):193-8

[574] Sanlioglu S, Luleci G, Thomas KW. Simultaneous inhibition of Rac1 and IKK pathways sensitizes lung cancer cells to TNFalpha-mediated apoptosis. *Cancer Gene Ther* 2001 Nov;8(11):897-905

[575] Javelaud D, Poupon MF, Wietzerbin J, Besancon F. Inhibition of constitutive NF-kappa B activity suppresses tumorigenicity of Ewing sarcoma EW7 cells. *Int J Cancer* 2002 Mar 10;98(2):193-8

[576] Takada M, Koizumi T, Toyama H, Suzuki Y, Kuroda Y. Differential expression of RAGE in human pancreatic carcinoma cells. *Hepatogastroenterology* 2001 Nov-Dec;48(42):1577-8

[577] Beppu M, Ikebe T, Shirasuna K. The inhibitory effects of immunosuppressive factors, dexamethasone and interleukin-4, on NF kappaB-mediated protease production by oral cancer. *Biochim Biophys Acta* 2002 Jan 2;1586(1):11-22

[578] Jones DR, Broad RM, Comeau LD, Parsons SJ, Mayo MW. Inhibition of nuclear factor kappaB chemosensitizes non-small cell lung cancer through cytochrome c release and caspase activation. *J Thorac Cardiovasc Surg* 2002 Feb;123(2):310-7

[579] Sugita S, Kohno T, Yamamoto K, Imaizumi Y, Nakajima H, Ishimaru T, Matsuyama T. Induction of macrophage-inflammatory protein-3alpha gene expression by TNF-dependent NF kappaB activation. *J Immunol* 2002 Jun 1;168(11):5621-8

[580] Tharappel JC, Lee EY, Robertson LW, Spear BT, Glauert HP. Regulation of cell proliferation, apoptosis, and transcription factor activities during the promotion of liver carcinogenesis by polychlorinated biphenyls. *Toxicol Appl Pharmacol* 2002 Mar 15;179(3):172-84

[581] Szabo G, Catalano D, Bellerose G, Mandrekar P. Interferon alpha and alcohol augment nuclear regulatory factor-kappaB activation in HepG2 cells, and interferon alpha increases pro-inflammatory cytokine production. *Alcohol Clin Exp Res* 2001 Aug;25(8):1188-97

[582] Wright G, Singh IS, Hasday JD, Farrance IK, Hall G, Cross AS, Rogers TB. Endotoxin stress-response in cardiomyocytes: NF kappaB activation and tumor necrosis factor-alpha expression. *Am J Physiol Heart Circ Physiol* 2002 Mar;282(3):H872-9

[583] Ginis I, Jaiswal R, Klimanis D, Liu J, Greenspon J, Hallenbeck JM. TNF-alpha-induced tolerance to ischemic injury involves differential control of NF kappaB transactivation: the role of NF kappaB association with p300 adaptor. *J Cereb Blood Flow Metab* 2002 Feb;22(2):142-52

[584] Bouloumie A, Marumo T, Lafontan M, Busse R. Leptin induces oxidative stress in human endothelial cells. *FASEB J* 1999 Jul;13(10):1231-8

[585] Viita H, Sen CK, Roy S, Siljamaki T, Nikkari T, Yla-Herttuala S. High expression of human 15-lipoxygenase induces NF kappaB-mediated expression of vascular cell adhesion molecule 1, intercellular adhesion molecule 1, and T-cell adhesion on human endothelial cells. *Antioxid Redox Signal* 1999 Spring;1(1):83-96

[586] Napoleone E, Di Santo A, Bastone A, Peri G, Mantovani A, de Gaetano G, Donati MB, Lorenzet R. Long pentraxin PTX3 upregulates tissue factor expression in human endothelial cells: a novel link between vascular inflammation and clotting activation. *Arterioscler Thromb Vasc Biol* 2002 May 1;22(5):782-7

[587] Ialenti A, Ianaro A, Maffia P, Carnuccio R, D'Acquisto F, Maiello FM, Di Rosa M. Role of nuclear factor-kappaB in a rat model of vascular injury. *Naunyn Schmiedebergs Arch Pharmacol* 2001 Oct;364(4):343-50

[588] Mattson MP, Culmsee C, Yu Z, Camandola S. Roles of nuclear factor kappaB in neuronal survival and plasticity. *J Neurochem* 2000 Feb;74(2):443-56

[589] Del Rio MJ, Velez-Pardo C. Monoamine neurotoxins-induced apoptosis in lymphocytes by a common oxidative stress mechanism: involvement of hydrogen peroxide (H(2)O(2)), caspase-3, and nuclear factor kappa-B (NF kappaB), p53, c-Jun transcription factors. *Biochem Pharmacol* 2002 Feb 15;63(4):677-88

[590] Paganelli R, Di Iorio A, Patricelli L, Ripani F, Sparvieri E, Faricelli R, Iarlori C, Porreca E, Di Gioacchino M, Abate G. Pro-inflammatory cytokines in sera of elderly patients with dementia: levels in vascular injury are higher than those of mild-moderate Alzheimer's disease patients. *Exp Gerontol* 2002 Jan-Mar;37(2-3):257-63

[591] Perry RT, Collins JS, Wiener H, Acton R, Go RC. The role of TNF and its receptors in Alzheimer's disease. *Neurobiol Aging* 2001 Nov-Dec;22(6):873-83

[592] Grammas P, Ovase R. Inflammatory factors are elevated in brain microvessels in Alzheimer's disease. *Neurobiol Aging* 2001 Nov-Dec;22(6):837-42

[593] McGeer PL, McGeer EG. Polymorphisms in inflammatory genes and the risk of Alzheimer disease. *Arch Neurol* 2001 Nov;58(11):1790-2

[594] Bruunsgaard H, Andersen-Ranberg K, Jeune B, Pedersen AN, Skinhoj P, Pedersen BK. A high plasma concentration of TNF-alpha is associated with dementia in centenarians. *J Gerontol A Biol Sci Med Sci* 1999 Jul;54(7):M357-64

[595] Knight DS, Mahajan DK, Qiao X. Dietary fat up-regulates the apolipoprotein E mRNA level in the Zucker lean rat brain. *Neuroreport* 2001 Oct 8;12(14):3111-5

[596] Calderon-Garciduenas L, Azzarelli B, Acuna H, Garcia R, Gambling TM, Osnaya N, Monroy S, DEL Tizapantzi MR, Carson JL, Villarreal-Calderon A, Rewcastle B. Air pollution and brain damage. *Toxicol Pathol* 2002 May-Jun;30(3):373-89

[597] Campbell A, Yang EY, Tsai-Turton M, Bondy SC. Pro-inflammatory effects of aluminum in human glioblastoma cells. *Brain Res* 2002 Apr 12;933(1):60-5

[598] Carpenter DO. Effects of metals on the nervous system of humans and animals. *Int J Occup Med Environ Health* 2001;14(3):209-18

[599] Busso N, So A, Chobaz-Peclat V, Morard C, Martinez-Soria E, Talabot-Ayer D, Gabay C. Leptin signaling deficiency impairs humoral and cellular immune responses and attenuates experimental arthritis. *J Immunol* 2002 Jan 15;168(2):875-82

[600] Nguyen VT, Benveniste EN. Critical role of tumor necrosis factor-alpha and NF-kappa B in interferon-gamma -induced CD40 expression in microglia/macrophages. *J Biol Chem* 2002 Apr 19;277(16):13796-803

[601] Brennan FM, Hayes AL, Ciesielski CJ, Green P, Foxwell BM, Feldmann M. Evidence that rheumatoid arthritis synovial T cells are similar to cytokine-activated T cells: involvement of phosphatidylinositol 3-kinase and nuclear factor kappaB pathways in tumor necrosis factor alpha production in rheumatoid arthritis. *Arthritis Rheum* 2002 Jan;46(1):31-41

[602] Kwok BH, Koh B, Ndubuisi MI, Elofsson M, Crews CM. The anti-inflammatory natural product parthenolide from the medicinal herb Feverfew directly binds to and inhibits IkappaB kinase. *Chem Biol* 2001 Aug;8(8):759-66

[603] Reuter U, Chiarugi A, Bolay H, Moskowitz MA. Nuclear factor-kappaB as a molecular target for migraine therapy. *Ann Neurol* 2002 Apr;51(4):507-16

[604] Kang BY, Chung SW, Kim TS. Inhibition of interleukin-12 production in lipopolysaccharide-activated mouse macrophages by parthenolide, a predominant sesquiterpene lactone in Tanacetum parthenium: involvement of nuclear factor-kappaB. *Immunol Lett* 2001 Jul 2;77(3):159-63

[605] Kang SN, Kim SH, Chung SW, Lee MH, Kim HJ, Kim TS. Enhancement of 1 alpha,25-dihydroxyvitamin D(3)-induced differentiation of human leukaemia HL-60 cells into monocytes by parthenolide via inhibition of NF-kappa B activity. *Br J Pharmacol* 2002 Mar;135(5):1235-44

[606] Patel NM, Nozaki S, Shortle NH, Bhat-Nakshatri P, Newton TR, Rice S, Gelfanov V, Boswell SH, Goulet RJ Jr, Sledge GW Jr, Nakshatri H.Paclitaxel sensitivity of breast cancer cells with constitutively active NF kappaB is enhanced by IkappaBalpha super-repressor and parthenolide. *Oncogene* 2000 Aug 24;19(36):4159-69

[607] Li-Weber M, Giaisi M, Baumann S, Treiber MK, Krammer PH. The anti-inflammatory sesquiterpene lactone parthenolide suppresses CD95-mediated activation-induced-cell-death in T-cells. *Cell Death Differ* 2002 Nov;9(11):1256-65

[608] Mogensen TH, Paludan SR. Virus-cell interactions: impact on cytokine production, immune evasion and tumor growth. *Eur Cytokine Netw* 2001 Jul-Sep;12(3):382-90

[609] Hiscott J, Kwon H, Genin P. Hostile takeovers: viral appropriation of the NF kappaB pathway. *J Clin Invest* 2001 Jan;107(2):143-51

610 Tai DI, Tsai SL, Chang YH, Huang SN, Chen TC, Chang KS, Liaw YF. Constitutive activation of nuclear factor kappaB in hepatocellular carcinoma. *Cancer* 2000 Dec 1;89(11):2274-81

611 Tai DI, Tsai SL, Chen YM, Chuang YL, Peng CY, Sheen IS, Yeh CT, Chang KS, Huang SN, Kuo GC, Liaw YF. Activation of nuclear factor kappaB in hepatitis C virus infection: implications for pathogenesis and hepatocarcinogenesis. *Hepatology* 2000 Mar;31(3):656-64

612 Liu X, Zou S, Qiu F. NF-kappa B expression in cholangiocarcinoma transfected with hepatitis C virus core gene. [Article in Chinese] *Zhonghua Zhong Liu Za Zhi* 2002 Jan;24(1):20-3

613 Huo TI, Wang XW, Forgues M, Wu CG, Spillare EA, Giannini C, Brechot C, Harris CC. Hepatitis B virus X mutants derived from human hepatocellular carcinoma retain the ability to abrogate p53-induced apoptosis. *Oncogene* 2001 Jun 21;20(28):3620-8

614 Diao J, Garces R, Richardson CD. X protein of hepatitis B virus modulates cytokine and growth factor related signal transduction pathways during the course of viral infections and hepatocarcinogenesis. *Cytokine Growth Factor Rev* 2001 Jun-Sep;12(2-3):189-205

615 Vockerodt M, Tesch H, Kube D. Epstein-Barr virus latent membrane protein-1 activates CD25 expression in lymphoma cells involving the NF kappaB pathway. *Genes Immun* 2001 Dec;2(8):433-41

616 Portis T, Harding JC, Ratner L. The contribution of NF-kappa B activity to spontaneous proliferation and resistance to apoptosis in human T-cell leukemia virus type I Tax-induced tumors. *Blood* 2001 Aug 15;98(4):1200-8

617 Mahieux R, Pise-Masison C, Gessain A, Brady JN, Olivier R, Perret E, Misteli T, Nicot C. Arsenic trioxide induces apoptosis in human T-cell leukemia virus type I- and type II-infected cells by a caspase-3-dependent mechanism involving Bcl-2 cleavage. *Blood* 2001 Dec 15;98(13):3762-9

618 Vancurova I, Wu R, Miskolci V, Sun S. Increased p50/p50 NF kappaB activation in human papillomavirus type 6- or type II-induced laryngeal papilloma tissue. *J Virol* 2002 Feb;76(3):1533-6

619 Shepard LW, Yang M, Xie P, Browning DD, Voyno-Yasenetskaya T, Kozasa T, Ye RD. Constitutive activation of NF-kappa B and secretion of interleukin-8 induced by the G protein-coupled receptor of Kaposi's sarcoma-associated herpesvirus involve G alpha(13) and RhoA. *J Biol Chem* 2001 Dec 7;276(49):45979-87

620 Esposito E, Rotilio D, Di Matteo V, Di Giulio C, Cacchio M, Algeri S. A review of specific dietary antioxidants and the effects on biochemical mechanisms related to neurodegenerative processes. *Neurobiol Aging* 2002 Sep-Oct;23(5):719

621 Cadenas S, Cadenas AM. Fighting the stranger-antioxidant protection against endotoxin toxicity. *Toxicology* 2002 Oct 30;180(1):45-63

622 Carcamo JM, Pedraza A, Borquez-Ojeda O, Golde DW. Vitamin C suppresses TNF alpha-induced NF kappa B activation by inhibiting I kappa B alpha phosphorylation. *Biochemistry* 2002 Oct 29;41(43):12995-3002

623 Fletcher RH, Fairchild KM Vitamins for chronic disease prevention in adults:clinical applications. *JAMA* June 19, 2002;287:3217-3219

624 Mundy GR. Directions of drug discovery in osteoporosis. *Annu Rev Med* 2002;53:337-54

625 Wolf AS. The overweight and underweight girl: from findings to prevention *Zentralbl Gynakol* 2002 Mar;124(3):146-52

626 Espallargues M, Sampietro-Colom L, Estrada MD, Sola M, del Rio L, Setoain J, Granados A. Identifying bone-mass-related risk factors for fracture to guide bone

densitometry measurements: a systematic review of the literature. *Osteoporos Int* 2001;12(10):811-22

[627] Barker ME, Blumsohn A. Is weight loss in obese pre-menopausal women associated with a decline in bone mass? *J Bone Miner Res* 2002 Apr;17(4):746-9

[628] Morley JE. Anorexia, body composition, and ageing. *Curr Opin Clin Nutr Metab Care* 2001 Jan;4(1):9-13

[629] Laharrague P, Truel N, Fontanilles AM, Corberand JX, Penicaud L, Casteilla L. Regulation by cytokines of leptin expression in human bone marrow adipocytes. *Horm Metab Res* 2000 Oct;32(10):381-5

[630] Holloway WR, Collier FM, Aitken CJ, Myers DE, Hodge JM, Malakellis M, Gough TJ, Collier GR, Nicholson GC. Leptin inhibits osteoclast generation. *J Bone Miner Res* 2002 Feb;17(2):200-9

[631] Amling M, Schilling AF, Haberland M, Rueger JM. Leptin: factor in the central nervous system regulation of bone mass. Development of a new understanding of bone remodeling, skeletal reconstruction, skeletal preservation and skeletal repair. *Orthopade* 2001 Jul;30(7):418-24

[632] Karsenty G. Leptin controls bone formation through a hypothalamic relay. *Recent Prog Horm Res* 2001;56:401-15

[633] Watkins BA, Li Y, Seifert MF. Nutraceutical fatty acids as biochemical and molecular modulators of skeletal biology. *J Am Coll Nutr* 2001 Oct;20(5 Suppl):410S-416S; discussion 417S-420S

[634] Romas E, Gillespie MT, Martin TJ. Involvement of receptor activator of NF kappaB ligand and tumor necrosis factor-alpha in bone destruction in rheumatoid arthritis. *Bone* 2002 Feb;30(2):340-6

[635] Kim MS, Chae HJ, Shin TY, Kim HM, Kim HR. Estrogen regulates cytokine release in human mast cells. *Immunopharmacol Immunotoxicol* 2001 Nov;23(4):495-504

[636] Roggia C, Gao Y, Cenci S, Weitzmann MN, Toraldo G, Isaia G, Pacifici R. Up-regulation of TNF-producing T cells in the bone marrow: a key mechanism by which estrogen deficiency induces bone loss in vivo. *Proc Natl Acad Sci U S A* 2001 Nov 20;98(24):13960-5

[637] Ota N, Hunt SC, Nakajima T, Suzuki T, Hosoi T, Orimo H, Shirai Y, Emi M. Linkage of human tumor necrosis factor-alpha to human osteoporosis by sib pair analysis. *Genes Immun* 2000;1(4):260-4

[638] Habtezion A, Silverberg MS, Parkes R, Mikolainis S, Steinhart AH. Risk factors for low bone density in Crohn's disease. *Inflamm Bowel Dis* 2002 Mar;8(2):87-92

[639] Hansen CM, Hansen D, Holm PK, Binderup L. Vitamin D compounds exert anti-apoptotic effects in human osteosarcoma cells in vitro. *J Steroid Biochem Mol Biol* 2001 Apr;77(1):1-11

[640] Farmer PK, He X, Schmitz ML, Rubin J, Nanes MS. Inhibitory effect of NF kappaB on 1,25-dihydroxyvitamin D(3) and retinoid X receptor function. *Am J Physiol Endocrinol Metab* 2000 Jul;279(1):E213-20

[641] Norazlina M, Ima-Nirwana S, Abul Gapor MT, Abdul Kadir Khalid B. Tocotrienols are needed for normal bone calcification in growing female rats. *Asia Pac J Clin Nutr* 2002;11(3):194-9

[642] Rude RK, Gruber HE, Wei LY, Frausto A, Mills BG. Magnesium Deficiency: Effect on Bone and Mineral Metabolism in the Mouse. *Calcif Tissue Int* 2002 Oct 10;

[643] Tucker KL, Hannan MT, Kiel DP. The acid-base hypothesis: diet and bone in the Framingham Osteoporosis Study. Eur J Nutr 2001 Oct;40(5):231-7

[644] Hsing AW, Chua S Jr, Gao YT, Gentzschein E, Chang L, Deng J, Stanczyk FZ. Prostate cancer risk and serum levels of insulin and leptin: a population-based study. *J Natl Cancer Inst* 2001 May 16;93(10):783-9

[645] Stattin P, Soderberg S, Hallmans G, Bylund A, Kaaks R, Stenman UH, Bergh A, Olsson T. Leptin is associated with increased prostate cancer risk: a nested case-referent study. *J Clin Endocrinol Metab* 2001 Mar;86(3):1341-5

[646] Chang S, Hursting SD, Contois JH, Strom SS, Yamamura Y, Babaian RJ, Troncoso P, Scardino PS, Wheeler TM, Amos CI, Spitz MR. Leptin and prostate cancer. *Prostate* 2001 Jan 1;46(1):62-7

[647] Gurumurthy S, Vasudevan KM, Rangnekar VM. Regulation of apoptosis in prostate cancer. *Cancer Metastasis Rev* 2001;20(3-4):225-43

[648] Chen CD, Sawyers CL. NF-kappa B activates prostate-specific antigen expression and is upregulated in androgen-independent prostate cancer. *Mol Cell Biol* 2002 Apr;22(8):2862-70

[649] Gasparian AV, Yao YJ, Kowalczyk D, Lyakh LA, Karseladze A, Slaga TJ, Budunova IV. The role of IKK in constitutive activation of NF kappaB transcription factor in prostate carcinoma cells. *J Cell Sci* 2002 Jan 1;115(Pt 1):141-51

[650] Maliner-Stratton MS, Klein RD, Udayakumar TS, Nagle RB, Bowden GT. Interleukin-1beta-induced promatrilysin expression is mediated by NF kappaB-regulated synthesis of interleukin-6 in the prostate carcinoma cell line, LNCaP. Neoplasia 2001 Nov-Dec;3(6):509-20

[651] Catz SD, Johnson JL. Transcriptional regulation of bcl-2 by nuclear factor kappa B and its significance in prostate cancer. *Oncogene* 2001 Nov 1;20(50):7342-51

[652] Kimura K, Markowski M, Bowen C, Gelmann EP. Androgen blocks apoptosis of hormone-dependent prostate cancer cells. *Cancer Res* 2001 Jul 15;61(14):5611-8

[653] Lindholm PF, Bub J, Kaul S, Shidham VB, Kajdacsy-Balla A. The role of constitutive NF kappaB activity in PC-3 human prostate cancer cell invasive behavior. *Clin Exp Metastasis* 2000;18(6):471-9

[654] Huang S, Pettaway CA, Uehara H, Bucana CD, Fidler IJ. Blockade of NF kappaB activity in human prostate cancer cells is associated with suppression of angiogenesis, invasion, and metastasis. *Oncogene* 2001 Jul 12;20(31):4188-97

[655] Muenchen HJ, Lin DL, Walsh MA, Keller ET, Pienta KJ. Tumor necrosis factor-alpha-induced apoptosis in prostate cancer cells through inhibition of nuclear factor-kappaB by an IkappaBalpha "super-repressor". *Clin Cancer Res* 2000 May;6(5):1969-77

[656] Uzzo RG, Leavis P, Hatch W, Gabai VL, Dulin N, Zvartau N, Kolenko VM. Zinc Inhibits Nuclear Factor-kappaB Activation and Sensitizes Prostate Cancer Cells to Cytotoxic Agents. *Clin Cancer Res* 2002 Nov;8(11):3579-83

[657] Verhoeven, D.T.H., Verhagen, H., Goldbohm, R.A., van den Brandt, P.A., and van Poppel, G. 1997 A review of mechanisms underlying anticarcinogenicity by brassica vegetables. *Chem. Bio. Interactions.* 103:79-129.

[658] Cohen JH, Kristal AR, Stanford JL. Fruit and vegetable intakes and prostate cancer risk. *J Natl Cancer Inst* 2000 Jan 5;92(1):61-8

[659] Chinni SR, Sarkar FH. Akt Inactivation Is a Key Event in Indole-3-carbinol-induced Apoptosis in PC-3 Cells. *Clin Cancer Res* 2002 Apr;8(4):1228-36

[660] Chinni SR, Li Y, Upadhyay S, Koppolu PK, Sarkar FH. Indole-3-carbinol (I3C) induced cell growth inhibition, G1 cell cycle arrest and apoptosis in prostate cancer cells. *Oncogene* 2001 May 24;20(23):2927-36

[661] Mukhopadhyay A, Bueso-Ramos C, Chatterjee D, Pantazis P, Aggarwal BB. Curcumin downregulates cell survival mechanisms in human prostate cancer cell lines. *Oncogene* 2001 Nov 15;20(52):7597-609

[662] Hour TC, Chen J, Huang CY, Guan JY, Lu SH, Pu YS. Curcumin enhances cytotoxicity of chemotherapeutic agents in prostate cancer cells by inducing

p21(WAF1/CIP1) and C/EBPbeta expressions and suppressing NF kappaB activation. *Prostate* 2002 May 15;51(3):211-8

[663] Dhanalakshmi S, Singh RP, Agarwal C, Agarwal R. Silibinin inhibits constitutive and TNFalpha-induced activation of NF kappaB and sensitizes human prostate carcinoma DU145 cells to TNFalpha-induced apoptosis. *Oncogene* 2002 Mar 7;21(11):1759-67

[664] Tozawa K, Okamoto T, Hayashi Y, Sasaki S, Kawai N, Kohri K. N-acetyl-L-cysteine enhances chemotherapeutic effect on prostate cancer cells. Urol Res 2002 Mar;30(1):53-8

[665] O'brien SN, Welter BH, Price TM. Presence of leptin in breast cell lines and breast tumors. *Biochem Biophys Res Commun* 1999 Jun 16;259(3):695-8

[666] Tessitore L, Vizio B, Jenkins O, De Stefano I, Ritossa C, Argiles JM, Benedetto C, Mussa A. Leptin expression in colorectal and breast cancer patients. *Int J Mol Med* 2000 Apr;5(4):421-6

[667] Petridou E, Papadiamantis Y, Markopoulos C, Spanos E, Dessypris N, Trichopoulos D. Leptin and insulin growth factor I in relation to breast cancer (Greece). *Cancer Causes Control* 2000 May;11(5):383-8

[668] Dieudonne MN, Machinal-Quelin F, Serazin-Leroy V, Leneveu MC, Pecquery R, Giudicelli Y. Leptin mediates a proliferative response in human MCF7 breast cancer cells. Biochem Biophys Res Commun 2002 Apr 26;293(1):622-8

[669] Laud K, Gourdou I, Pessemesse L, Peyrat JP, Djiane J. Identification of leptin receptors in human breast cancer: functional activity in the T47-D breast cancer cell line. *Mol Cell Endocrinol* 2002 Feb 25;188(1-2):219-26

[670] Okumura M, Yamamoto M, Sakuma H, Kojima T, Maruyama T, Jamali M, Cooper D, Yasuda K. Leptin and high glucose stimulate cell proliferation in MCF-7 human breast cancer cells: reciprocal involvement of PKC-alpha and PPAR expression. *Biochim Biophys Acta* 2002 Oct 21;1592(2):107

[671] Bhat-Nakshatri P, Sweeney CJ, Nakshatri H. Identification of signal transduction pathways involved in constitutive NF kappaB activation in breast cancer cells. *Oncogene* 2002 Mar 27;21(13):2066-78

[672] Toillon RA, Descamps S, Adriaenssens E, Ricort JM, Bernard D, Boilly B, Le Bourhis X. Normal breast epithelial cells induce apoptosis of breast cancer cells via Fas signaling. *Exp Cell Res* 2002 Apr 15;275(1):31-43

[673] Marttunen MB, Andersson S, Hietanen P, Karonen SL, Koistinen HA, Koivisto VA, Tiitinen A, Ylikorkala O. Antiestrogenic tamoxifen and toremifene increase serum leptin levels in postmenopausal breast cancer patients. Maturitas 2000 May 29;35(2):175-9

[674] Ozet A, Arpaci F, Yilmaz MI, Ayta H, Ozturk B, Komurcu S, Yavuz AA, Tezcan Y,Acikel C. Effects of tamoxifen on the serum leptin level in patients with breast cancer. *Jpn J Clin Oncol* 2001 Sep;31(9):424-7

[675] Goodwin PJ, Ennis M, Pritchard KI, Trudeau ME, Koo J, Madarnas Y, Hartwick W, Hoffman B, Hood N. Fasting insulin and outcome in early-stage breast cancer: results of a prospective cohort study. *J Clin Oncol* 2002 Jan 1;29(1):42-51.

[676] Nishino M, Hayakawa K, Nakamura Y, Morimoto T, Mukaihara S. Effects of tamoxifen on hepatic fat content and the development of hepatic steatosis in patients with breast cancer: high frequency of involvement and rapid reversal after completion of tamoxifen therapy. *AJR Am J Roentgenol* 2003 Jan;180(1):129-34

[677] Wang H, Isaksson E, Von Schoultz B, Cline JM, Sahlin L. The effect of long-term treatment with steroid hormones or tamoxifen on oestrogen receptors (alpha and beta) in the endometrium of ovariectomized cynomolgus macaques. *J Endocrinol* 2002 Dec;175(3):673-81

[678] The ATAC Trialists' Group. Arimidex, tamoxifen alone or in combination. Anastrozole alone or in combination with tamoxifen versus tamoxifen alone for adjuvant treatment of postmenopausal women with early breast cancer: first results of the ATAC randomised trial. *Lancet* 2002 Jun 22;359(9324):2131-9

[679] Baum M. Has tamoxifen had its day? *Breast Cancer Res* 2002;4(6):213-7

[680] Gadd SL, Hobbs G, Miller MR. Acetaminophen-induced proliferation of estrogen-responsive breast cancer cells is associated with increases in c-myc RNA expression and NF kappaB activity. *Toxicol Sci* 2002 Apr;66(2):233-43

[681] Schwenke DC. Does lack of tocopherols and tocotrienols put women at increased risk of breast cancer? *J Nutr Biochem* 2002 Jan;13(1):2-20

[682] Sylvester PW, Nachnani A, Shah S, Briski KP. Role of GTP-binding proteins in reversing the antiproliferative effects of tocotrienols in preneoplastic mammary epithelial cells. *Asia Pac J Clin Nutr* 2002 Oct;11 Suppl 7:S452-S459

[683] Nesaretnam K, Dorasamy S, Darbre PD. Tocotrienols inhibit growth of ZR-75-1 breast cancer cells. *Int J Food Sci Nutr* 2000;51 Suppl:S95-103

[684] McIntyre BS, Briski KP, Gapor A, Sylvester PW. Antiproliferative and apoptotic effects of tocopherols and tocotrienols on preneoplastic and neoplastic mouse mammary epithelial cells. *Proc Soc Exp Biol Med* 2000 Sep;224(4):292-301

[685] Yu W, Simmons-Menchaca M, Gapor A, Sanders BG, Kline K. Induction of apoptosis in human breast cancer cells by tocopherols and tocotrienols. *Nutr Cancer* 1999;33(1):26-32

[686] Nesaretnam K, Stephen R, Dils R, Darbre P. Tocotrienols inhibit the growth of human breast cancer cells irrespective of estrogen receptor status. *Lipids* 1998 May;33(5):461-9

[687] Guthrie N, Gapor A, Chambers AF, Carroll KK. Inhibition of proliferation of estrogen receptor-negative MDA-MB-435 and -positive MCF-7 human breast cancer cells by palm oil tocotrienols and tamoxifen, alone and in combination. *J Nutr* 1997 Mar;127(3):544S-548S

[688] Theriault A, Chao JT, Gapor A.Tocotrienol is the most effective vitamin E for reducing endothelial expression of adhesion molecules and adhesion to monocytes. *Atherosclerosis* 2002 Jan;160(1):21-30

[689] Ip C, Chin SF, Scimeca JA, Pariza MW. Mammary cancer prevention by conjugated dienoic derivative of linoleic acid. *Cancer Res* 1991 Nov 15;51(22):6118-24

[690] Choi Y, Park Y, Storkson JM, Pariza MW, Ntambi JM. Inhibition of stearoyl-CoA desaturase activity by the cis-9,trans-11 isomer and the trans-10,cis-12 isomer of conjugated linoleic acid in MDA-MB-231 and MCF-7 human breast cancer cells. *Biochem Biophys Res Commun* 2002 Jun 21;294(4):785-90

[691] Devery R, Miller A, Stanton C. Conjugated linoleic acid and oxidative behaviour in cancer cells. *Biochem Soc Trans* 2001 May;29(Pt 2):341-4

[692] Hubbard NE, Lim D, Summers L, Erickson KL. Reduction of murine mammary tumor metastasis by conjugated linoleic acid. *Cancer Lett* 2000 Mar 13;150(1):93-100

[693] O'Shea M, Devery R, Lawless F, Murphy J, Stanton C. Milk fat conjugated linoleic acid (CLA) inhibits growth of human mammary MCF-7 cancer cells. *Anticancer Res* 2000 Sep- Oct;20(5B):3591-601

[694] Park Y, Allen KG, Shultz TD. Modulation of MCF-7 breast cancer cell signal transduction by linoleic acid and conjugated linoleic acid in culture. *Anticancer Res* 2000 Mar-Apr;20(2A):669-76

[695] Aro A, Mannisto S, Salminen I, Ovaskainen ML, Kataja V, Uusitupa M. Inverse association between dietary and serum conjugated linoleic acid and risk of breast cancer in postmenopausal women. *Nutr Cancer* 2000;38(2):151-7

[696] Majumder B, Wahle KW, Moir S, Schofield A, Choe SN, Farquharson A, Grant I, Heys SD. Conjugated linoleic acids (CLAs) regulate the expression of key apoptotic genes in human breast cancer cells. *FASEB J* 2002 Sep;16(11):1447-9

[697] Suganuma M, Sueoka E, Sueoka N, Okabe S, Fujiki H. Mechanisms of cancer prevention by tea polyphenols based on inhibition of TNF-alpha expression. *Biofactors* 2000;13(1-4):67-72

[698] Pianetti S, Guo S, Kavanagh KT, Sonenshein GE. Green tea polyphenol epigallocatechin-3 gallate inhibits Her-2/neu signaling, proliferation, and transformed phenotype of breast cancer cells. *Cancer Res* 2002 Feb 1;62(3):652-5

[699] Vergote D, Cren-Olive C, Chopin V, Toillon RA, Rolando C, Hondermarck H, Le Bourhis X. (-)-Epigallocatechin (EGC) of green tea induces apoptosis of human breast cancer cells but not of their normal counterparts. *Breast Cancer Res Treat* 2002 Dec;76(3):195-201

[700] Brownson DM, Azios NG, Fuqua BK, Dharmawardhane SF, Mabry TJ. Flavonoid effects relevant to cancer. *J Nutr* 2002 Nov;132(11 Suppl):3482S-3489S

[701] Banerjee S, Bueso-Ramos C, Aggarwal BB. Suppression of 7,12-dimethylbenz(a)anthracene-induced mammary carcinogenesis in rats by resveratrol: role of nuclear factor-kappaB, cyclooxygenase 2, and matrix metalloprotease 9. *Cancer Res* 2002 Sep 1;62(17):4945-54

[702] Bhat KP, Lantvit D, Christov K, Mehta RG, Moon RC, Pezzuto JM. Estrogenic and antiestrogenic properties of resveratrol in mammary tumor models. *Cancer Res* 2001 Oct 15;61(20):7456-63

[703] Serrero G, Lu R. Effect of resveratrol on the expression of autocrine growth modulators in human breast cancer cells. *Antioxid Redox Signal* 2001 Dec;3(6):969-79

[704] Bove K, Lincoln DW, Tsan MF. Effect of resveratrol on growth of 4T1 breast cancer cells in vitro and in vivo. *Biochem Biophys Res Commun* 2002 Mar 8;291(4):1001-5

[705] Waffo-Teguo P, Hawthorne ME, Cuendet M, Merillon JM, Kinghorn AD, Pezzuto JM, Mehta RG. Potential cancer-chemopreventive activities of wine stilbenoids and flavans extracted from grape (Vitis vinifera) cell cultures. *Nutr Cancer* 2001;40(2):173-9

[706] Choi JA, Kim JY, Lee JY, Kang CM, Kwon HJ, Yoo YD, Kim TW, Lee YS, Lee SJ. Induction of cell cycle arrest and apoptosis in human breast cancer cells by quercetin. *Int J Oncol* 2001 Oct;19(4):837-44

[707] Han D, Tachibana H, Yamada K. Inhibition of environmental estrogen-induced proliferation of human breast carcinoma MCF-7 cells by flavonoids. *In Vitro Cell Dev Biol Anim* 2001 May;37(5):275-82

[708] Scambia G, Ranelletti FO, Benedetti Panici P, et al. Quercetin inhibits the growth of a multidrug-resistant estrogen-receptor-negative MCF-7 human breast-cancer cell line expressing type II estrogen-binding sites. *Cancer Chemother Pharmacol* (Germany) 28:255-258; 1991.

[709] Piantelli M, Tatone D, Castrilli G, Savini F, Maggiano N, Larocca LM, Ranelletti FO, Natali PG. Quercetin and tamoxifen sensitize human melanoma cells to hyperthermia. *Melanoma Res* 2001 Oct;11(5):469-76

[710] Michnoviez JJ, Bradlow HL. Altered estrogen metabolism and excretion in humans following consumption of indole-3-carbinol. *Nutr Cancer.* 1991; 16(1): 59-66.

[711] Michnoviez JJ., Bradlow HL. Induction of estradiol metabolism by dietary indole-3-carbinol in humans. *J Natl Cancer Inst.* 1990; 82(11):947-949.

[712] Michnoviez JJ, Bradlow HL. Altered estrogen metabolism and excretion in humans following consumption of indole-3-carbinol. *Nutr Cancer.* 1991; 16(1): 59-66.

[713] Cover CM, Hsieh SJ, Tran SH, Hallden G, Kim GS, Bjeldanes LF and Firestone GL. Indole-3-Carbinol inhibits the expression of cyclin-dependent kinase-6 and induces a G1 cell cycle arrest of human breast cancer cells independent of estrogen receptor signaling. *J Biol Chem.* 1998; 273:3838-3847.

[714] Cover CM, Hsieh SJ, Cram EJ, Hong C, Riby JE, Bjeldanes LF, and Firestone GL. Indole-3-carbinol and tamoxifen cooperate to arrest the cell cycle of MCF-7 human breast cancer cells. *Cancer Research* 1999; 59:1244-1251.

[715] Fujiki H, Suganuma M, Okabe S, Kurusu M, Imai K, Nakachi K. Involvement of TNF-alpha changes in human cancer development, prevention and palliative care. *Mech Ageing Dev* 2002 Nov;123(12):1655-63